TOTAL FITNESS *and* WELLNESS

Brief Edition

TOTAL FITNESS *and* WELLNESS

SCOTT K. POWERS ☀ STEPHEN L. DODD
University of Florida

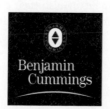

Benjamin
Cummings

San Francisco Boston New York
Cape Town Hong Kong London Madrid Mexico City
Montreal Munich Paris Singapore Sydney Tokyo Toronto

Publisher: Daryl Fox
Sponsoring Editor: Deirdre McGill
Developmental Editor: Claire Brassert
Project Editor: Susan Teahan
Publishing Assistant: Marie Beaugureau
Managing Editor: Wendy Earl
Production Editor: Janet Vail
Photo Researcher: Diane Austin
Cover and Text Design: Kathleen Cunningham
Copyeditor: Alan Titche
Compositor: The Left Coast Group
Manufacturing Buyer: Stacey Weinberger
Marketing Manager: Sandy Lindelof

Photography and illustration credits appear on p. 309

Library of Congress Cataloging-in-Publication Data
Powers, Scott K. (Scott Kline), 1950–
     Total fitness and wellness / Scott K. Powers, Stephen L. Dodd.—Brief ed.
        p. cm.
     Includes bibliographical references and index.
     ISBN 0-8053-6505-2
        1. Exercise. 2. Physical fitness. 3. Health. I. Dodd, Stephen L.
     II. Title.

     RA781 .P66 2003b
     613.7—dc21

                                                        2002067467

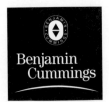

ISBN 0-8053-6505-2
1 2 3 4 5 6 7 8 9 10—CRK—06 05 04 03 02

www.aw.com/bc

☀ To my family Haney, Will, Mom, and Dad. Your love and encouragement have always meant more than you will ever know.
    Stephen L. Dodd

☀ To my mother who encouraged me to pursue academic endeavors.
    Scott K. Powers

RELATED BENJAMIN CUMMINGS KINESIOLOGY TITLES

Anshel, *Sport Psychology: From Theory to Practice,* Fourth Edition (2003)

Bishop, *Fitness through Aerobics,* Fifth Edition (2002)

Darst/Pangrazi, *Dynamic Physical Education for Secondary School Students,* Fourth Edition (2002)

Darst/Pangrazi, *Lesson Plans for Dynamic Physical Education for Secondary School Students,* Fourth Edition (2002)

Freeman, *Physical Education and Sport in a Changing Society,* Sixth Edition (2001)

Fronske, *Teaching Cues for Sport Skills,* Second Edition (2001)

Fronske/Wilson, *Teaching Cues for Basic Sports Skills for Elementary and Middle School Children* (2002)

Hastie, *Teaching for Lifetime Physical Activity Through Quality High School Education* (2003)

Harris/Pitman/Waller/Park, *Social Dance from Dance a While,* Second Edition (2003)

Horvat/Eichstaedt/Kalakian/Croche, *Developmental and Adapted Physical Education,* Fourth Edition (2003)

Housh/Housh/Johnson, *Introduction to Exercise Science,* Second Edition (2003)

Lacy/Hastad, *Measurement and Evaluation in Physical Education and Exercise Science,* Fourth Edition (2003)

Mosston/Ashworth, *Teaching Physical Education,* Fifth Edition (2002)

Pangrazi, *Dynamic Physical Education for Elementary School Children,* Thirteenth Edition (2001)

Pangrazi, *Lesson Plans for Dynamic Physical Education for Elementary School Children,* Thirteenth Edition (2001)

Plowman/Smith, *Exercise Physiology for Health, Fitness, and Performance,* Second Edition (2003)

Powers/Dodd, *Total Fitness and Wellness,* Third Edition (2003)

Schmottlach/McManama, *Physical Education Activity Handbook,* Tenth Edition (2002)

Silva/Stevens, *Psychological Foundations of Sport* (2002)

RELATED BENJAMIN CUMMINGS HEALTH TITLES

Anspaugh/Ezell, *Teaching Today's Health,* Sixth Edition (2001)

Barr, *Introduction to U. S. Health Policy* (2002)

Buckingham, *Primer on International Health* (2001)

Cottrell/Girvan/McKenzie, *Principles and Foundations of Health Promotion and Education,* Second Edition (2002)

Donatelle, *Access to Health,* Seventh Edition (2002)

Donatelle, *Health: The Basics,* Fifth Edition (2003)

Donnelly/Elburne/Kittleson, *Mental Health: Dimensions of Self-Esteem and Emotional Well-Being* (2001)

Girdano/Dusek/Everly, *Controlling Stress and Tension,* Sixth Edition (2001)

Karren/Hafen/Smith/Frandsen, *Mind/Body Health,* Second Edition (2002)

McKenzie/Smeltzer, *Planning, Implementing, and Evaluating Health Promotion Programs: A Primer,* Third Edition (2001)

Neutens/Rubinson, *Research Techniques for the Health Sciences,* Third Edition (2002)

Reagan/Brookins-Fisher, *Community Health in the 21st Century,* Second Edition (2002)

Seaward, *Health of the Human Spirit: Spiritual Dimensions for Personal Health and Well-Being* (2001)

Skinner, *Promoting Health through Organizational Change* (2002)

Check out these and other Benjamin Cummings health and kinesiology titles at www.aw.com/bc.

☀ Brief Contents

✸ Contents

Chapter 3: General Principles of Exercise for Health and Fitness   63

☀ Preface

Good health is our most precious possession. Although it is usually only in times of illness or injury that we really appreciate good health, more and more people are realizing that health is not simply the lack of disease. Indeed, there are degrees of health, or wellness, on which lifestyle can have a major impact.

Intended for an introductory college course in physical fitness and wellness, *Total Fitness and Wellness* focuses on how lifestyle can be altered to achieve a high degree of physical fitness and wellness. Two major aspects of daily life that most affect our level of wellness are exercise and diet. Hence, the interaction of exercise and diet and the essential role of regular exercise and good nutrition in achieving total fitness and wellness are major themes of the text.

Total Fitness and Wellness, Brief Edition, was built on a strong foundation of both exercise physiology and nutrition. The text provides clear and objective research-based information to college students during their first course in physical fitness and wellness. By offering a research-based text, we hope to dispel many myths associated with exercise, nutrition, weight loss, and wellness. For the evaluation of various wellness components such as fitness levels and nutritional status, a how-to approach is used. Ways to change your lifestyle that will improve wellness (e.g., designing a fitness program, altering food choices) are described. Indeed, the title of the book, "Total Fitness and Wellness" reflects our goals.

Numerous physical fitness and wellness texts are available today. Our motivation in writing *Total Fitness and Wellness,* Brief Edition, was to create a unique physical fitness text, one that not only covers primary concepts of physical fitness and wellness but also addresses important issues such as behavior change, exercise-related injuries, exercise and the environment, and exercise for special populations.

FOUNDATION IN EXERCISE PHYSIOLOGY

We believe it is imperative that students develop an understanding of the basic physiological adaptations that occur in response to both acute exercise and regular exercise training. Without this understanding, it is impossible to plan, modify, and properly execute a lifetime exercise program.

STRONG EMPHASIS ON NUTRITION

Because we feel so strongly about the important interaction between nutrition and exercise, a nutritional theme is incorporated throughout the text. Each chapter includes Nutritional Links to Fitness boxes, which explain how nutrition affects health and wellness in areas such as cardiorespiratory fitness, muscular strength and endurance, and prevention of cardiovascular disease. We put major emphasis on and provide comprehensive coverage of basic nutrition and weight control by dedicating separate chapters to each topic: Chapter 7, Nutrition, Health, and Fitness (includes a new section on nutritional supplements) and Chapter 8, Exercise, Diet, and Weight Control.

COVERAGE OF THE LATEST SCIENTIFIC RESEARCH ON PHYSICAL FITNESS, NUTRITION, AND WELLNESS

We firmly believe that college physical fitness and wellness texts should contain the latest scientific information and include references for scientific studies to support key information about physical fitness, nutrition, and wellness. Our approach is to provide current scientific references that document the validity of facts presented. Accordingly, source information and suggested readings are placed at the end of each chapter.

The most current research in the arena of fitness and wellness is offered in *Total Fitness and Wellness,* Brief Edition. For example, it is now clear that exercise plays a role in reducing the risk of some cancers and can contribute to a longer life. While there has long been speculation about the health benefits of exercise, evidence that supports the exercise and wellness connection has only recently become available. In the area of nutrition, scientific data now suggest that vitamins may play a new role in preventing certain diseases and combating the aging process. In addition, while it is well accepted that fat in the diet increases our risk of heart disease, it has just lately been shown that dietary fat plays a greater role than other nutrients in weight gain.

With any attempt to present the most current information, there is always the danger of presenting ideas that are not fully substantiated by good research. We have made a concerted effort to avoid such a risk by using information from the most highly respected scientific journals and consulting with experts in the field.

Layout and Features

While many topic and organization options have to be considered when developing a text, the best way to determine content and order is to ask instructors. Therefore, with input from instructors across the country, we have included the following coverage, layout, and features:

- **Coverage:** *Total Fitness and Wellness,* Brief Edition is a shortened version of *Total Fitness and Wellness,* Third Edition. The brief edition contains all of the lab activities and special features of our larger text, but it lacks the 5 chapters on special topics: exercise and the environment; exercise for special populations; prevention and rehabilitation of exercise-related injuries; prevention of cancer; and sexually transmitted diseases and drug abuse. This shorter text works for classes that don't cover special topics, but do need the depth in the basic fitness and wellness material. All of the supplements for the main version of our text are available with this text as well, including the Behavior Change Log Book.

- **Informational Boxes:** Each chapter contains informational boxes, called **A Closer Look,** which offer extended coverage of concepts discussed in the body of the text with suggestions for practical application. **Nutritional Links to Health and Fitness** boxes emphasize the importance of nutrition to physical fitness. For this edition, three new types of boxes have been developed: **Ask an Expert, Fitness and Wellness for All,** and **Fitness-Wellness Consumer.** Ask an Expert boxes provide the latest information from internationally known experts in the fields of resistance training, exercise and nutrition, obesity and weight loss, and adherence to regular exercise. Fitness and Wellness for All boxes contain fitness, wellness, and nutritional information with respect to diversity. Fitness-Wellness Consumer boxes provide exercise and wellness information related to consumer issues.

- **Lab Exercises:** Most chapters contain easy-to-follow, application-based lab exercises such as fitness testing, nutritional evaluation, and cardiovascular risk assessment.

- **Healthy People 2010 Objectives:** National health promotion and disease prevention initiatives are reflected in selected Healthy People 2010 goals listed in Appendix A.

- **Food Appendices:** To assist students in tracking and modifying food intake, caloric and nutrient content of common foods and fast foods is offered in Appendices B and C.

- **Pedagogical Aids:** To stimulate students' interest and alert them to the significance of the material to be covered, Learning Objectives open each chapter. In Summary lists, found throughout the text, recapitulate the more difficult sections, prompting students to recall and process main concepts covered. To emphasize and support understanding of material, important terms are boldfaced in the text and defined in a running glossary at the bottom of text pages. Also, several features are offered at the end of each chapter to reinforce learning. For students' review, the Chapter Summary sections succinctly restate the most significant ideas presented in the chapter. Study Questions encourage analysis of chapter discussions and prepare students for tests. Suggested Readings and References offer quality information sources for further study of fitness and wellness.

Supplements

The following is a list of supplements included with this text:

BEHAVIOR CHANGE LOG BOOK
(0-321-11219-9)
The Behavior Change Log Book is a tool to help students change behavior patterns, institute new, more healthy diet plans, and develop and adhere to a fitness prescription. Sections on behavior change, nutrition and weight management, and fitness offer key information on major topics in fitness and wellness. The log book is packaged free with every new copy of the textbook.

EXPANDED INSTRUCTOR'S MANUAL
AND TEST BANK (0-321-10657-1)
The Instructor's Manual includes lecture outlines, chapter summaries, student activities, a new extensive media section, and a new section offering 15 labs.

COMPUTERIZED TEST BANK
(0-321-10655-5)
Available in computerized and printed versions, the Test Bank provides multiple-choice, true/false, short answer, matching, and discussion questions for each chapter. Instructors can pick and choose to create custom made tests and quizzes that fit the specific needs of their course.

POWERPOINT® PRESENTATION CD-ROM
(0-321-11217-2)
The PowerPoint® Presentation Slides provide instructors with a multimedia presentation for their classroom or a lecture hall. Presented on a CD-ROM, the presentation is easily run and allows instructors to download lecture notes and images from over 200 slides.

TRANSPARENCY ACETATES
(0-321-10656-3)
Over 140 transparency acetates show figures, graphs, and tables from the main text. The transparencies are excellent for presentation of information in a clear manner consistent with that of the text.

NUTRIFIT® SOFTWARE
(0-321-11218-0)

NutriFit® software provides students with the means to track and analyze their daily food intake and exercise. Instructors can use the software to assign a variety of assessment activities to students for evaluation of nutrient balance and calorie expenditure. This supplement, included with every new copy of the text, is also available for purchase separately.

STUDENTBODY101.COM
www.StudentBody101.com

StudentBody101.com, accredited by Health on the Net (HON), focuses on alcohol, drugs, stress, fitness, nutrition, tobacco, and sexuality and facilitates active learning by posting current journal articles, self-assessments, online discussions, and personalized behavior change tips. This supplement is included with every new copy of the text.

STUDY GUIDE FOR
STUDENTBODY101.COM (0-8053-4793-3)

The Study Guide for StudentBody101.com provides several activities to ensure maximum use of the website, www.StudentBody101.com.

INSTRUCTOR'S GUIDE TO
STUDENTBODY101.COM (0-205-35084-4)

Incorporating journal articles and online resources featured on StudentBody101.com, Instructor's Guide for StudentBody101.com offers tips for conducting discussion sessions, assigning writing activities, spurring debates, and encouraging self-assessment.

BENJAMIN CUMMINGS HEALTH VIDEO PROGRAM

Available for qualified adopters. Ask your local Benjamin Cummings sales representative for a complete list of videos.

Changes in the Third Edition

Each chapter of the third edition has been revised to include the newest research developments in exercise, wellness, and health-related nutrition. In addition to the changes listed in the paragraphs above, several other features have been added. These include

- expanded nutrition coverage and a detailed discussion of nutritional supplements and ergogenic aids;
- new and improved art and photos throughout the text;
- new and updated references in every chapter.

Acknowledgments

An enormous number of people have made great contributions to *Total Fitness and Wellness*. Ted Bolen was the driving force behind the first edition. Elisa Adams deserves much credit for her unique editing skills in the initial development of the book. Brian Urichko, Vicki Sullivan, Natasha Staron, Kelly Hinson, Karen Devault, and Dr. Robert Herb also deserve to be recognized for their contributions to various aspects of the first two editions of this book.

The third edition of *Total Fitness and Wellness* was published by Benjamin Cummings. The book has been greatly improved by the important contributions of Claire Brassert, Development Editor, and Deirdre McGill, Sponsoring Editor. Their organization, insight, and encouragement are greatly appreciated. Susan Teahan, Project Editor, and Marie Beaugureau, Publishing Assistant, expertly shepherded our manuscript to production. Marie also ensured the supplements, including the Behavior Change Log Book, came out with fresh ideas and on schedule. Janet Vail, Production Editor, guided the manuscript through production with aplomb.

Jennifer Del Toro and Jenna Jones at the University of Florida have both made important and unique contributions to the third edition of this book. There are also several professionals whose reviews of the content and style have shaped every part of this book. We owe them a tremendous debt of gratitude:

Debra L. Power	Iowa State University
Eugene Sessoms	College of Charleston
Donna Chun	Brigham Young University—Hawaii
Nicholas J. DiCicco	Camden County College
Richard A. Washburn	University of Illinois—Urbana-Champaign
David Rider	Bloomsburg University

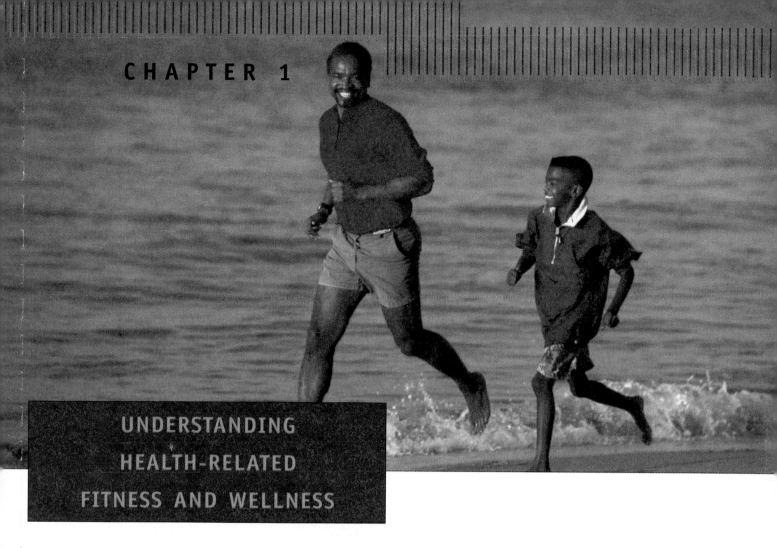

CHAPTER 1

UNDERSTANDING
HEALTH-RELATED
FITNESS AND WELLNESS

After studying this chapter, you should be able to:

1. Describe the health benefits of exercise.

2. Define the terms *coronary artery disease* and *myocardial infarction*.

3. Compare the goals of health-related fitness programs and sport performance conditioning programs.

4. Describe the components of health-related physical fitness.

5. Discuss the wellness concept.

6. Outline the components of wellness.

Congratulations! By reading this chapter, you are taking the first step toward improving your physical fitness and maintaining good health. By deciding to improve your personal fitness, you will join millions of people worldwide who are becoming interested in maintaining good health through daily exercise, improved health behaviors, and proper diet.

This book contains the latest scientific information on how to develop and maintain a physical fitness program. A major theme is that good nutrition and exercise work together to improve health and overall well-being. Additional chapters discuss issues such as preventing and treating exercise-related injuries, environmental effects on exercise, stress reduction, and modifying unhealthy behavior. Careful reading of the material throughout will provide answers to hundreds of diet- and exercise-related questions.

In this first chapter, we discuss the health benefits of exercise, outline the major components of physical fitness, present the concept of wellness, and introduce exercise goal setting. Understanding the role that exercise plays in the maintenance of good health is a strong motivation for developing and sustaining a lifetime physical fitness program.

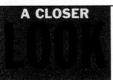 ## Health Benefits of Exercise

Why exercise? Almost all of us ask this question at some time in our lives. The answer is simple: Exercise is good for you. Indeed, regular exercise makes us feel better

and look better, and provides added vitality and energy to achieve everyday tasks. And perhaps more importantly, it can improve your health (1–7). The importance of regular exercise in promoting good health is emphasized in a report by the Surgeon General. This report concludes that a lack of physical activity is a major public health problem in the United States, and that all Americans can improve their health by engaging in regular exercise. The Surgeon General's report recognizes numerous health benefits of exercise. A summary of these benefits is illustrated in Figure 1.1. A brief discussion of the major health benefits of exercise follows.

EXERCISE REDUCES THE RISK OF HEART DISEASE

Cardiovascular diseases (i.e., ailments of the heart and blood vessels) are a major cause of death in the United States (A Closer Look). In fact, one of every two Americans dies of cardiovascular disease (8). It is well established, however, that regular exercise can significantly reduce your risk of developing cardiovascular disease (1–4, 6–13). Further, strong evidence suggests that regular physical activity reduces the risk of death during a heart attack (14–17). The protective effect of exercise training during a heart attack is illustrated in Figure 1.2. Notice that exercise training can reduce the magnitude of cardiac injury during a heart attack by 66% (15, 16). Many preventive medicine specialists

---

A CLOSER LOOK

Coronary Heart Disease and Heart Attacks

Coronary heart disease (CHD) is a form of cardiovascular disease that results from a blockage of one or more of the arteries in the heart. The most common cause of coronary artery blockage is the formation of a fatty deposit (called *plaque*) composed of cholesterol, calcium, and fibrous tissue (9). Narrowing of coronary arteries due to plaque buildup can vary from a partial to a severe blockage.

Numerous influences contribute to the development of CHD. Damage

to the interior of a coronary artery creates an area that is vulnerable to the collection of cholesterol, and the formation of plaque begins. The factor(s) that create the original damage to the artery continue to be debated; stress and high blood pressure are potential causes (9). Once the plaque collection begins, elevated blood cholesterol increases the buildup and therefore accelerates the progress of disease.

Blockage of coronary arteries by plaque can reduce the blood flow to

the working heart muscle during heavy exercise, thereby depriving the heart of needed oxygen and nutrients. Inadequate heart blood flow can result in chest pain (called *angina*), and advanced CHD can result in complete blockage of a coronary artery. When the heart is deprived of blood flow for several minutes, a heart attack or **myocardial infarction (MI)** occurs, resulting in the death of heart muscle cells. Mild MIs result in the death of only a few heart cells, while severe MIs can destroy hundreds or even thousands of heart cells. Damage to a large portion of the heart reduces its effectiveness as a pump, and in severe cases can result in death.

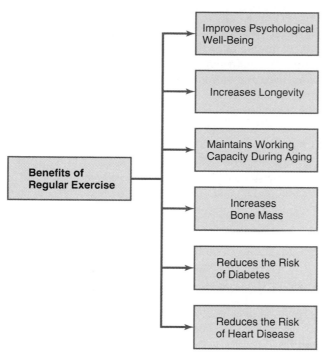

FIGURE 1.1
Benefits of regular exercise.

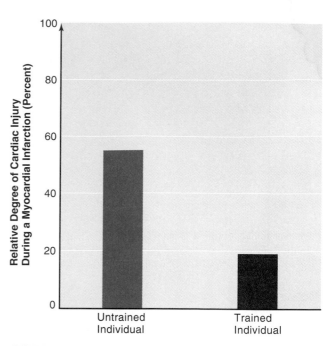

FIGURE 1.2
Regular endurance exercise protects the heart against injury during a heart attack. This figure illustrates that during a myocardial infarction (i.e., heart attack), exercise-trained individuals suffer less cardiac (i.e., heart) injury compared to the untrained individuals. Data are from research by Yamashita et al. (16).

argue that these facts alone are reason enough to exercise regularly (3, 9, 18). Chapter 9 provides a detailed discussion of exercise and cardiovascular disease.

EXERCISE REDUCES THE RISK OF DIABETES

Diabetes is a disease characterized by high blood sugar (glucose) levels. Untreated diabetes can result in numerous health problems, including blindness and kidney dysfunction. Regular exercise can reduce the risk of a specific type of diabetes, called type II (or "adult-onset" diabetes). Specifically, exercise reduces the risk of type II diabetes by improving the regulation of blood glucose (5, 19, 20). More is said about diabetes in Chapter 9 and Chapter 12.

EXERCISE INCREASES BONE MASS

The primary functions of the skeleton are to provide a mechanical lever system of interconnected bones to permit movement, and to protect internal organs. Given these roles, it is important to maintain strong and healthy bones. The loss of bone mass and strength (called **osteoporosis**) increases the risk of bone fractures. Although osteoporosis can occur in men and women of all ages, it is more common in the elderly, particularly among women.

Is there a link between exercise and maintenance of good bone health? Yes! A key factor in regulating bone mass and strength is mechanical force applied by muscular activity. Indeed, numerous studies have dem-

onstrated that regular exercise increases bone mass and strength in young adults (21–23). Further, research on osteoporosis suggests that regular exercise can prevent bone loss in the elderly and is also useful in the treatment of the osteoporotic patient (21).

EXERCISE MAINTAINS PHYSICAL WORKING CAPACITY DURING AGING

Human aging is characterized by a gradual loss of physical working capacity. As we grow older, there is a progressive decline in our ability to perform strenuous activities (e.g., running, cycling, or swimming). Although this process may begin as early as the 20s, the most dramatic changes occur after approximately 60 years of age (1, 24–26). It is well established that regular exercise training can reduce the rate of decline in

myocardial infarction (MI)   Damage to the heart due to a reduction in blood flow, resulting in the death of heart muscle cells.
diabetes   A metabolic disorder characterized by high blood glucose levels. Chronic elevation of blood glucose is associated with increased incidence of heart disease, kidney disease, nerve dysfunction, and eye damage.
osteoporosis   The loss of bone mass and strength, which increases the risk of bone fractures.

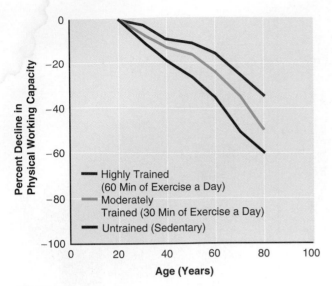

FIGURE 1.3
The relationship among age, physical activity, and decline in physical working capacity.

physical working capacity during aging (24, 27, 28). This fact is illustrated in Figure 1.3. Notice the differences in physical working capacity among highly trained, moderately trained, and inactive individuals during the aging process. The key point is that although a natural decline of physical working capacity occurs with age, regular exercise can reduce the rate of this decline, resulting in an increased ability to enjoy a lifetime of physical recreation. Indeed, perhaps the most important benefit of regular exercise may be the improved quality of life associated with being physically fit.

EXERCISE INCREASES LONGEVITY

Although it is controversial, growing evidence suggests that regular exercise (combined with a healthy lifestyle) increases longevity (1, 3, 4, 17, 29–31). For example, a classic study of Harvard alumni over the past 30 years reported that men with a sedentary (i.e., physically inactive) lifestyle have a 31% greater risk of death from all causes than men who exercise regularly (4). This translates into a longer life span for those who exercise. What factors are responsible for the increased longevity due to regular exercise? The primary factor is that individuals who exercise have a lower risk of both heart attack and cancer (3, 4) (Chapters 9 and 14).

EXERCISE IMPROVES PSYCHOLOGICAL WELL-BEING

Strong evidence indicates that regular exercise improves psychological well-being in people of all ages. Specifically, the mental health benefits of regular exer-

cise include a reduction in anxiety, depression, and reactivity to stress (1). These mental benefits of exercise lead to an improved sense of well-being in the physically active individual. We will further discuss the role of exercise as a method for reducing psychological stress in Chapter 10.

☼ IN SUMMARY

- Regular exercise reduces the risk of both heart disease and diabetes.
- Exercise increases bone mass in young people and reduces bone loss in the elderly.
- Systematic physical activity maintains physical working capacity during aging.
- Regular exercise has been shown to increase longevity and improve quality of life.
- Exercise promotes psychological well-being and reduces feelings of depression and anxiety.

☼ Exercise Does Not Guarantee Good Health

We have seen that there are many good reasons for engaging in regular exercise. While it is well established that exercise can lower risk of CHD, reduce the loss in physical working capacity due to aging, and generally improve the quality of life, exercise alone does not guarantee good health. Indeed, good health is the complex interaction of many variables. Factors such as age, gender, genetics, diet, lifestyle, smoking habits, and environment all contribute to the risk of disease (1, 3–7). The interaction among exercise, nutrition, and factors that increase the risk of disease is discussed throughout this text.

☼ Exercise Training for Health-Related Fitness

In general, exercise conditioning programs can be divided into two broad categories defined by their goals: exercise training to improve sport performance and health-related physical fitness. This textbook focuses on health-related fitness.

The overall goal of a total health-related physical fitness program is to optimize the quality of life (1, 2, 10). The specific goals of this type of fitness program are to reduce the risk of disease and to improve total physical fitness so that daily tasks can be completed with less effort and fatigue.

Although some conditioning programs aimed at improving sport performance may reduce the risk of disease, this is not their primary purpose. By contrast, the single goal of sport conditioning is to improve physical performance in a specific sport. However, the "weekend" athlete who engages in a total health-related physical fitness program could also improve his or her physical performance in many sports. Specifically, a health-related fitness program improves sport performance by increasing muscular strength and endurance, improving flexibility, and reducing the risk of injury, as we see in the chapters that follow.

⚙ Components of Health-Related Physical Fitness

Exercise scientists (i.e., experts in exercise and physical fitness) do not always agree on all of the basic components of physical fitness. However, most do agree that the five major components of total health-related physical fitness (Figure 1.4) are

1. cardiorespiratory endurance
2. muscular strength
3. muscular endurance
4. flexibility
5. body composition

In addition to these, many people also include motor skill performance as a sixth component. Motor skills are those movement qualities, such as agility and coordination, that are required to achieve success in athletics. Although motor skills are important to sport performance, they are not directly linked to improvement of health in young adults and are therefore not considered a major component of health-related physical fitness.

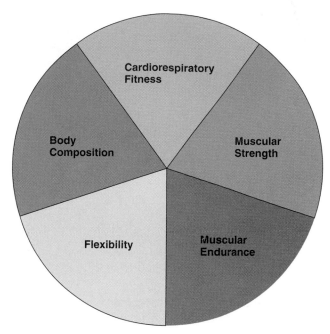

FIGURE 1.4
Components of health-related physical fitness.

CARDIORESPIRATORY FITNESS

Cardiorespiratory fitness (sometimes called *aerobic fitness* or *cardiorespiratory endurance*) is considered to be a key component of health-related physical fitness. It is a measure of the heart's ability to pump oxygen-rich blood to the working muscles during exercise. It is also a measure of the muscles' ability to take up and use the delivered oxygen to produce the energy needed to continue exercising. In practical terms, cardiorespiratory endurance is the ability to perform endurance-type

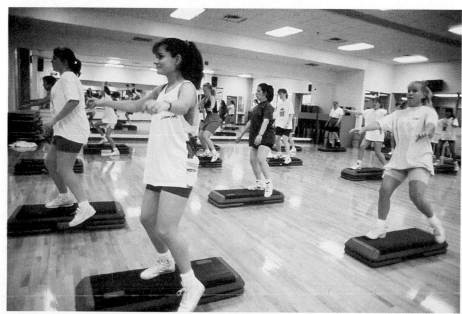

Regular exercise can prevent loss of bone mass.

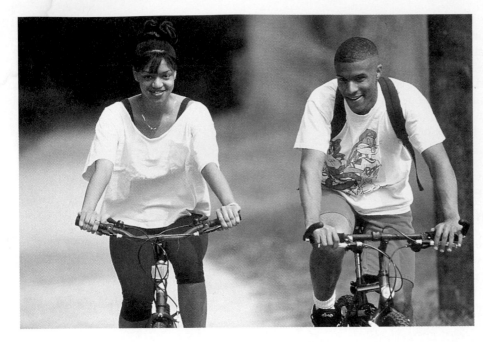

Individuals who have achieved a high level of cardiorespiratory fitness are capable of performing 30 to 60 minutes of vigorous exercise without undue fatigue.

exercises (distance running, cycling, swimming, etc.). The individual that has achieved a high measure of cardiorespiratory endurance is generally capable of performing 30 to 60 minutes of vigorous exercise without undue fatigue. Chapter 4 discusses the details of exercise training designed to improve cardiorespiratory fitness.

MUSCULAR STRENGTH

Muscular strength is the maximal ability of a muscle to generate force (32–34). It is evaluated by how much force a muscle (or muscle group) can generate during a single maximal contraction. Practically, this means how much weight an individual can lift during one maximal effort.

Muscular strength is important in almost all sports. Sports such as football, basketball, and events in track and field require a high level of muscular strength. Even nonathletes require some degree of muscular strength to function in everyday life. For example, routine tasks around the home, such as lifting bags of groceries and moving furniture, require muscular strength. Weight training (also called *strength training*) results in an increase in the size and strength of muscles. The principles of developing muscular strength are presented in Chapter 5.

MUSCULAR ENDURANCE

Muscular endurance is defined as the ability of a muscle to generate force over and over again. Although muscular strength and muscular endurance are related, they are not the same. These two terms can be best distinguished by examples. An excellent example of muscular strength is a person lifting a heavy barbell during one maximal muscular effort. In contrast, muscular endurance is illustrated by a weight lifter performing multiple lifts or repetitions of a lighter weight.

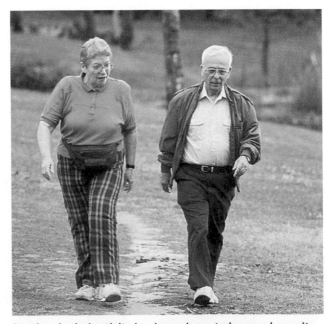

Regular physical activity has been shown to improve longevity.

> **muscular strength**   The maximal ability of a muscle to generate force.
> **muscular endurance**   The ability of a muscle to generate force over and over again.

Most successfully played sports require muscular endurance. For instance, tennis players, who must repeatedly swing their racquets during a match, require a high level of muscular endurance. Many everyday activities (e.g., waxing your car) also require some level of it. Techniques of developing muscular endurance are discussed in Chapter 5.

FLEXIBILITY

Flexibility is the ability to move joints freely through their full range of motion. Flexible individuals can bend and twist at their joints with ease. Without routine stretching, muscles and tendons shorten and become tight; this can retard the range of motion around joints and impair flexibility.

Individual needs for flexibility vary. Certain athletes (such as gymnasts and divers) require great flexibility in order to accomplish complex movements. The average individual requires less flexibility than an athlete; however, everyone needs some flexibility in order to perform activities of daily living. Research suggests that flexibility is useful in preventing some types of muscle–tendon injuries and may be useful in reducing low back pain (35, 36). Techniques for improving flexibility are discussed in Chapter 6.

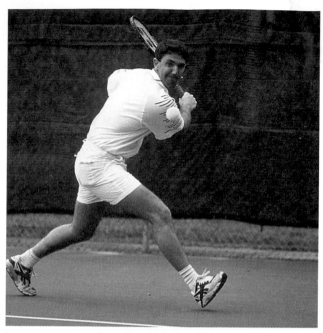

Tennis players require a high level of muscular endurance to play long matches.

BODY COMPOSITION

The term **body composition** refers to the relative amounts of fat and lean body tissue (muscle, organs, bone) found in your body. The rationale for including body composition as a component of health-related physical fitness is that having a high percentage of body fat (a condition known as obesity) is associated with an increased risk of CHD. Obesity increases the risk of development of type II diabetes and contributes to joint stress during movement. In general, being "over-fat" elevates the risk of medical problems.

Lack of physical activity has been shown to play a major role in gaining body fat. Conversely, regular exercise is an important factor in promoting the loss of body fat. Assessment of body composition is discussed in Chapter 2, and the relationship between exercise and weight loss is discussed in Chapter 8.

☼ IN SUMMARY

Health-related physical fitness comprises five components:

- cardiorespiratory fitness
- muscular strength

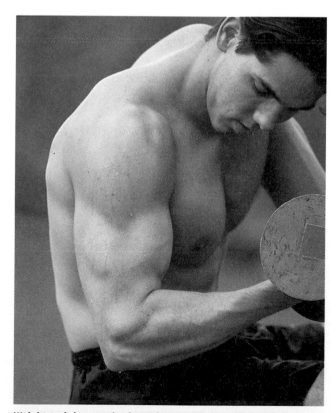

Weight training results in an increase in muscular strength.

flexibility   The ability to move joints freely through their full range of motion.
body composition   The relative amounts of fat and lean body tissue (muscle, organs, bone) found in the body.

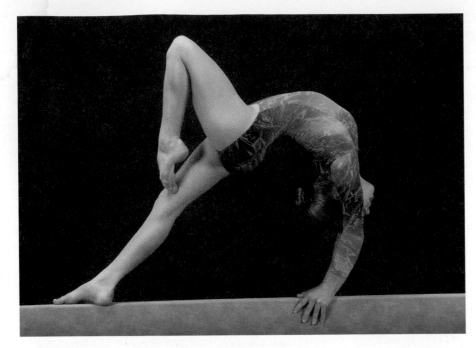

Gymnasts require great flexibility to be successful.

- muscular endurance
- flexibility
- body composition

Wellness Concept

Good health was once defined as the absence of disease. In the 1970s and 1980s many exercise scientists and health educators became dissatisfied with this limited definition of good health. These futuristic thinkers believed that health was not only an absence of disease but included physical fitness and emotional and spiritual health as well. This new concept of good health is called **wellness** (2). In a broad sense, the term *wellness* means "healthy living." This state of healthy living is achieved by the practice of a healthy lifestyle that includes regular physical activity, proper nutrition (Nutritional Links to Health and Fitness), eliminating unhealthy behaviors (avoiding high-risk activities such as reckless driving, smoking, and drug use), and maintaining good emotional and spiritual health (2). Given the importance of wellness, let's discuss wellness and a healthy lifestyle in more detail.

wellness   A state of healthy living. This state is achieved by the practice of a healthy lifestyle, which includes regular physical activity, proper nutrition, eliminating unhealthy behaviors, and maintaining good emotional and spiritual health.

Wellness: A Healthy Lifestyle

A healthy lifestyle refers to health behaviors aimed at reducing one's risk of disease and accidents, achieving optimal physical health, and maximizing emotional, social, intellectual, and spiritual health (2, 3, 7). It can be achieved by eliminating unhealthy behavior to reach a state of wellness. *Wellness* is defined specifically as a state of optimal health that includes physical, emotional, intellectual, spiritual, and social health (Figure 1.5).

PHYSICAL HEALTH

Physical health means not only freedom from disease but includes physical fitness as well. Physical fitness can positively affect your health by reducing your risk of disease and improving your quality of life.

EMOTIONAL HEALTH

Emotions play an important role in how you feel about yourself and others. Emotional health (also called *mental health*) includes your social skills and interpersonal relationships. Also included are your levels of self-esteem and your ability to cope with the routine stress of daily living.

The cornerstone of emotional health is emotional stability, which describes how well you deal with the day-to-day stresses of personal interactions and the physical environment. Although it is normal to experience some range of emotional highs and lows, the

Nutritional Links
TO HEALTH AND FITNESS

Good Nutrition Is Essential to Achieving Physical Fitness and Wellness

A major theme of this book is that good nutrition is essential for developing and maintaining physical fitness and a state of wellness. Good nutrition means that an individual's diet provides all of the components of food (called *nutrients*) needed to promote growth and repair body tissues. Additionally, a proper diet supplies the energy required to meet the body's daily needs.

Consuming too little of any nutrient can impair physical fitness and potentially result in disease (32). Therefore, achieving good nutrition should be a goal for everyone. In many of the chapters that follow, we provide nutritional information in the form of informational boxes such as this one. In addition, Chapter 7 is devoted entirely to nutrition.

Although consuming inadequate nutrients increases your risk of disease, consuming too much food energy (overeating) can be problematic as well. Overeating on a regular basis can result in large amounts of fat gain, resulting in obesity. As mentioned earlier, obesity increases your risk of heart disease and type II diabetes. Chapter 8 discusses the relationship among nutrition, exercise, and weight loss.

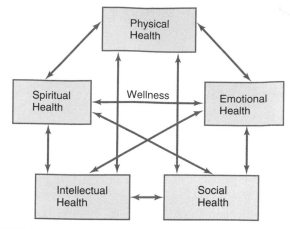

FIGURE 1.5
The wellness components and their interactions.

SPIRITUAL HEALTH

Spiritual health is often called the glue that holds an individual together. The term *spiritual* means different things to different people, but regardless of whether you define spiritual health as religious beliefs or the establishment of personal values, it is an important aspect of wellness and is closely linked to emotional health (34).

Optimal spiritual health is often described as the development of spiritual makeup to its fullest potential. This includes the ability to understand the basic purpose in life and to experience love, joy, pain, peace, and sorrow, and to care for and respect all living things (34). Anyone who has experienced a beautiful sunset or smelled the first scents of spring can appreciate the pleasure of maintaining optimal spiritual health (34).

SOCIAL HEALTH

Social health is defined as the development and maintenance of meaningful interpersonal relationships. This results in the creation of a support network of friends and family. Good social health results in feelings of confidence in social interactions and provides you with a feeling of emotional security.

INTERACTION OF WELLNESS COMPONENTS

None of the components of wellness work in isolation; a strong interaction must occur among the five. For example, poor physical health can lead to poor emotional health. Similarly, a lack of spiritual health can contribute to poor emotional health as well as poor physical

objective of achieving emotional wellness is to maintain emotional stability somewhere between an extreme high and an extreme low.

INTELLECTUAL HEALTH

Intellectual health can be maintained by keeping your mind active through life-long learning. Although there are many ways to maintain an active mind, attending lectures, engaging in thoughtful discussions with friends or teachers, and reading are obvious ways to promote intellectual health. Maintaining good intellectual health can improve your quality of life by increasing your ability to define and solve problems. Further, continuous learning and thinking can provide you with a sense of fulfillment that accompanies an active mind.

Wellness Issues Across the Population

The steps required to achieve wellness are the same across all populations. However, some individuals may experience difficulties in achieving wellness due to factors related to ethnicity, gender, age, and socioeconomic status. For example, compared to the U.S. population as a whole, the risk of developing hypertension (high blood pressure) is greater among African Americans. Similarly, diabetes is more common in Native Americans or people with a Latino heritage. Further, men and women differ in their risk for heart disease, osteoporosis, and certain types of cancer. Aging can also affect the ability of people to fulfill wellness. For instance, the risk of many diseases (e.g., heart disease and cancer) increases with age. Finally, people earning low incomes experience a higher incidence of obesity, heart disease, and drug abuse. Therefore, although wellness goals are similar across all populations, individual differences among people can present special challenges in achieving wellness. This important issue will be discussed throughout this book.

and intellectual health. These mind–body interactions are illustrated in Figure 1.5. Total wellness can be achieved only by a balance of physical, intellectual, social, emotional, and spiritual health.

LIVING A HEALTHY LIFESTYLE

How does one practice a healthy lifestyle? A good place to begin is with a personal assessment of your health risk status. Laboratory 1.1 on page 15 is a lifestyle assessment inventory designed to increase your awareness of factors that affect your health. As you work on Laboratory 1.1, keep in mind that you have control over each of these factors, but that awareness alone does not bring about change. A decision to alter your lifestyle to achieve total wellness is necessary and is a decision that only you can make. Make a commitment today to improve the quality of your life by practicing a healthy lifestyle.

Physical fitness, good nutrition and weight control, proper stress management, and healthy behavior are all key components of a lifestyle that leads to wellness. Each of these issues is discussed in detail in Chapters 3 through 16.

WELLNESS GOALS FOR THE NATION

Healthy people are one of a nation's greatest resources. Poor health drains national resources by reducing worker productivity and increasing the amount of government money spent on health care. Because of this fact, the U.S. government has established wellness goals for the nation. The government's nationwide Healthy People Initiative seeks to prevent unnecessary disease and to improve the quality of life for all Americans. The wellness goals for the nation are discussed in Healthy

People reports first published in 1980 and revised every 10 years. Each report includes a broad range of health and wellness objectives based on 10-year agendas. For example, major objectives contained in the current report ("Healthy People 2010") include increasing the span of healthy life of all Americans and reducing health disparities across special populations of our society (Fitness and Wellness For All). For more details on the goals and objectives of Healthy People 2010, see Appendix A or visit the Healthy People website listed at the end of this chapter.

☼ IN SUMMARY

- Wellness is defined as a state of optimal health achieved by living a healthy lifestyle.
- Wellness is composed of five interacting components: physical health, emotional health, intellectual health, spiritual health, and social health.

☼ Motivation and Setting Exercise Goals

Achieving physical fitness requires time and effort. Unfortunately, many people who begin an exercise program stop before much progress has been achieved. Fitness cannot be achieved in a matter of a few days. In general, 3 to 6 weeks of regular exercise is required for noticeable improvements in muscle tone or muscular endurance. After beginning your personal fitness program, be patient; improvement will come, and you will like the changes.

The key to maintaining a long-term exercise program is personal motivation. Motivation, in this case, can be viewed as the *energy required to maintain your drive* to engage in daily exercise (33). The motivation to change from a sedentary lifestyle to an active lifestyle requires behavior modification and establishing goals. Without question, goal-setting is the cornerstone of any successful exercise program. Establishing realistic goals provides a target for your fitness efforts.

Table 1.1 contains some helpful information concerning exercise goal-setting. Note that it is important to establish both short-term and long-term goals. Short-term goals permit you to achieve a goal in a few weeks or months, whereas long-term goals are designed to provide motivation for years to come. Achievement of a short-term goal delivers great personal satisfaction and provides the needed incentive to pursue another fitness goal.

An additional point to notice in Table 1.1 is that goals should be written down. Putting exercise goals on paper is an excellent means of establishing a "contract" with yourself to maintain regular exercise habits. Another important aspect of goal-setting is that goals should be measurable. For example, your short-term goal for weight loss might be to lose 5 pounds during a period of 6 weeks. Because body weight is easily measured, you can assess your progress toward the attainment of your goal by periodic weighing. After achieving a fitness goal, it is important to set new goals to provide the incentive and motivation to continue your fitness program. More guidance in exercise goal-setting is provided in Chapters 3 and 16.

> **TABLE 1.1**
> **Strategies for Setting Exercise Goals**
>
> Establish achievable goals.
> Put goals in writing and in a place where you can see them every day.
> Establish both short-term and long-term goals.
> Establish goals that are measurable.
> Set target dates for achieving goals.
> After you achieve a goal, establish another achievable goal.
> Reward yourself after achieving each goal.

☀ Physical Fitness and Wellness: A Final Word

In this chapter we discussed the benefits of regular exercise and the importance of a healthy lifestyle to achieve wellness. The remainder of this book will present information that will help you set goals to increase your physical fitness, enrich your diet, and improve your health. Simply reading this book, however, will not accomplish these goals. Achieving physical fitness and wellness requires a personal commitment to regular exercise and wise lifestyle choices. Indeed, there is no "magic pill" that you can take to make you healthy or improve your physical fitness. Start today and become an exercise convert; your body will love you for it!

Summary

1. Exercise offers many health benefits. Regular exercise has been shown to reduce risk of CHD and diabetes, increase bone mass, and maintain physical working capacity during normal aging.

2. The five major components of "total" health-related physical fitness are
   a. cardiorespiratory endurance
   b. muscular strength
   c. muscular endurance
   d. flexibility
   e. body composition

3. The term *wellness* means "healthy living." This state is achieved by the practice of a positive healthy lifestyle, which includes regular physical activity, proper nutrition, eliminating unhealthy behaviors (avoiding high-risk activities such as reckless driving, smoking, and drug use), and maintaining good emotional and spiritual health.

4. Total wellness can be achieved only by a balance of physical, emotional, intellectual, spiritual, and social health. The components of wellness do not work in isolation; the five components interact strongly. For example, poor physical health can lead to poor emotional health. Similarly, a lack of spiritual health can contribute to poor emotional health as well as poor physical health.

5. Setting exercise goals is a key component in the maintenance of a lifetime fitness program.

Study Questions

1. Define the term *body composition*.
2. What is cardiorespiratory endurance?
3. Discuss the wellness concept.
4. Define osteoporosis.
5. List and discuss four major health benefits of regular exercise.

6. Discuss fitness training for sport performance versus training for health-related fitness.
7. List and discuss the five components of health-related fitness.
8. Outline the seven strategies for setting exercise goals.
9. What causes a myocardial infarction?
10. List and discuss the five components of wellness.

Suggested Reading

Armbruster, B., and L. Gladwin. More than fitness for older adults. *ACSM's Health and Fitness Journal* 5:6–12, 2001.

Blair, S., and M. Moore. Surgeon General's report on physical fitness: The inside story. *ACSM's Health and Fitness Journal* 1:14–18, 1997.

Franklin, B. Improved fitness = Increased longevity. *ACSM's Health and Fitness Journal* 5:32–33, 2001.

Maughan, R., ed. *Basic and Applied Sciences for Sports Medicine.* Oxford, England: Butterworth-Heinemann, 1999.

Powers, S., and E. Howley. *Exercise Physiology: Theory and Application to Fitness and Performance,* 4th ed. St. Louis: McGraw-Hill, 2001.

For links to the Web sites below visit Web Links at www.aw.com/fitness and choose Powers/Dodd Web Links from the drop-down menu.

American Heart Association

Contains latest information about ways to reduce your risk of heart and vascular diseases. Site includes information about exercise, diet, and heart disease.

American College of Sports Medicine

Contains information about exercise, health, and fitness.

WebMD

Contains the latest information on a variety of health-related topics including diet, exercise, and stress. Links to nutrition, fitness, and wellness topics.

Healthy People

Contains information about the U.S. government's initiative to improve health and wellness for the American people.

References

1. Bouchard, C., R. Shephard, T. Stephens, J. Sutton, and B. McPherson, eds. *Exercise, Fitness, and Health: A Consensus of Current Knowledge.* Champaign, IL: Human Kinetics, 1990.
2. Margen, S., et al., eds. *The Wellness Encyclopedia.* Boston: Houghton Mifflin, 1992.
3. Paffenbarger, R., J. Kampert, I-Min Lee, R. Hyde, R. Leung, and A. Wing. Changes in physical activity and other lifeway patterns influencing longevity. *Medicine and Science in Sports and Exercise* 26:857–865, 1994.
4. Paffenbarger, R., R. Hyde, A. Wing, and C. Hsieh. Physical activity, all cause mortality, longevity of college alumni. *New England Journal of Medicine* 314:605–613, 1986.
5. Helmrich, S., D. Ragland, and R. Paffenbarger. Prevention of non-insulin-dependent diabetes mellitus with physical activity. *Medicine and Science in Sports and Exercise* 26:824–830, 1994.
6. Wood, P. Physical activity, diet, and health: Independent and interactive effects. *Medicine and Science in Sports and Exercise* 26:838–843, 1994.
7. Morris, J. Exercise in the prevention of coronary heart disease: Today's best buy in public health. *Medicine and Science in Sports and Exercise* 26:807–814, 1994.
8. American Heart Association. *Heart and Stroke Facts.* Dallas: 2000.
9. Barrow, M. *Heart Talk: Understanding Cardiovascular Diseases.* Gainesville, FL: Cor-Ed Publishing, 1992.
10. Pollock, M., and J. Wilmore. *Exercise in Health and Disease.* Philadelphia: W. B. Saunders, 1990.
11. Williams, P. T. Relationship between distance run per week to coronary heart disease risk factors in 8283 male runners. The National Runners Health Study. *Archives of Internal Medicine* 157:191–198, 1997.
12. Fagard, R. Physical activity in the prevention and treatment of hypertension in the obese. *Medicine and Science in Sports and Exercise* 31:S624–S630, 1999.
13. Williams, P. Physical fitness and activity as separate heart disease risk factors: A meta-analysis. *Medicine and Science in Sports and Exercise* 33:754–761, 2001.
14. Powers, S., H. A. Demirel, et al. Exercise training improves myocardial tolerance to in vivo ischemia-reperfusion in the rat. *American Journal of Physiology* 275:R1468–1477, 1998.
15. Powers, S., M. Locke, and H. Demirel. Exercise, heat shock proteins, and myocardial protection from I-R injury. *Medicine and Science in Sports and Exercise* 33:386–392, 2001.
16. Yamashita, N., S. Hoshida, K. Otsu, M. Asahi, T. Kuzuya, and M. Hori. Exercise provides direct biphasic cardioprotection via manganese superoxide dismutase activation. *Journal of Experimental Medicine* 189:1699–1706, 1999.
17. Lee, I. M., and R. Paffenbarger. Associations of light, moderate, and vigorous intensity physical activity with longevity: The Harvard Alumni Health Study. *American Journal of Epidemiology* 151:293–299, 2000.
18. Powell, K., and S. Blair. The public health burdens of sedentary living habits: Theoretical but realistic estimates. *Medicine and Science in Sports and Exercise* 26:851–856, 1994.
19. Rodnick, K., J. Holloszy, C. Mondon, and D. James. Effects of exercise training on insulin-regulatable glucose-transporter protein levels in rat skeletal muscle. *Diabetes* 39:1425–1429, 1990.

20. Pan, X. R., et al. Effects of diet and exercise in preventing NIDDM in people with impaired glucose tolerance. *Diabetes Care* 20:537–544, 1997.

21. Rankin, J. Diet, exercise, and osteoporosis. *Certified News (American College of Sports Medicine)* 3:1–4, 1993.

22. Wheeler, D., J. Graves, G. Miller, R. Vander Griend, T. Wronski, S. K. Powers, and H. Park. Effects of running on the torsional strength, morphometry, and bone mass on the rat skeleton. *Medicine and Science in Sports and Exercise* 27:520–529, 1995.

23. Taaffe, D., T. Robinson, C. Snow, and R. Marcus. High impact exercise promotes bone gain in well-trained female athletes. *Journal of Bone and Mineral Research* 12:255–260, 1997.

24. Hagberg, J. Effect of training in the decline of $\dot{V}O_{2max}$ with aging. *Federation Proceedings* 46:1830–1833, 1987.

25. Fleg, J., and E. Lakatta. Role of muscle loss in the age-associated reduction in $\dot{V}O_{2max}$. *Journal of Applied Physiology* 65:1147–1151, 1988.

26. Nakamura, E., T. Moritani, and A. Kanetaka. Effects of habitual physical exercise on physiological age in men and women aged 20–85 years as estimated using principal component analysis. *European Journal of Applied Physiology* 73:410–418, 1996.

27. Hammeren, J., S. Powers, J. Lawler, D. Criswell, D. Martin, D. Lowenthal, and M. Pollock. Exercise training–induced alterations in skeletal muscle oxidative and antioxidant enzyme activity in senescent rats. *International Journal of Sports Medicine* 13:412–416, 1992.

28. Powers, S., J. Lawler, D. Criswell, Fu-Kong Lieu, and D. Martin. Aging and respiratory muscle metabolic plasticity: Effects of endurance training. *Journal of Applied Physiology* 72:1068–1073, 1992.

29. Holloszy, J. Exercise increases average longevity of female rats despite increased food intake and no growth retardation. *Journal of Gerontology* 48:B97–B100, 1993.

30. Lee, I., R. Paffenbarger, and C. Hennekens. Physical activity, physical fitness, and longevity. *Aging-Milano* 9:2–11, 1997.

31. Franklin, B. Improved fitness = Increased longevity. *ACSM's Health and Fitness Journal* 5:32–33, 2001.

32. Powers, S., and E. Howley. *Exercise Physiology: Theory and Application to Fitness and Performance,* 4th ed. St. Louis: McGraw-Hill, 2001.

33. Robergs, R., and S. Roberts. *Fundamental Principles of Exercise Physiology: For Fitness, Performance, and Health.* St. Louis: McGraw-Hill, 2000.

34. Williams, M. *Lifetime Fitness and Wellness.* Dubuque, IA: Wm. C. Brown, 1996.

35. Cady, L., D. Bischoff, E. O'Connell, P. Thomas, and J. Allan. Strength and fitness and subsequent back injuries in fire-fighters. *Journal of Occupational Medicine* 4:269–272, 1979.

36. Cady, L., P. Thomas, and R. Karasky. Programs for increasing health and physical fitness of fire-fighters. *Journal of Occupational Medicine* 2:111–114, 1985.

37. U.S. Department of Health and Human Services. Physical activity and health: A report of the Surgeon General. U.S. Department of Health and Human Services, Centers for Disease Control and Prevention, National Center for Chronic Disease Prevention and Health Promotion, Atlanta, GA, 1996.

38. Armbruster, B., and L. Gladwin. More than fitness for older adults. *ACSM's Health and Fitness Journal* 5:6–12, 2001.

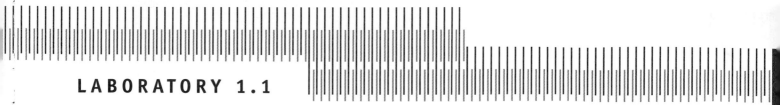

LABORATORY 1.1

Lifestyle Assessment Inventory

NAME _____ DATE _____

The purpose of this lifestyle assessment inventory is to increase your awareness of areas in your life that increase your risk of disease, injury, and possibly premature death. A key point to remember is that you have control over each of the lifestyle areas discussed.

Awareness is the first step in making change. After identifying the areas that require modification, you will be able to use the behavior modification techniques presented in Chapter 10 to bring about positive lifestyle changes.

DIRECTIONS

Put a check by each statement that applies to you. You may select more than one choice per category.

A. PHYSICAL FITNESS

_____ I exercise for a minimum of 20 to 30 minutes at least 3 days per week.
_____ I play sports routinely (2 to 3 times per week).
_____ I walk for 15 to 30 minutes (3 to 7 days per week).

B. BODY FAT

_____ There is no place on my body where I can pinch more than 1 inch of fat.
_____ I am satisfied with the way my body appears.

C. STRESS LEVEL

_____ I find it easy to relax.
_____ I rarely feel tense or anxious.
_____ I am able to cope with daily stresses without undue emotional stress.

D. CAR SAFETY

_____ I have not had an auto accident in the past 4 years.
_____ I always use a seat belt when I drive.
_____ I rarely drive above the speed limit.

E. SLEEP

_____ I always get 7 to 9 hours of sleep.
_____ I do not have trouble going to sleep.
_____ I generally do not wake up during the night.

F. RELATIONSHIPS

_____ I have a happy and satisfying relationship with my spouse or boy/girl friend.
_____ I have a lot of close friends.
_____ I get a great deal of love and support from my family.

(continued on next page)

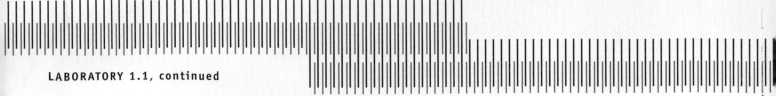

G. DIET

_____ I generally eat three balanced meals per day.
_____ I rarely overeat.
_____ I rarely eat large quantities of fatty foods and sweets.

H. ALCOHOL USE

_____ I consume fewer than two drinks per day.
_____ I never get intoxicated.
_____ I never drink and drive.

I. TOBACCO USE

_____ I never smoke (cigarettes, pipe, cigars, etc.).
_____ I am not exposed to second-hand smoke on a regular basis.
_____ I do not use smokeless tobacco.

J. DRUG USE

_____ I never use illicit drugs.
_____ I never abuse legal drugs such as diet or sleeping pills.

K. SEXUAL PRACTICES

_____ I always practice safe sex (e.g., always using condoms or being involved in a monoga-
mous relationship).

SCORING

1. **Individual areas:** If there are any unchecked areas in categories A through K, you can
improve those aspects of your lifestyle.

2. **Overall lifestyle:** Add up your total number of checks. Scoring can be interpreted as follows:

   23–29   Very healthy lifestyle
   17–22   Average healthy lifestyle
   ≤16   Unhealthy lifestyle (needs improvement)

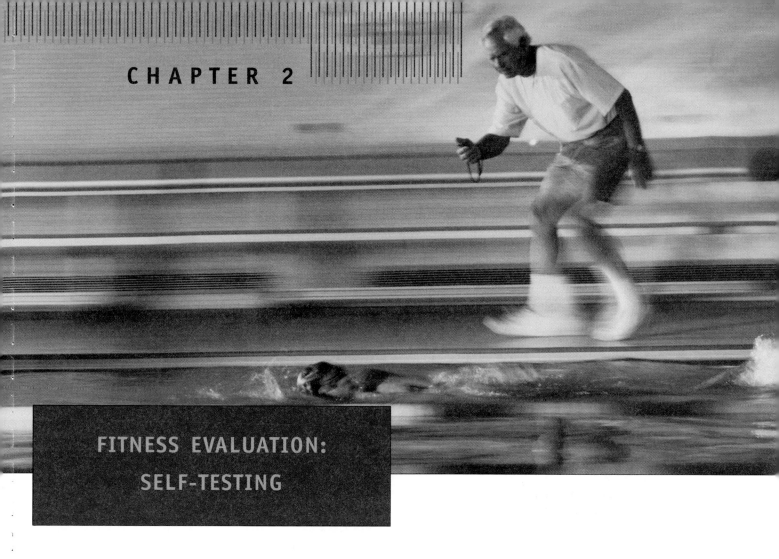

CHAPTER 2

FITNESS EVALUATION: SELF-TESTING

After studying this chapter, you should be able to:

1. Explain the principle behind field testing of cardiorespiratory fitness using the 1.5-mile run test, the 1-mile walking test, the cycle ergometer exercise test, and the step test.

2. Outline the design of the one-repetition maximum test for measurement of muscular strength.

3. Compare the push-up and sit-up tests as a means of evaluating muscular endurance.

4. Define the term *flexibility* and discuss two field tests used to assess it.

5. Discuss why assessment of body composition is important in health-related fitness testing.

6. Explain how body composition is assessed using hydrostatic weighing, the skinfold test, body mass index, and waist-to-hip circumference ratio.

An objective evaluation of your current fitness status is important prior to beginning an exercise training program (1–7). This evaluation provides valuable information concerning your fitness strengths and weaknesses and enables you to set reasonable fitness goals. Further, testing your initial fitness level also provides a benchmark against which you can compare future evaluations. Periodic re-testing (e.g., every 3 to 6 months) provides motivating feedback as your fitness program progresses.

This chapter presents a battery of physical fitness tests you can use to assess your fitness level. These tests are designed to evaluate each of the major components of health-related physical fitness: cardiorespiratory fitness, muscular strength, muscular endurance, flexibility, and body composition.

Although the risks associated with regular exercise are generally less than the risks associated with living a sedentary lifestyle, it is important to evaluate your health status before engaging in any physical fitness test. A brief discussion of the need for medical clearance prior to beginning an exercise program follows.

☀ Evaluating Health Status

Is a medical exam required before beginning a fitness program? The answer is probably "no" for healthy college-age individuals (1, 2). Although regular medical exams are encouraged for everyone, most people under 29 years of age generally do not require special medical clearance before beginning a low-to-moderate intensity exercise program. However, if you have any concerns about your health, an examination by a physician is prudent prior to starting an exercise program. Laboratory 2.1 on page 45 is a useful screening questionnaire for people of all ages who are beginning an exercise program. An answer of "yes" to any of the questions in

Laboratory 2.1 suggests that a medical problem may exist and that a complete medical exam is required.

Should individuals over 30 years old have a medical exam at the beginning of an exercise program? The most conservative answer is "yes." This is particularly true for obese and/or sedentary individuals. The following general guidelines apply:

18–29 years (men and women): You should have had a medical checkup within the last 2 years and completed Laboratory 2.1.

30–39 years (men) and 30–44 years (women): You should have had a medical checkup within the last year and completed Laboratory 2.1.

40 years and above (men): You should have had a medical checkup and a physician-supervised stress test within the last year (A Closer Look).

45 years and above (women): You should have had a medical checkup and a physician-supervised stress test within the last year (A Closer Look).

☀ IN SUMMARY

- Prior to beginning a fitness program you should evaluate your health status.
- An evaluation of your current fitness status provides valuable information regarding fitness strengths and weaknesses and enables you to set fitness goals.

☀ Measuring Cardiorespiratory Fitness

As we saw in Chapter 1, cardiorespiratory fitness is the ability to perform endurance-type exercises (e.g., running, cycling, swimming) and is considered a key component of health-related physical fitness. The most

---

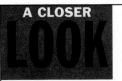

A CLOSER LOOK

The Exercise ECG

The electrocardiogram (ECG, or sometimes EKG) is a common medical test that measures the electrical activity of the heart and can be used to diagnose several types of heart disease (7, 8). Although a resting ECG is useful for determining the heart's function, ECG monitoring during exercise is particularly useful in diagnosing hidden heart problems, because heart abnormalities often appear during periods of emotional or exercise stress (7). An exercise ECG, commonly called an **exercise stress test,** is generally performed on a treadmill while a physician monitors heart rate, blood pressure, and ECG. The test begins with a brief warm-up period followed by a progressive increase in exercise intensity until the patient cannot continue or the physician stops the test for medical reasons. In general, the duration of the test varies as a function of the subject's fitness level. For example, poorly conditioned people may exercise for only 10 to 12 minutes, whereas well-conditioned subjects may work for up to 25 or 30 minutes. Therefore, the exercise stress test not only provides data about your cardiovascular health, but also provides information about cardiorespiratory fitness.

TABLE 2.1
Fitness Categories for Cooper's 1.5-Mile Run Test to Determine Cardiorespiratory Fitness

Fitness Category	Age (years)					
	13–19	20–29	30–39	40–49	50–59	60+
Men						
Very poor	>15:30	>16:00	>16:30	>17:30	>19:00	>20:00
Poor	12:11–15:30	14:01–16:00	14:46–16:30	15:36–17:30	17:01–19:00	19:01–20:00
Average	10:49–12:10	12:01–14:00	12:31–14:45	13:01–15:35	14:31–17:00	16:16–19:00
Good	9:41–10:48	10:46–12:00	11:01–12:30	11:31–13:00	12:31–14:30	14:00–16:15
Excellent	8:37–9:40	9:45–10:45	10:00–11:00	10:30–11:30	11:00–12:30	11:15–13:59
Superior	<8:37	<9:45	<10:00	<10:30	<11:00	<11:15
Women						
Very poor	>18:30	>19:00	>19:30	>20:00	>20:30	>21:00
Poor	16:55–18:30	18:31–19:00	19:01–19:30	19:31–20:00	20:01–20:30	20:31–21:31
Average	14:31–16:54	15:55–18:30	16:31–19:00	17:31–19:30	19:01–20:00	19:31–20:30
Good	12:30–14:30	13:31–15:54	14:31–16:30	15:56–17:30	16:31–19:00	17:31–19:30
Excellent	11:50–12:29	12:30–13:30	13:00–14:30	13:45–15:55	14:30–16:30	16:30–18:00
Superior	<11:50	<12:30	<13:00	<13:45	<14:30	<16:30

Times are given in minutes and seconds. (> = greater than; < = less than)

From Cooper, K. The aerobics program for total well-being. Bantam Books, New York, 1982. Copyright © 1982 by Kenneth H. Cooper. Used by permission of Bantam Books, a division of Bantam Doubleday Dell Publishing Group, Inc.

accurate means of measuring cardiorespiratory fitness is the laboratory assessment of maximal oxygen consumption (9, 10) (called $\dot{V}O_{2max}$). In simple terms, $\dot{V}O_{2max}$ is a measure of the endurance capacity of both the cardiorespiratory system and exercising skeletal muscles. Because direct measurement of $\dot{V}O_{2max}$ requires expensive laboratory equipment and is very time consuming, it is impractical for general use. Fortunately, researchers have developed numerous methods for estimating $\dot{V}O_{2max}$ using simple field tests (11–13). In the following paragraphs we describe several types of field exercise tests designed to evaluate cardiorespiratory fitness.

THE 1.5-MILE RUN TEST

One of the simplest and most accurate means of evaluating cardiorespiratory fitness is the **1.5-mile run test.** This test, popularized by Dr. Kenneth Cooper, works on the physiological principle that people with a high level of cardiorespiratory fitness can run 1.5 miles in less time than less-fit individuals (11, 12).

The 1.5-mile run test is excellent for physically active college-age individuals. Due to its intensity, however, the 1.5-mile run test is not well suited for sedentary people over 30 years of age, severely deconditioned people, individuals with joint problems, and obese individuals.

The objective of the test is to complete a 1.5-mile distance (preferably on a track) in the shortest possible time. The test is best conducted in moderate weather conditions (avoiding very hot or very cold days). For a reasonably physically fit individual, the 1.5-mile distance can be covered by running or jogging. For less fit individuals, the test becomes a run/walk test. A good strategy is to try to keep a steady pace during the entire distance. In this regard, it may be beneficial to perform a practice test in order to determine the optimal pace that you can maintain. Accurate timing of the test is essential, and use of a stop watch is best. Laboratory 2.2 on page 47 provides instructions for performing the test and recording the score.

Interpreting your test results is simple. Table 2.1 contains norms for cardiorespiratory fitness using the

exercise stress test A diagnostic text designed to determine if a patient's cardiovascular system has a normal response to exercise. The test is generally performed on a treadmill while a physician monitors heart rate, blood pressure, and ECG.

1.5-mile run test A fitness test designed to evaluate cardiorespiratory fitness. The objective of the test is to complete a 1.5-mile distance (preferably on a track) in the shortest possible time.

> **TABLE 2.2**
> **Fitness Classification for 1-Mile Walk Test**
>
> | Fitness Category | Age (years) | | | |
> |---|---|---|---|---|
> | | 13–19 | 20–29 | 30–39 | 40+ |
> | *Men* | | | | |
> | Very poor | >17:30 | >18:00 | >19:00 | >21:30 |
> | Poor | 16:01–17:30 | 16:31–18:00 | 17:31–19:00 | 18:31–21:30 |
> | Average | 14:01–16:00 | 14:31–16:30 | 15:31–17:30 | 16:01–18:30 |
> | Good | 12:30–14:00 | 13:00–14:30 | 13:30–15:30 | 14:00–16:00 |
> | Excellent | <12:30 | <13:00 | <13:30 | <14:00 |
> | *Women* | | | | |
> | Very poor | >18:01 | >18:31 | >19:31 | >20:01 |
> | Poor | 16:31–18:00 | 17:01–18:30 | 18:01–19:30 | 19:31–20:00 |
> | Average | 14:31–16:30 | 15:01–17:00 | 16:01–18:00 | 18:01–19:30 |
> | Good | 13:31–14:30 | 13:31–15:00 | 14:01–16:00 | 14:31–18:00 |
> | Excellent | <13:30 | <13:30 | <14:00 | <14:30 |
>
> *Because the 1-mile walk test is designed primarily for older or less conditioned individuals, the fitness categories listed here do not include a "superior" category.*
>
> *Modified from Rockport Fitness Walking Test. Copyright © 1993. The Rockport Company, Inc. All rights reserved. Reprinted by permission of The Rockport Company, Inc.*

1.5-mile run test. Find your sex, age group, and finish time in the table and then locate your fitness category on the left side of the table. Consider the following example: Johnny Jones is 21 years old and completes the 1.5-mile run in 13 minutes and 25 seconds (13:25). Using Table 2.1 on page 19, locate Johnny's age group and time column. Note that a finish time of 13:25 for the 1.5-mile run would place Johnny in the "average" fitness category.

THE 1-MILE WALK TEST

Another field test to determine cardiorespiratory fitness is the **1-mile walk test,** which is particularly useful for sedentary individuals (14–16). It is a weight-bearing test, however, so individuals with joint problems should not participate.

The 1-mile walk test works on the same principle as the 1.5-mile run test. That is, individuals with high

levels of cardiorespiratory fitness will complete a 1-mile walk in a shorter time than those who are less conditioned. This test is also best conducted in moderate weather conditions, preferably on a track. Subjects should try to maintain a steady pace over the distance. Again, because test scores are based on time, accurate timing is essential.

Laboratory 2.3 on page 49 provides instructions for performing the test and for recording your score. Table 2.2 contains norms for scoring cardiorespiratory fitness using the 1-mile walk test. Find your age group and finish time in the table and then locate your fitness category on the left side of it.

THE CYCLE ERGOMETER FITNESS TEST

For those with access to a cycle ergometer (a stationary exercise bicycle that provides pedaling resistance via friction applied to the wheel), a **cycle ergometer fitness test** is an excellent means of evaluating cardiorespiratory fitness. It offers advantages over running or walking tests for individuals with joint problems due to the non-weight-bearing nature of cycling. Further, because this type of test can be performed indoors, it has advantages over outdoor fitness tests during very cold or hot weather.

Although numerous types of cycle ergometers exist, the most common type is friction braked, which

1-mile walk test A fitness test designed to evaluate cardiorespiratory fitness. The objective of the test is to complete a 1-mile walk (preferably on a track) in the shortest possible time.
cycle ergometer fitness test A submaximal exercise test designed to evaluate cardiorespiratory fitness.

TABLE 2.3
Work Rates for Submaximal Cycle Ergometer Fitness Test

Gender	Age (years)	Pedal Speed (RPM)	Load (watts)
Male	Up to 29	60	150 (900 KPM)
	30 and up	60	50 (300 KPM)
Female	Up to 29 (or poorly conditioned)	60	100 (600 KPM)
	30 and up (or poorly conditioned)	60	50 (300 KPM)

---

incorporates a belt wrapped around the wheel. The belt can be loosened or tightened to provide a change in resistance (pedaling difficulty). The work performed on a cycle ergometer is commonly expressed either in units called *kilopond meters per minute (KPM)* or in watts. It is not important that you understand the details of these units, but you should recognize that KPMs and watts are measurement units that represent how much work is performed. For example, a workload of 300 KPM (50 watts) on the cycle ergometer would be considered a submaximal (involving a light load) work rate for almost everyone, whereas a load of 3000 KPM (500 watts) would represent a high work rate for even highly conditioned individuals.

The cycle ergometer fitness test is conducted as follows:

1. Warm up for 3 minutes while pedaling the cycle at 60 revolutions per minute (RPM) with no load against the pedals.

2. After completion of the warm-up, begin the fitness test. Set the load on the cycle ergometer using Table 2.3 and perform 5 minutes of exercise.

3. During the last minute of exercise, measure your heart rate for 15 seconds. This can be achieved by palpation of the pulse in your wrist (radial artery) or by gentle palpation of the pulse in your neck (carotid artery) (Figure 2.1). Note that accurate

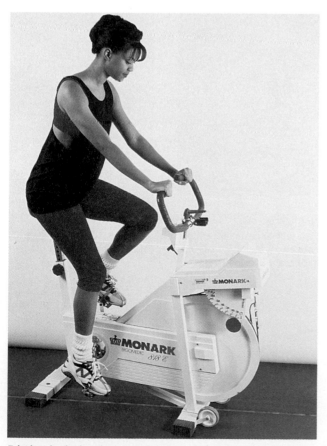

Friction-braked cycle ergometer (exercise cycle) can be used to evaluate cardiorespiratory fitness.

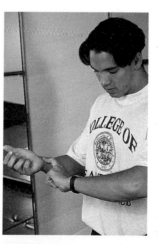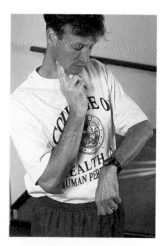

FIGURE 2.1
Subjects counting heart rate for 15 seconds using the radial or carotid artery. Palpation of the radial artery (wrist) or carotid artery (neck) is a simple means of determining heart rate. The procedure is performed as follows. Locate your radial or carotid artery using your index finger. After finding your radial or carotid pulse, count the number of heart beats (pulses) that occur during a 15-second period. Heart rate for 1 minute is computed by multiplying the number of heart beats counted in 15 seconds by 4. For example, a 15-second heart rate count of 30 beats would indicate that the heart rate was 120 beats/min (i.e., 30 × 4 = 120). When palpating the carotid artery, take care to apply limited pressure on the neck. Application of too much force on the carotid artery will result in a reflexic lowering of your heart rate and will therefore bias heart rate measurement.

measurement of heart rate is critical for this test to be a valid assessment of cardiorespiratory fitness.

This type of submaximal cycle test works on the principle that individuals with high cardiorespiratory fitness levels have a lower exercise heart rate at a standard workload than less fit individuals (8, 13).

After completing the test, use your 15-second heart rate count to find your estimated $\dot{V}O_{2max}$ as instructed in Table 2.4. For example, a 21-year-old woman with a 15-second heart rate of 36 would have an estimated $\dot{V}O_{2max}$ of 27 ml/kg/min. (See A Closer Look on page 23 for a discussion of $\dot{V}O_2$ units.) Now use Table 2.5 on page 24 to find the corresponding fitness category. A $\dot{V}O_{2max}$ of 27 ml/kg/min for a 21-year-old woman would place her in the "very poor" cardiorespiratory fitness category. Laboratory 2.4 on page 51 permits recording of your score on this test.

☼ The Step Test

An alternative test to determine your cardiorespiratory fitness level is the **step test.** The step test works on the principle that individuals with a high level of cardiorespiratory fitness will have a lower heart rate during recovery from 3 minutes of standardized exercise (bench stepping) than less conditioned individuals (4, 9). Although the step test is not considered the best field method to estimate cardiorespiratory fitness, it does have advantages in that it can be performed indoors and can be used by people at all fitness levels. Further, the step test does not require expensive equipment and can be performed in a short amount of time.

Step height for both men and women should be approximately 18 inches. In general, locker room benches or sturdy chairs can be used as stepping devices. The test is conducted as follows:

1. Select a partner to assist you in the step test. Your partner is responsible for timing the test and assisting you in maintaining the proper stepping cadence. The exercise cadence is 30 complete steps (up and down) per minute during a 3-minute exer-

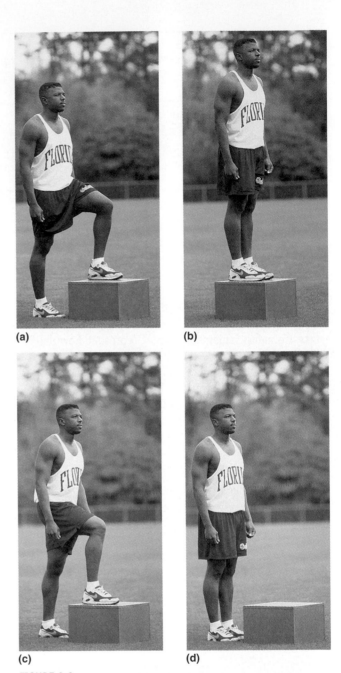

(a)　　　　(b)

(c)　　　　(d)

FIGURE 2.2
Step test to evaluate cardiorespiratory fitness. Subjects step up onto an 18-inch high surface (a), (b), and then down (c), (d) once every 2 seconds.

---

step test　A submaximal exercise test designed to evaluate cardiorespiratory fitness. The step test works on the principle that individuals with a high level of cardiorespiratory fitness will have a lower heart rate during recovery from 3 minutes of standardized exercise (bench stepping) than less-conditioned individuals.

---

cise period, which can be maintained by a metronome or voice cues from your friend ("up, up, down, down"). Thus you need to make one complete step cycle every 2 seconds (i.e., set the metronome at 60 tones/min and step up and down with each sound). Note that it is important that you straighten your knees during the "up" phase of the test (Figure 2.2).

2. After completing the test, sit quietly in a chair or on the step bench. Find your pulse and count your

---

TABLE 2.4
Cycle Ergometer Fitness Index for Men and Women

Locate your 15-second heart rate in the left-hand column; then find your estimated $\dot{V}O_{2max}$ in the appropriate column on the right. For example, the second column from the left contains the absolute $\dot{V}O_{2max}$ (expressed in ml/min) for male subjects using the 900-KPM work rate. The third column from the left contains the absolute $\dot{V}O_{2max}$ (expressed in ml/min) for women using the 600-KPM work rate, and so on. After determination of your absolute $\dot{V}O_{2max}$, calculate your relative $\dot{V}O_{2max}$ (ml/kg/min) by dividing your $\dot{V}O_{2max}$ expressed in ml/min by your body weight in kilograms (1 kilogram = 2.2 pounds). For example, if your body weight is 70 kilograms and your absolute $\dot{V}O_{2max}$ is 2631 ml/min, your relative $\dot{V}O_{2max}$ is approximately 38 ml/kg/min (i.e., 2631 divided by 70 = 37.6). After computing your relative $\dot{V}O_{2max}$, use Table 2.5 to identify your fitness category.

	Estimated Absolute $\dot{V}O_{2max}$ (ml/mn)		
15-Second Heart Rate	Men: 900-KPM Work Rate (ml/min)	Women: 600-KPM Work Rate (ml/min)	Men or Women: 300-KPM Work Rate (ml/min)
28	3560	2541	1525
29	3442	2459	1475
30	3333	2376	1425
31	3216	2293	1375
32	3099	2210	1325
33	2982	2127	1275
34	2865	2044	1225
35	2748	1961	1175
36	2631	1878	1125
37	2514	1795	1075
38	2397	1712	1025
39	2280	1629	—
40	2163	1546	—
41	2046	1463	—
42	1929	1380	—
43	1812	1297	—
44	1695	1214	—
45	1578	1131	—

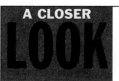
A CLOSER LOOK

Maximum Oxygen Uptake ($\dot{V}O_{2max}$)

As discussed earlier, $\dot{V}O_{2max}$ is the maximal capacity to transport and utilize oxygen during exercise, and it is considered to be the most valid measurement of cardiorespiratory fitness (9, 10). In cardiorespiratory fitness testing, it is common to express $\dot{V}O_{2max}$ as a function of body weight (called relative $\dot{V}O_{2max}$). This means that the "absolute" $\dot{V}O_{2max}$ (expressed in milliliters per minute; commonly written as ml/min) is divided by the subject's body weight in kilograms (1 kilogram = 2.2 pounds). Therefore, relative $\dot{V}O_{2max}$ is expressed in milliliters (ml) of oxygen consumed per minute per kilogram of body weight (ml/kg/min). Expressing $\dot{V}O_{2max}$ relative to body weight is particularly appropriate when describing an individual's fitness status during weight-bearing activities such as running, walking, climbing steps, or ice skating (9).

The higher the relative $\dot{V}O_{2max}$, the greater the cardiorespiratory fitness. For example, a 20-year-old female college student with a relative $\dot{V}O_{2max}$ of 53 ml/kg/min would be classified in the "superior" cardiorespiratory fitness category. In contrast, a 20-year-old woman with a $\dot{V}O_{2max}$ of 29 ml/kg/min would be classified in the "very poor" fitness category (17) (Table 2.5).

TABLE 2.5

Cardiorespiratory Fitness Norms for Men and Women Based on Estimated $\dot{V}O_{2max}$ Values Determined by the Bicycle Ergometer Fitness Test

After determining your relative $\dot{V}O_{2max}$ (ml/kg/min) in Table 2.4, find your appropriate fitness category.

Age Group (years)	Fitness Categories Based on $\dot{V}O_{2max}$ (ml/kg/min)					
	Very Poor	Poor	Average	Good	Excellent	Superior
Men						
13–19	<35	36–39	40–46	47–53	54–59	>60
20–29	<33	34–38	39–45	46–52	53–58	>59
30–39	<32	33–37	38–43	44–49	50–53	>54
40–49	<30	31–36	37–41	42–48	49–52	>53
50–59	<28	29–32	33–38	39–45	46–49	>50
60+	<24	25–29	30–34	35–39	40–44	>45
Women						
13–19	<28	29–34	35–40	41–44	45–52	>52
20–29	<30	31–33	34–38	39–42	43–51	>51
30–39	<28	29–31	32–36	37–42	43–45	>45
40–49	<25	26–28	29–34	35–39	40–42	>42
50–59	<23	24–25	26–30	31–34	35–38	>38
60+	<22	23–24	25–29	30–34	35–36	>36

Modified from Golding, L., C. Myers, and W. Sinning. Y's way to physical fitness: The complete guide to fitness testing and instruction. *3rd ed. Human Kinetics, Champaign, IL, 1989.*

---

heart rate for 30-second periods during the following recovery times:

1 to 1.5 minutes post exercise

2 to 2.5 minutes post exercise

3 to 3.5 minutes post exercise

Your partner should assist you in timing the recovery period and recording your recovery heart rates. Note that the accuracy of this test depends on both the faithful execution of 30 steps per minute during the test and the valid measurement of heart rate during the appropriate recovery times.

Laboratory 2.5 on page 53 provides a place to record your recovery heart rates and fitness category. To determine your fitness category, add the three 30-second heart rates obtained during recovery; this is called the **recovery index.** Table 2.6 contains norms for step test results in a college-age population (18–25 years). For example, a male student with a recovery in-

dex of 165 beats would be classified as having average cardiorespiratory fitness.

CARDIORESPIRATORY FITNESS: HOW DO YOU RATE?

After completing the cardiorespiratory fitness test of your choice, the next step is to interpret your results and set goals for improvement. If your cardiorespiratory fitness test score placed you in the "very poor" or "poor" classification, your current fitness level is below average compared with that of other healthy men or women of similar age in North America. On the other hand, a fitness test score in the "good" category means that your current cardiorespiratory fitness level is above average for your gender and age group. The fitness category "excellent" means that your level of cardiorespiratory conditioning is well above average. The "superior" rating is reserved for those individuals whose cardiorespiratory fitness level ranks in the top 15% of people in their age group. A key point here is that regardless of how low your current cardiorespiratory fitness level may be, you can improve by adherence to a regular exercise training program.

As mentioned earlier, testing your initial cardiorespiratory fitness level provides a benchmark against

---

recovery index   Measurement of heart rate during three 30-second recovery periods following a submaximal step test. (See the text for complete details.)

TABLE 2.6
Norms for Cardiorespiratory Fitness Using the Sum of Three Recovery Heart Rates Obtained Following the Step Test

Fitness Category	3-Minute Step Test Recovery Index	
	Women	Men
Superior	95–120	95–117
Excellent	121–135	118–132
Good	136–153	133–147
Average	154–174	148–165
Poor	175–204	166–192
Very poor	205–233	193–217

Fitness categories are for college-age men and women (ages 18–25 years) at the University of Florida who performed the test on an 18-inch bench.

which you can compare future evaluations. Performing additional fitness tests as your fitness level improves is important because this type of positive feedback provides motivation to maintain regular exercise habits (3–5, 18).

☀ IN SUMMARY

- Cardiorespiratory fitness is the ability to perform endurance exercises (e.g., running, cycling) and is a key component of health-related physical fitness.

- Individuals with superior cardiorespiratory fitness have the ability to perform high levels of endurance-type activities.

- Field tests to evaluate cardiorespiratory fitness include the 1.5-mile run test, the 1-mile walk test, the cycle ergometer fitness test, and the step test.

☀ Evaluation of Muscular Strength

As discussed in Chapter 1, muscular strength is defined as the maximum amount of force you can produce during one contraction (19). Muscular strength not only is important for success in athletics, but also is useful for the average person in performing routine tasks at work or home. Strength can be measured by the **one-repetition maximum (1 RM) test,** which measures the maximum amount of weight that can be lifted one time. It is also possible to estimate the 1 RM by performing multiple repetitions using a submaximal weight. Methods for directly measuring and for estimating the 1 RM are discussed in the following sections.

Nutritional Links
TO HEALTH AND FITNESS

Dehydration Can Negatively Impact a Cardiorespiratory Fitness Test

Approximately 60–70% of the body is water. Heavy sweating and/or the failure to drink enough fluids during the day can lower body water levels and result in dehydration. Water is involved in every vital process of the body, so dehydration can impair exercise performance. For example, dehydration results in reduced blood volume and elevated heart rates during submaximal exercise. This dehydration-induced high heart rate during submaximal exercise will result in an underestimation of $\dot{V}O_{2max}$ during submaximal fitness tests (e.g., a cycle ergometer or step fitness test) (9). Further, dehydration can negatively impact endurance performance during field tests of $\dot{V}O_{2max}$ (e.g., 1.5-mile run) (9, 19). Therefore, because dehydration can impair exercise performance, cardiorespiratory fitness tests should be performed only when the test subjects are adequately hydrated. See Chapter 7 for more details on the maintenance of normal body water levels.

THE 1 RM TEST

Although the 1 RM test for muscular strength is widely accepted (7), it has been criticized as unsuitable for use with older individuals or highly deconditioned people. The major concern is the risk of injury. The 1 RM test should therefore be attempted only after several weeks of strength training, which will result in improvements in both skill and strength and reduce the risk of injury during the test. An older or sedentary individual would probably require 6 weeks of exercise training prior to the 1 RM test, whereas a physically active college-age student could probably perform the 1 RM test after 1 to 2 weeks of training.

The 1 RM test is designed to test muscular strength in selected muscle groups and is performed in the following manner. Begin with a 5- to 10-minute warm-up using the muscles to be tested. For each muscle group, select an initial weight that you can lift without undue stress. Then gradually add weight until you reach the maximum weight that you can lift one time.

one-repetition maximum (1 RM) test   Measurement of the maximum amount of weight that can be lifted one time.

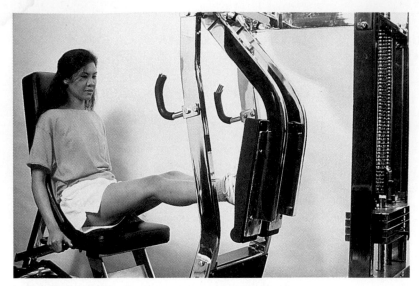

FIGURE 2.3
A leg press to evaluate muscular strength.

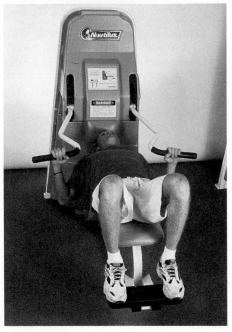

FIGURE 2.4
The bench press to evaluate muscular strength.

If you can lift the weight more than once, add additional weight until you reach a level of resistance such that you can perform only one repetition. Remember that a true 1 RM is the maximum amount of weight that you can lift one time.

Figures 2.3 through 2.6 illustrate four common lifts used to measure strength. Three of these (bench press, biceps curl, and shoulder press) use upper body muscle groups; the fourth lift (leg press) measures leg strength. Your muscle strength score is your percentage of body weight lifted in each exercise. To compute your strength score in each lift, divide your 1 RM weight in pounds by your body weight in pounds and then multiply by 100. For example, suppose a 150-pound man has a bench press 1 RM of 180 pounds. This individual's muscle strength score for the bench press is computed as

$$\frac{1\ RM\ weight}{body\ weight} \times 100 = muscle\ strength\ score$$

Therefore,

$$muscle\ strength\ score = \frac{180\ pounds}{150\ pounds} \times 100 = 120$$

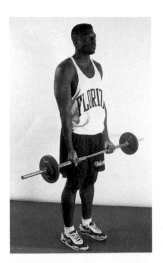
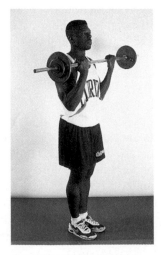

FIGURE 2.5
A biceps curl to evaluate muscular strength.

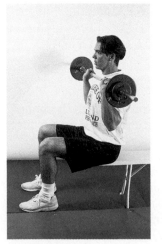
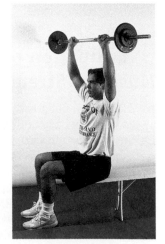

FIGURE 2.6
The shoulder or "military" press to evaluate muscular strength.

TABLE 2.7
Norms for Muscle Strength Scores Using a 1 RM Test

In this table, use your muscle strength score to locate your fitness level.

Exercise	Fitness Category					
	Very Poor	**Poor**	**Average**	**Good**	**Excellent**	**Superior**
Men						
Bench press	<50	50–99	100–110	111–130	131–149	>149
Biceps curl	<30	30–40	41–54	55–60	61–79	>79
Shoulder press	<40	41–50	51–67	68–80	81–110	>110
Leg press	<160	161–199	200–209	210–229	230–239	>239
Women						
Bench press	<40	41–69	70–74	75–80	81–99	>99
Biceps curl	<15	15–34	35–39	40–55	56–59	>59
Shoulder press	<20	20–46	47–54	55–59	60–79	>79
Leg press	<100	100–130	131–144	145–174	175–189	>189

Norms are from ref. 7.

Table 2.7 contains strength score norms for college-age men and women in each of these lifts. Using Table 2.7, a muscle strength score of 120 on the bench press places a college-age man in the "good" category. You can record your muscle strength scores in Laboratory 2.6 on page 55.

ESTIMATING THE 1 RM USING A 10 RM TEST

Determining the 1 RM is relatively easy for an experienced weight lifter, but measurement of the 1 RM for an inexperienced lifter is often difficult and can present a risk for injury. To reduce the possibility of injury during strength testing, researchers developed a method to estimate the 1 RM using a series of submaximal lifts. Although the use of submaximal lifts to estimate the 1 RM is slightly less accurate, the advantage of this technique is the reduced risk of injury.

Estimation of the 1 RM in any particular lift (e.g., bench press) is achieved using the following procedure (19). Testing begins with the individual performing a set of 10 repetitions using a light weight. Depending on the ease with which these repetitions are completed, the instructor then adds additional weight, and the individual performs another set of 10 repetitions. This process continues until a weight is reached that can only be lifted 10 times (called the 10 RM). In general, an experienced instructor can aid the individual by supervising the process so that the 10 RM weight can be discovered in fewer than five trials (19). Note that a rest period of approximately 5 minutes should separate these trials to permit adequate time for recovery.

After determining the 10 RM, the 1 RM can be estimated using Table 2.8 on pages 28 and 29. For example, if an individual's 10 RM for a particular lift is 100 pounds, then the estimate for the 1 RM would be 135 pounds. This was determined by locating the number closest to 100 pounds in the 10 repetitions column (i.e., 99.2 pounds) in Table 2.8 and then locating the 1 RM weight in the left-hand column for this row.

Note that the 1 RM can also be estimated using fewer than 10 repetitions (i.e., 7–9 repetitions). For example, a beginning weight lifter can sometimes develop muscle fatigue and fail to complete 10 repetitions during a testing period. In this case, if the individual completes as many as 7–9 repetitions with a given weight, the 1 RM can be still estimated using Table 2.8. For instance, if an individual completes 7 repetitions with 110 pounds, the estimate for 1 RM is 135 pounds. As in the previous example, the estimated 1 RM was determined by locating the number closest to 110 pounds in the 7 repetitions column (i.e., 109.4 pounds) in Table 2.8, and then locating the 1 RM weight in the left-hand column for this row.

After determining the estimated 1 RM, the individual's muscle strength score is determined using the formula discussed in the previous section. That is,

$$\text{muscle strength score} = \frac{1 \text{ RM weight}}{\text{body weight}} \times 100$$

After calculating your muscle strength score, record your strength scores in Laboratory 2.6 on page 55.

TABLE 2.8
Estimating the 1 RM from the 10 RM

Estimated 1 RM (pounds)	Weight (pounds) Lifted During 7 Repetitions	Weight (pounds) Lifted During 8 Repetitions	Weight (pounds) Lifted During 9 Repetitions	Weight (pounds) Lifted During 10 Repetitions
5.0	4.1	3.9	3.8	3.7
10.0	8.2	7.9	7.6	7.4
15.0	12.2	11.8	11.4	11.0
20.0	16.2	15.7	15.2	14.7
25.0	20.2	19.6	19.0	18.4
30.0	24.3	23.6	22.8	22.1
35.0	28.4	27.5	26.6	25.7
40.0	32.4	31.4	30.4	29.4
45.0	36.5	35.3	34.2	33.1
50.0	40.5	39.3	38.0	36.8
55.0	44.6	43.2	41.8	40.4
60.0	48.6	47.1	45.6	44.1
65.0	52.7	51.0	49.4	47.8
70.0	56.7	55.0	53.2	51.5
75.0	60.8	58.9	57.0	55.1
80.0	64.8	62.8	60.8	58.8
85.0	68.9	66.7	64.6	62.5
90.0	72.9	70.7	68.4	66.2
95.0	77.0	74.6	72.2	69.8
100.0	81.0	78.5	76.0	73.5
105.0	85.1	82.4	79.8	77.2
110.0	89.1	86.4	83.6	80.9
115.0	93.2	90.3	87.4	84.5
120.0	97.2	94.2	91.2	88.2
125.0	101.3	98.1	95.0	91.9
130.0	105.3	102.1	98.8	95.6
135.0	109.4	106.0	102.6	99.2
140.0	113.4	109.9	106.4	102.9
145.0	117.5	113.8	110.2	106.6
150.0	121.5	117.8	114.0	110.3
155.0	125.6	121.7	117.8	113.9
160.0	129.6	125.6	121.6	117.6
165.0	133.7	129.5	125.4	121.3
170.0	137.7	133.5	129.2	125.0
175.0	141.8	137.4	133.0	128.6
180.0	145.8	141.3	136.8	132.3
185.0	149.9	145.2	140.6	136.0
190.0	153.9	149.2	144.4	139.7
195.0	158.0	153.1	148.2	143.3
200.0	162.0	157.0	152.0	147.0
205.0	166.1	160.9	155.8	150.7
210.0	170.1	164.9	159.6	154.4
215.0	174.2	168.8	163.4	158.0
220.0	178.2	182.7	167.2	161.7
225.0	182.3	176.6	171.0	165.4

Data are from ref. 20.

TABLE 2.8
Estimating the 1 RM from the 10 RM (continued)

Estimated 1 RM (pounds)	Weight (pounds) Lifted During 7 Repetitions	Weight (pounds) Lifted During 8 Repetitions	Weight (pounds) Lifted During 9 Repetitions	Weight (pounds) Lifted During 10 Repetitions
230.0	186.3	180.6	174.8	169.1
235.0	190.4	184.5	178.6	172.7
240.0	194.4	188.4	182.4	176.4
245.0	198.5	192.3	186.2	180.1
250.0	202.5	196.3	190.0	183.8
255.0	206.6	200.2	193.8	187.4
260.0	210.6	204.1	197.6	191.2
265.0	214.7	208.1	201.4	194.8
270.0	218.7	212.0	205.2	198.5
275.0	222.8	215.9	209.0	202.1
280.0	226.8	219.8	212.8	205.8
285.0	230.9	223.7	216.6	209.5
290.0	234.9	227.7	220.4	213.2
295.0	239.0	231.6	224.2	216.8
300.0	243.0	235.5	228.0	220.5
305.0	247.1	239.4	231.8	224.2
310.0	251.1	243.4	235.6	227.9
315.0	255.2	247.3	239.4	231.5
320.0	259.2	251.2	243.2	235.2
325.0	263.3	255.1	247.0	238.9
330.0	267.3	259.1	250.8	242.6
335.0	271.4	263.0	254.6	246.2
340.0	275.4	266.9	258.4	249.9
345.0	279.5	270.8	262.2	253.6
350.0	283.6	274.8	266.0	257.3
355.0	287.6	278.7	269.8	260.9
360.0	291.6	282.6	273.6	264.6
365.0	295.7	286.5	277.4	268.3
370.0	299.7	290.5	281.2	272.0
375.0	303.8	294.4	285.0	275.6
380.0	307.8	298.3	288.8	279.3
385.0	311.9	302.0	292.6	283.0
390.0	315.9	306.2	296.4	286.7
395.0	320.0	310.1	300.2	290.3
400.0	324.0	314.0	304.0	294.0
405.0	328.1	317.9	307.8	297.7
410.0	332.1	321.9	311.6	301.4
415.0	336.2	325.8	315.4	305.0
420.0	340.2	329.7	319.2	308.7
425.0	344.3	333.6	323.0	312.4
430.0	348.3	337.6	326.8	316.1
435.0	352.4	341.5	330.6	319.7
440.0	356.4	345.4	334.4	323.4
445.0	360.5	349.3	338.2	327.1
450.0	364.5	353.3	342.0	330.8
455.0	368.6	357.2	345.8	334.4

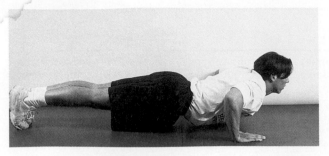
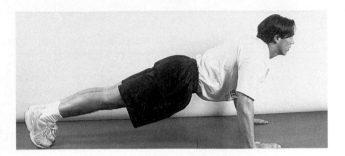

FIGURE 2.7
The standard push-up.

MUSCULAR STRENGTH: HOW DO YOU RATE?

When you have completed your muscular strength test, the next step is to interpret your results (Table 2.7) and set goals for improvement. Similar to the fitness categories used for cardiorespiratory fitness, the fitness categories for muscular strength range from very poor (lowest) to superior (highest). If your current strength level is classified as average or below, don't be discouraged; you can improve! A key point in maintaining your motivation to exercise regularly is the establishment of goals. Record both short-term and long-term goals for improvement. After 6 to 12 weeks of training, perform a retest to evaluate your progress. Reaching a short-term goal provides added incentive to continue your exercise program.

☀ IN SUMMARY

- Muscular strength is the maximum amount of force you can produce during one contraction.
- A common method of evaluating muscular strength is the one-repetition maximum (1 RM) test. However, it is possible to estimate the 1 RM by using the 10 RM (submaximal) test. Compared to the 1 RM test, the 10 RM poses less risk of injury to an inexperienced weight lifter.

☀ Measurement of Muscular Endurance

Muscular endurance is the ability of a muscle or muscle group to generate force over and over again. Although an individual might have sufficient strength to lift a heavy box from the ground to the back of a truck, he or she might not have sufficient muscular endurance to perform this task multiple times. Because many every-

day tasks require submaximal but repeated muscular contractions, muscular endurance is an important facet of health-related physical fitness.

Although numerous methods exist to evaluate muscular strength, two simple tests to assess muscular endurance involve the performance of push-ups and either sit-ups or curl-ups. Push-ups are a measure of muscular endurance using the shoulder, arm, and chest muscles, whereas sit-ups and curl-ups primarily evaluate abdominal muscle endurance.

THE PUSH-UP TEST

The standard **push-up test** to evaluate muscular endurance is performed in the following way. Start by positioning yourself on the ground in push-up position (Figure 2.7). Your hands should be approximately shoulder width, and your legs should be extended in a straight line with your weight placed on your toes. Lower your body until your chest is within 1 to 2 inches of the ground and raise yourself back to the up position. It is important to keep your back straight and to lower your entire body to the ground as a unit.

The push-up test is performed as follows:

1. Select a partner to count your push-ups and assist in the timing of the test (test duration is 60 seconds). Warm up with a few push-ups. Give yourself a 2- to 3-minute recovery period after the warm-up and prepare to start the test.

2. On the command "go," start performing push-ups. Your partner counts your push-ups aloud and informs you of the amount of time remaining in the test period (e.g., at 15-second intervals). Remember only those push-ups that are performed correctly will be counted toward your total; therefore, use the proper form and make every push-up count.

3. After completion of the push-up test, use Table 2.9 on page 32 to determine your fitness classification, and then record your scores in Laboratory 2.7 on page 57.

push-up test A fitness test designed to evaluate muscular endurance of shoulder and arm muscles.

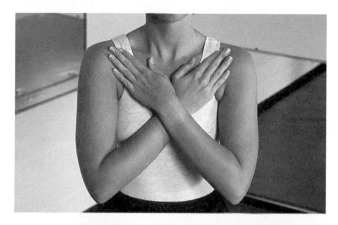

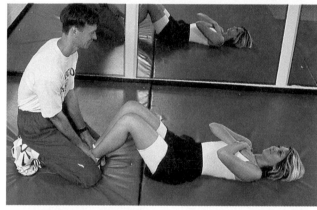

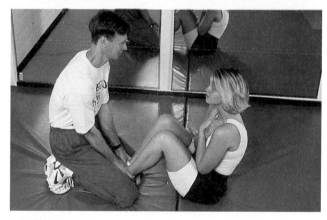

FIGURE 2.8
The proper position for the performance of sit-ups.

THE SIT-UP TEST

The bent-knee **sit-up test** is probably the best-known field test available to evaluate abdominal muscle endurance (4, 6). Figure 2.8 illustrates the correct position for performance of bent-knee sit-ups. Begin by lying on your back with your arms crossed on your chest. Your knees should be bent at approximately 90-degree angles, with your feet flat on the floor. The complete sit-up is performed by bringing your chest up to touch your knees and returning to the original lying position.

Note that although the abdominal muscles are very active during the performance of a bent-leg sit-up, leg muscles such as hip flexors also play a role. Therefore, this test evaluates not only abdominal muscle endurance but hip muscle endurance as well (21).

Sit-up tests are generally considered to be relatively safe fitness tests, but two precautions should be mentioned. First, avoid undue stress on your neck during the "up" phase of the exercise. That is, let your abdominal muscles do the work; do not whip your neck during the sit-up movement. Second, avoid hitting the back of your head on the floor during the "down" phase of the sit-up. Performance of the test on a padded mat is helpful.

The protocol for the sit-up test is as follows:

1. Select a partner to count your sit-ups, to hold your feet on the floor by grasping your ankles, and to assist in the timing of the test.

sit-up test A field test to evaluate abdominal and hip muscle endurance.

TABLE 2.9
Norms for Muscular Endurance Using the Push-Up Test
Find your age group on the left and then locate your fitness category in the appropriate column to the right.

Age Group (years)	Fitness Category Based on Push-Ups (1 min)					
	Very Poor	Poor	Average	Good	Excellent	Superior
Men						
15–19	<20	20–24	25–34	35–44	45–53	>53
20–29	<19	19–23	24–33	34–43	44–52	>52
30–39	<15	15–20	21–24	25–34	35–44	>44
40–49	<12	12–14	15–19	20–29	30–39	>39
50–59	<8	8–11	12–15	16–24	25–34	>34
60+	<5	5–7	8–9	10–19	20–29	>29
Women						
15–19	<5	5–9	10–12	13–14	15–19	>19
20–29	<4	4–8	9–10	11–12	13–18	>18
30–39	<3	3–7	8–11	12–13	14–16	>16
40–49	<2	2–5	6–9	10–12	13–15	>15
50–59	1	2–3	4–5	6–9	10–11	>11
60+	0	1–2	2–3	4–5	6–8	>8

Men's norms are modified from Pollock, M., J. Wilmore, and S. Fox. Health and fitness through physical activity. *John Wiley and Sons, New York, 1978. Women's norms are unpublished data from the University of Florida.*

2. Warm up with a few sit-ups. Give yourself a 2- to 3-minute recovery period after the warm-up and prepare to start the test.

3. On the command "go," start performing sit-ups and continue for 60 seconds. Your partner should count your sit-ups aloud and inform you of the time remaining in the test period (perhaps by called-out 15-second intervals). Remember that only sits-ups performed correctly will be counted toward your total.

4. After completing the sit-up test, use Table 2.10 to determine your fitness classification. Record your scores in Laboratory 2.7 on page 57.

THE CURL-UP TEST

As mentioned earlier, although sit-up tests utilize abdominal muscles, leg muscles are also recruited to move the trunk upward. Use of these leg muscles can be eliminated by performing a partial sit-up or a curl-up. The curl-up differs from the sit-up in that the trunk is not raised more than 30 to 40 degrees above the mat (attained when the shoulders are lifted approximately

6–10 inches above the mat; Figure 2.9) (21, 22). There are two advantages of the curl-up over the sit-up. First, the curl-up recruits only abdominal muscles, whereas the sit-up test involves both abdominal muscles and hip flexors. Second, research suggests that the curl-up provides less stress on the lower back than the conventional sit-up (20). For these reasons, the **curl-up test** is growing in popularity and is often used instead of the sit-up test to evaluate abdominal muscle endurance.

The protocol for the curl-up test is as follows:

1. Select a partner to count your curl-ups; lie on your back with knees bent 90 degrees.

2. Extend your arms so that your fingertips touch a strip of tape perpendicular to the body (Figure 2.9). A second strip of tape is located toward the feet and parallel to the first (8 centimeters or 3 inches apart). The curl-up is accomplished by raising your trunk (i.e., curling upward) until your fingertips touch the second strip of tape and then returning to the starting position.

3. The curl-up test is not timed and is performed at a slow and controlled cadence of 20 curl-ups per minute. This cadence is guided by the aid of a metronome set at 40 beats per minute (curl up on one beat and down on the second).

4. On the command "go," start performing curl-ups in cadence with the metronome. Perform as many

curl-up test   A field test to evaluate abdominal muscle endurance.

TABLE 2.10
Norms for Muscular Endurance Using the 1-Minute Sit-Up Test

Find your gender and age group on the left and then locate your fitness category in the appropriate column to the right.

Age Group (years)	Fitness Category Based on Sit-Ups (1 min)					
	Very Poor	Poor	Average	Good	Excellent	Superior
Men						
17–29	<17	17–35	36–41	42–47	48–50	>50
30–39	<13	13–26	27–32	33–38	39–48	>48
40–49	<12	12–22	23–27	28–33	34–43	>43
50–59	<8	8–16	17–21	22–28	29–38	>38
60+	<6	6–12	13–17	18–24	25–35	>35
Women						
20–29	<14	14–28	29–32	33–35	36–47	>47
30–39	<11	11–22	23–28	29–34	35–45	>45
40–49	<9	9–18	19–23	24–30	31–40	>40
50–59	<6	6–12	13–17	18–24	25–35	>35
60+	<5	5–10	11–14	15–20	21–30	>30

Modified from Pollock, M., J. Wilmore, and S. Fox. Health and fitness through physical activity. *John Wiley and Sons, New York, 1978.*

---

curl-ups as you can to a maximum of 75 without missing a beat. See Table 2.11 on page 34 to determine your fitness category, and then record your score in Laboratory 2.7 on page 57.

MUSCULAR ENDURANCE: HOW DO YOU RATE?

The fitness categories for muscular endurance range from very poor (lowest) to superior (highest). If your muscular endurance test score placed you in the "very poor" or "poor" classification, your present muscular endurance level is below average compared with other men or women of your age group. On the other hand, a fitness test score in the "good" category means that your current muscular endurance is above average. The fitness category "excellent" means that your muscular endurance level is well above average. Finally, the fitness category labeled "superior" is reserved for those individuals whose muscular endurance ranks in the top 15% of men or women in your age group.

If you scored poorly on either the push-up or sit-up test, do not be discouraged. Establish your goals and begin doing sit-ups and push-ups on a regular basis (see Chapter 5 for the exercise prescription for muscular strength). Your ability to perform both sit-ups and push-ups will increase within the first 3 to 4 weeks of training and will continue to improve for weeks to come.

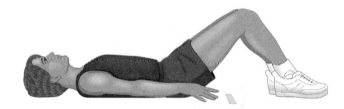

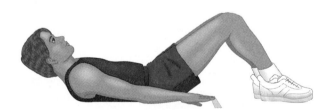

FIGURE 2.9
The proper position and movement pattern for the performance of a curl-up.

☀ IN SUMMARY

- Muscular endurance is the ability of a muscle or muscle group to generate force over and over again during repeated contractions.
- Two common methods to evaluate muscular endurance are the push-up and sit-up tests.

TABLE 2.11
Norms for Muscular Endurance Using the Curl-Up Test

Find your gender and age group on the left and locate the fitness category closest to your score in the columns to the right.

Age Group (years)	Fitness Category Based on Curl-Ups Performed				
	Poor	Average	Good	Excellent	Superior
Men					
<35	15	30	45	60	75
35–44	10	25	40	50	60
>44	5	15	25	40	50
Women					
<35	10	25	40	50	60
35–44	6	15	25	40	50
>44	4	10	15	30	40

Modified from Faulkner, R. A., et al. A partial curl-up protocol for adults based on two procedures. Canadian Journal of Sports Sciences 14:135–141, 1989.

☀ Assessment of Flexibility

Flexibility, the ability to move joints freely through their full range of motion, can decrease over time due to tightening of muscles and/or tendons. Loss of flexibility can occur due to both muscle disuse and muscular training. The key to maintaining flexibility is a program of regular stretching exercises (Chapter 6).

Individual needs for flexibility are variable. Some athletes, such as gymnasts, require great flexibility in order to perform complex movements in competition (3, 5, 10, 18). In general, the nonathlete requires less flexibility than the athlete. Some flexibility, however, is required for everyone in order to perform common activities of daily living or recreational pursuits.

It is important to understand that flexibility is joint specific. That is, a person might be flexible in one joint but lack flexibility in another. Although no single test is representative of total body flexibility, measurements of trunk and shoulder flexibility are commonly evaluated.

TRUNK FLEXIBILITY

The **sit and reach test** measures the ability to flex the trunk, which means stretching the lower back muscles and the muscles in the back of the thigh (hamstrings). Figure 2.10 illustrates the sit and reach test using a sit and reach box. The test is performed in the following manner.

Start by sitting upright with your feet flat against the box. Keeping your feet flat on the box and your legs straight, extend your hands as far forward as possible and hold this position for 3 seconds. Repeat this procedure three times. Your score on the sit and reach test is the distance, measured in inches, between the edge of the sit and reach box closest to you and the tips of your fingers during the best of your three stretching efforts.

Note that a brief warm-up period consisting of a few minutes of stretching is recommended prior to

> **sit and reach test**   A fitness test that measures the ability to flex the trunk (i.e., stretching the lower back muscles and the muscles in the back of the thigh).

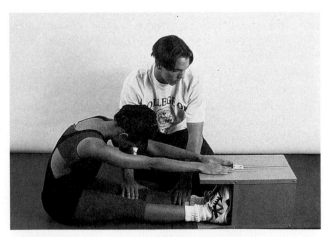

FIGURE 2.10
The sit and reach test to evaluate trunk flexibility.

TABLE 2.12
Physical Fitness Norms for Trunk Flexion Using the Sit and Reach Test

Note that these norms are for both men and women (ages 18–50 years). Units for the sit and reach score are inches and indicate the distance of your fingertips from the near edge of the sit and reach box. Negative numbers indicate that you cannot reach your toes, whereas positive numbers indicate the number of inches that you can reach past your toes.

Sit and Reach Score	Fitness Classification
−6 to −15	Very poor
−1 to −5	Poor
0 to +1	Average
+2 to +3	Good
+3 to +5	Excellent
+6 or above	Superior

Modified from Golding, L., C. Myers, and W. Sinning. Y's way to physical fitness: The complete guide to fitness testing and instruction. 3rd ed. Human Kinetics, Champaign, IL, 1989.

TABLE 2.13
Physical Fitness Norms for Shoulder Flexibility

Note that these norms are for both men and women of all ages. Units for the shoulder flexibility test score are inches and indicate the distance between the fingers of your right and left hands.

Right Hand Up Score	Left Hand Up Score	Fitness Classification
<0	<0	Very poor
0	0	Poor
+1	+1	Average
+2	+2	Good
+3	+3	Excellent
+4	+4	Superior

From Fox, E.L., Kirby, T.E., and Fox, A.R. Bases of fitness. Copyright © 1987. All rights reserved. Adapted by permission of Allyn and Bacon. Norms from ref. 4.

performance of the test. To reduce the possibility of injury, participants should avoid rapid or jerky movements during the test. It is often useful to have a partner help by holding your legs straight during the test and to assist in measuring the distance. After completing the test, consult Table 2.12 to locate your flexibility fitness category, and record your scores in Laboratory 2.8 on page 59.

SHOULDER FLEXIBILITY

As the name implies, the shoulder flexibility test evaluates shoulder range of motion (flexibility). The test is performed in the following manner. While standing, raise your right arm and reach down your back as far as possible (Figure 2.11). At the same time, extend your left arm behind your back and reach upward toward your right hand. The objective is to try to overlap your fingers as much as possible. Your score on the shoulder flexibility test is the distance, measured in inches, of finger overlap.

Measure the distance of finger overlap to the nearest inch. For example, an overlap of 3/4 inch would be recorded as 1 inch. If your fingers fail to overlap, record this score as minus one (−1). Finally, if your fingertips barely touch, record this score as zero (0).

After completing the test with the right hand up, repeat the test in the opposite direction (left hand up). Note that it is common to be more flexible on one side than on the other.

A brief warm-up period consisting of a few minutes of stretching is recommended prior to performance of the shoulder flexibility test. Again, to prevent injury, avoid rapid or jerky movements during the test. After

completion of the test, consult Table 2.13 to locate your shoulder flexibility category, and record your scores in Laboratory 2.8 on page 59.

FLEXIBILITY: HOW DO YOU RATE?

It is not uncommon for both active and inactive individuals to be classified as average or below for both trunk and shoulder flexibility. In fact, only individuals

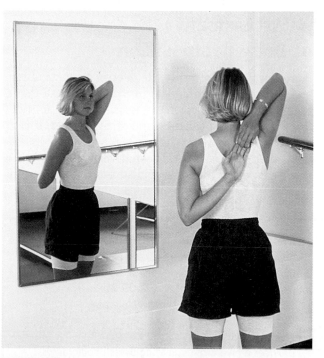

FIGURE 2.11
The shoulder flexibility test.

Nutritional Links

Can the Content of a Pre-Exercise Meal Improve the Results of a Fitness Test?

Many manufacturers of and "quick energy" candy bars claim that consumption of their products prior to exercise can improve performance. There is no scientific evidence, however, to support the idea that any type of meal eaten before exercise can improve physical performance (see ref. 23 for a review on this topic). In fact, consumption of high volumes of fluid or large solid meals immediately before exercising can negatively impact performance by creating abdominal discomfort (23). To avoid stomach cramps or other forms of abdominal discomfort during exercise, the pre-exercise meal should be relatively small and eaten at least 2 to 3 hours before exercise. This pre-exercise meal should contain primarily complex carbohydrates (complex sugars such as fruits and breads) and be low in fat. The rationale for this recommendation is based on the fact that carbohydrates are digested rapidly, whereas fat is broken down and absorbed slowly (9). See Cooper (1999) in the suggested reading list for details, and Chapter 7 for a complete discussion of nutrition and physical fitness.

---

who regularly perform stretching exercises are likely to possess flexibility levels that exceed the average. Regardless of your current flexibility classification, your flexibility goal should be to reach a classification of above average (i.e., good, excellent, or superior).

☀ IN SUMMARY

- Flexibility is defined as the ability to move joints freely through their full range of motion.
- Flexibility measurements are joint specific.
- Two popular tests to evaluate flexibility are the sit and reach test and the shoulder flexibility test.

☀ Assessment of Body Composition

Body composition refers to the relative amounts of fat and lean tissue (e.g., muscle) in the body. Recall that a high percentage of body fat is associated with an increased risk of heart disease and other diseases. It is therefore not surprising that several methods of assessing body composition have been developed. A technique considered to be the gold standard for laboratory assessment of body fat in humans is **hydrostatic**

> **hydrostatic weighing**   A method of determining body composition that involves weighing an individual both on land and in a tank of water.
>
> **skinfold test**   A field test to estimate body composition. The test works on the principle that over 50% of body fat lies just beneath the skin. Therefore, measurement of representative samples of subcutaneous fat provides a means of estimating overall body fatness.

---

weighing, which involves weighing the individual both on land and in a tank of water (7, 9, 24). The two body weights are then entered into a simple formula to calculate percent body fat. Unfortunately, underwater weighing is very time consuming and requires expensive equipment. Thus, this procedure is rarely employed to assess body composition in collegiate physical fitness courses. A rapid and inexpensive method to assess body composition involves measuring subcutaneous (beneath the skin) fat or fat and is called the *skinfold test.*

THE SKINFOLD TEST

Subcutaneous fat is measured using an instrument called a skinfold caliper. The **skinfold test** relies on the fact that over 50% of body fat lies just beneath the skin (7, 9, 25). Therefore, measurement of representative samples of subcutaneous fat provides a means of estimating overall body fatness. Skinfold measurements to determine body fat are reliable but generally have a ±3–4% margin of error (7, 9).

One of the most accurate skinfold tests to estimate body fatness for both men and women requires three skinfold measurements (25). The anatomical sites to be measured in men (chest, triceps, and subscapular skinfolds) are illustrated in Figure 2.12, and the measurement sites for women (triceps, suprailium, and abdominal skinfolds) are illustrated in Figure 2.13. Note that for standardization, all measurements should be made on the right side of the body.

1. To make each measurement, hold the skinfold between the thumb and index finger and slowly release the tension on the skinfold calipers so as to pinch the skinfold within 1/2 inch of your fingers. Continue to hold the skinfold with your fingers and fully release the tension on the calipers; then,

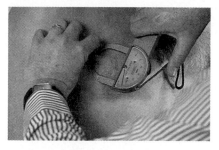
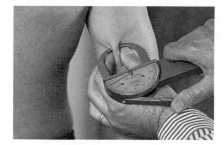
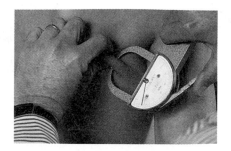

FIGURE 2.12
Skinfold measurement sites for men.

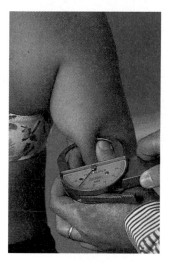
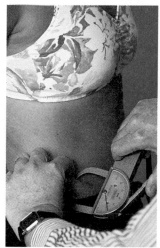
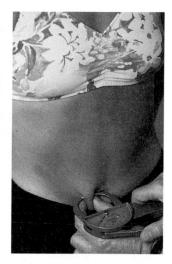

FIGURE 2.13
Skinfold measurement sites for women.

simply read the number (the skinfold thickness in millimeters) from the gauge. Release the skinfold and allow the tissue to relax. Repeat this procedure three times and average the three measurements.

2. After completing the three skinfold measurements, total the measurements and use Tables 2.14 and 2.15 on pages 38 and 39 to determine the percent body fat for women and men, respectively. After obtaining your percent body fat, refer to Table 2.16 (26) on page 40 to determine the body composition fitness category, and record your score in Laboratory 2.9 on page 61.

ESTIMATION OF BODY COMPOSITION: FIELD TECHNIQUES

Several quick and inexpensive field techniques exist to evaluate body composition and the risk of heart disease associated with over-fatness (18, 27, 28). Next we describe some of the more popular procedures currently in use.

WAIST-TO-HIP CIRCUMFERENCE RATIO   Recent evidence suggests that the waist-to-hip circumference ratio is an excellent index for determining the risk of

disease associated with high body fat (28). The rationale for this technique is that a high percentage of fat in the abdominal region is associated with an increased risk of disease (such as heart disease or hypertension). Therefore, an individual with a large fat deposit in the abdominal region would have a high waist-to-hip ratio and would have a higher risk of disease than someone with a lower waist-to-hip ratio. The procedure for assessing the **waist-to-hip circumference ratio** is as follows:

1. Both waist and hip circumference measurements should be made while standing, using a nonelastic

> **waist-to-hip circumference ratio**   An index for determining the risk of disease associated with high body fat. The rationale for this technique is that a high percentage of fat in the abdominal region is associated with an increased risk of disease (e.g., heart disease or hypertension). Therefore, an individual with a large fat deposit in the abdominal region would have a high waist-to-hip ratio and would have a higher risk of disease than someone with a lower waist-to-hip ratio.

TABLE 2.14
Percent Fat Estimate for Women

Sum of Triceps, Abdominal, and Suprailium Skinfolds

Sum of Skinfolds (mm)	Age (years) Sum of								
	18–22	23–27	28–32	33–37	38–42	43–47	48–52	53–57	>57
8–12	8.8	9.0	9.2	9.4	9.5	9.7	9.9	10.1	10.3
13–17	10.8	10.9	11.1	11.3	11.5	11.7	11.8	12.0	12.2
18–22	12.6	12.8	13.0	13.2	13.4	13.5	13.7	13.9	14.1
23–27	14.5	14.6	14.8	15.0	15.2	15.4	15.6	15.7	15.9
28–32	16.2	16.4	16.6	16.8	17.0	17.1	17.3	17.5	17.7
33–37	17.9	18.1	18.3	18.5	18.7	18.9	19.0	19.2	19.4
38–42	19.6	19.8	20.0	20.2	20.3	20.5	20.7	20.9	21.1
43–47	21.2	21.4	21.6	21.8	21.9	22.1	22.3	22.5	22.7
48–52	22.8	22.9	23.1	23.3	23.5	23.7	23.8	24.0	24.2
53–57	24.2	24.4	24.6	24.8	25.0	25.2	25.3	25.5	25.7
58–62	25.7	25.9	26.0	26.2	26.4	26.6	26.8	27.0	27.1
63–67	27.1	27.2	27.4	27.6	27.8	28.0	28.2	28.3	28.5
68–72	28.4	28.6	28.7	28.9	29.1	29.3	29.5	29.7	29.8
73–77	29.6	29.8	30.0	30.2	30.4	30.6	30.7	30.9	31.1
78–82	30.9	31.0	31.2	31.4	31.6	31.8	31.9	32.1	32.3
83–87	32.0	32.2	32.4	32.6	32.7	32.9	33.1	33.3	33.5
88–92	33.1	33.3	33.5	33.7	33.8	34.0	34.2	34.4	34.6
93–97	34.1	34.3	34.5	34.7	34.9	35.1	35.2	35.4	35.6
98–102	35.1	35.3	35.5	35.7	35.9	36.0	36.2	36.4	36.6
103–107	36.1	36.2	36.4	36.6	36.8	37.0	37.2	37.3	37.5
108–112	36.9	37.1	37.3	37.5	37.7	37.9	38.0	38.2	38.4
113–117	37.8	37.9	38.1	38.3	39.2	39.4	39.6	39.8	39.2
118–122	38.5	38.7	38.9	39.1	39.4	39.6	39.8	40.0	40.0
123–127	39.2	39.4	39.6	39.8	40.0	40.1	40.3	40.5	40.7
128–132	39.9	40.1	40.2	40.4	40.6	40.8	41.0	41.2	41.3
133–137	40.5	40.7	40.8	41.0	41.2	41.4	41.6	41.7	41.9
138–142	41.0	41.2	41.4	41.6	41.7	41.9	42.1	42.3	42.5
143–147	41.5	41.7	41.9	42.0	42.2	42.4	42.6	42.8	43.0
148–152	41.9	42.1	42.3	42.4	42.6	42.8	43.0	43.2	43.4
153–157	42.3	42.5	42.6	42.8	43.0	43.2	43.4	43.6	43.7
158–162	42.6	42.8	43.0	43.1	43.3	43.5	43.7	43.9	44.1
163–167	42.9	43.0	43.2	43.4	43.6	43.8	44.0	44.1	44.3
168–172	43.1	43.2	43.4	43.6	43.8	44.0	44.2	44.3	44.5
173–177	43.2	43.4	43.6	43.8	43.9	44.1	44.3	44.5	44.7
178–182	43.3	43.5	43.7	43.8	44.0	44.2	44.4	44.6	44.8

From Jackson, A., and M. Pollock. *Practical assessment of body composition.* Physician and Sports Medicine *13:76–90, 1985.*

tape. It is important that bulky clothing not be worn during the measurement, because it could bias the circumference measurement. During measurement, the tape should be placed snugly around the body but should not press into the skin. Record your measurements to the nearest millimeter or sixteenth of an inch.

2. Perform the waist measurement first. Begin by placing the tape at the level of the umbilicus (navel; Figure 2.14 (a)). Make your measurement at the end of a normal expiration.

3. To make the hip measurement, place the tape around the maximum circumference of the buttocks (Figure 2.14 (b)).

TABLE 2.15
Percent Fat Estimate for Men

Sum of Triceps, Chest, and Subscapular Skinfolds

Sum of Skinfolds (mm)	Age (years)								
	<22	23–27	28–32	33–37	38–42	43–47	48–52	53–57	>57
8–10	1.5	2.0	2.5	3.1	3.6	4.1	4.6	5.1	5.6
11–13	3.0	3.5	4.0	4.5	5.1	5.6	6.1	6.6	7.1
14–16	4.5	5.0	5.5	6.0	6.5	7.0	7.6	8.1	8.6
17–19	5.9	6.4	6.9	7.4	8.0	8.5	9.0	9.5	10.0
20–22	7.3	7.8	8.3	8.8	9.4	9.9	10.4	10.9	11.4
23–25	8.6	9.2	9.7	10.2	10.7	11.2	11.8	12.3	12.8
26–28	10.0	10.5	11.0	11.5	12.1	12.6	13.1	13.6	14.2
29–31	11.2	11.8	12.3	12.8	13.4	13.9	14.4	14.9	15.5
32–34	12.5	13.0	13.5	14.1	14.6	15.1	15.7	16.2	16.7
35–37	13.7	14.2	14.8	15.3	15.8	16.4	16.9	17.4	18.0
38–40	14.9	15.4	15.9	16.5	17.0	17.6	18.1	18.6	19.2
41–43	16.0	16.6	17.1	17.6	18.2	18.7	19.3	19.8	20.3
44–46	17.1	17.7	18.2	18.7	19.3	19.8	20.4	20.9	21.5
47–49	18.2	18.7	19.3	19.8	20.4	20.9	21.4	22.0	22.5
50–52	19.2	19.7	20.3	20.8	21.4	21.9	22.5	23.0	23.6
53–55	20.2	20.7	21.3	21.8	22.4	22.9	23.5	24.0	24.6
56–58	21.1	21.7	22.2	22.8	23.3	23.9	24.4	25.0	25.5
59–61	22.0	22.6	23.1	23.7	24.2	24.8	25.3	25.9	26.5
62–64	22.9	23.4	24.0	24.5	25.1	25.7	26.2	26.8	27.3
65–67	23.7	24.3	24.8	25.4	25.9	26.5	27.1	27.6	28.2
68–70	24.5	25.0	25.6	26.2	26.7	27.3	27.8	28.4	29.0
71–73	25.2	25.8	26.3	26.9	27.5	28.0	28.6	29.1	29.7
74–76	25.9	26.5	27.0	27.6	28.2	28.7	29.3	29.9	30.4
77–79	26.6	27.1	27.7	28.2	28.8	29.4	29.9	30.5	31.1
80–82	27.2	27.7	28.3	28.9	29.4	30.0	30.6	31.1	31.7
83–85	27.7	28.3	28.8	29.4	30.0	30.5	31.1	31.7	32.3
86–88	28.2	28.8	29.4	29.9	30.5	31.1	31.6	32.2	32.8
89–91	28.7	29.3	29.8	30.4	31.0	31.5	32.1	32.7	33.3
92–94	29.1	29.7	30.3	30.8	31.4	32.0	32.6	33.1	33.4
95–97	29.5	30.1	30.6	31.2	31.8	32.4	32.9	33.5	34.1
98–100	29.8	30.4	31.0	31.6	32.1	32.7	33.3	33.9	34.4
101–103	30.1	30.7	31.3	31.8	32.4	33.0	33.6	34.1	34.7
104–106	30.4	30.9	31.5	32.1	32.7	33.2	33.8	34.4	35.0
107–109	30.6	31.1	31.7	32.3	32.9	33.4	34.0	34.6	35.2
110–112	30.7	31.3	31.9	32.4	33.0	33.6	34.2	34.7	35.3
113–115	30.8	31.4	32.0	32.5	33.1	33.7	34.3	34.9	35.4
116–118	30.9	31.5	32.0	32.6	33.2	33.8	34.3	34.9	35.5

From Jackson, A., and M. Pollock. Practical assessment of body composition. Physician and Sports Medicine *13:76–90, 1985.*

4. After completing the measurements, divide the waist circumference by the hip circumference to determine the waist-to-hip ratio. Use Table 2.17 on page 41 to determine the waist-to-hip ratio rating. Your goal in terms of waist-to-hip ratio classification should be to reach the optimal classification that places you in the lowest risk category for heart disease.

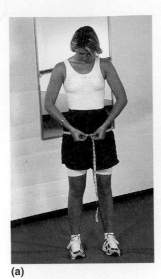 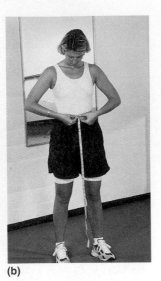

(a)   **(b)**

FIGURE 2.14
Illustration of the waist-to-hip circumference measurements.

BODY MASS INDEX Research has shown that the **body mass index** (BMI), despite its many limitations, is a useful technique for placing people into categories of normal or too much body fat (27, 28). The BMI is simply the ratio of the body weight (kilograms; kg) divided by height (in meters) squared (m^2):

$$BMI = weight\ (kg)/height\ (m)^2$$

(Note: 1 kg = 2.2 pounds, and 1 m = 39.25 inches.)

For example, if an individual weighs 64.5 kg and is 1.72 m tall, the BMI would be computed as follows:

$$64.5\ kg/(1.72\ m)^2 = 64.5/2.96 = 21.8$$

After calculating your BMI, use Table 2.18 to determine your degree of body fatness. The concept behind the BMI is that individuals with low percent body fat will have a low BMI. For example, men and women with a BMI of less than 25 and 27, respectively, are classified as having optimal body fat. In contrast, men and women with a BMI of greater than 40 are considered to be extremely obese.

Although BMI is a simple and inexpensive method for estimating body composition, this technique has limitations. Indeed, in some cases this method can over- or underestimate body fatness. For example, an individual with a low percentage of body fat but a high level of muscularity would typically have a relatively high BMI, which would incorrectly suggest a high per-

body mass index A useful technique for categorizing people with respect to their degree of body fat. The body mass index (BMI) is simply the ratio of body weight (kilograms; kg) divided by height squared (meters^2).

TABLE 2.16
Body Composition Fitness Categories for Men and Women

Percent Body Fat	Body Composition Fitness Category
Men	
<10%	Low body fat
10–20%	Optimal range of body fat
21–25%	Moderately high body fat
26–31%	High body fat
>31%	Very high body fat
Women	
<15%	Low body fat
15–25%	Optimal range of body fat
26–30%	Moderately high body fat
31–35%	High body fat
>35%	Very high body fat

Data from Lohman (29).

centage of body fat. Therefore, this technique should be used only when other more sensitive techniques (i.e., hydrostatic weighing and skinfold measurements) are not available.

HEIGHT/WEIGHT TABLES The Metropolitan Life Insurance Company has published a height/weight table designed to determine whether a person is overweight due to too much body fat. Although the idea that a simple table could be used to determine an individual's ideal body weight is attractive, several problems affect this procedure. The major problem with this approach is that the tables do not indicate how much of the body weight is fat. For example, an individual can exceed the ideal body weight on such a chart by being either heavily muscled or overfat. Therefore, this approach to a determination of an "ideal body weight" is not recommended.

BODY COMPOSITION: HOW DO YOU RATE?

The fitness categories presented for body composition differ from those earlier for the other components of health-related physical fitness. While "superior" was the highest fitness level presented that could be achieved for cardiorespiratory, strength, and muscular endurance fitness, the classification of "optimal" is the highest standard for body composition. Regardless of the body composition test employed to assess body fat, any category other than optimal is considered unsatisfactory for health-related fitness. Therefore, your goal should be to reach and maintain an optimal body composition.

TABLE 2.17
Waist-to-Hip Circumference Ratio Rating Scale

Men	Women	Classification (risk of disease)
>1.0	>0.85	High risk
0.90–1.0	0.80–0.85	Moderately high risk
<0.90	<0.80	Optimal low risk of disease

Modified from Van Itallie, T. Topography of body fat: Relationship to risk of cardiovascular and other diseases. In T. Lohman, et al., eds. Anthropometric standardization reference manual. Human Kinetics, Champaign, IL, 1988.

TABLE 2.18
Body Mass Index Classification of the Degree of Body Fatness

	BMI (weight/height^2)	
Body Fat Category	Men	Women
Optimal body fat	<25	<27
Moderately high body fat	25–30	27–30
High body fat	31–40	31–40
Very high body fat	>40	>40

Adapted from DiGirolamo, M. Body composition—roundtable. Physician and Sports Medicine (March):144–162, 1986.

The rationale for the concept of optimal body composition is as follows. Research suggests that a range of 10% to 20% body fat is an optimal health and fitness goal for men; the optimal range for women is 15% to 25%. These ranges in body fat provide little risk of disease associated with body fatness and permit individual differences in physical activity patterns and diet. Body fat levels above the optimal range are associated with an increased risk of disease and are therefore undesirable.

What is less obvious is that a body fat percentage that is lower than the recommended optimal range is also undesirable. Indeed, percentages of body fat below the optimal range may also increase the risk of health problems. This is because extremely low percentages of body fat are often associated with poor nutrition and a loss of muscle mass. This is clearly undesirable. The relationships among diet, exercise, and body composition are discussed in detail in Chapter 8.

☼ IN SUMMARY

- Body composition is an important part of health-related physical fitness because a high percentage of body fat is associated with an increased risk of disease.

- Field tests for estimating body composition include skinfold measurements, assessment of the body mass index, and/or examination of the waist-to-hip circumference ratio.

Summary

1. Prior to beginning a fitness program (or performing a fitness evaluation), you should have your health status evaluated by a physician.

2. An objective evaluation of your current fitness status is important before beginning an exercise training program. Further, periodic retesting can provide feedback about your training progress.

3. Cardiorespiratory fitness is the ability of the heart to pump oxygen-rich blood to exercising muscles; this translates into the ability to perform endurance-type exercise. Field tests to evaluate cardiorespiratory fitness include the 1.5-mile run test, the 1-mile walk test, the cycle ergometer fitness test, and the step test.

4. Muscular strength is the maximum amount of force you can produce during one contraction. The most popular method of evaluating muscular strength is the one-repetition maximum (1 RM) test.

5. Muscular endurance is the ability of a muscle group to generate force over and over again. Two commonly used methods of evaluating muscular endurance are the push-up and sit-up tests.

6. Flexibility is defined as the ability to move joints freely through their full range of motion. Although flexibility is joint specific, two popular means of evaluating flexibility are the sit and reach test and the shoulder flexibility test.

7. Body composition is an important component of health-related physical fitness because a high percentage of body fat is associated with an increased risk of disease. In the field, the amount of body fat can be estimated using skinfold measurements, assessment of the body mass index, or examination of the waist-to-hip circumference ratio.

Study Questions

1. Describe the following field tests used to evaluate cardiorespiratory fitness: the 1.5-mile run test, the 1-mile walk test, the cycle ergometer fitness test, and the step test.

2. Discuss the one-repetition maximum (1 RM) test for measuring muscular strength. What safety concerns are associated with this test?

3. Explain how the push-up and sit-up tests are used to evaluate muscular endurance.

4. Discuss the concept that flexibility is joint specific.

5. Identify two field tests used to examine flexibility.

6. Define the term *recovery index*.

7. Discuss the following techniques for assessing body composition: hydrostatic weighing and the skinfold test.

8. How can measurement of the waist-to-hip circumference ratio and body mass index be used to assess body composition?

Suggested Reading

American College of Sports Medicine. *Guidelines for Exercise Testing,* 6th ed. Philadelphia: Lea and Febiger, 2000.

Cooper, C. B. Medical aspects: Cardiopulmonary exercise testing. *ACSM's Health and Fitness Journal* 3(6):34, 41, 1999.

Powers, S., and E. Howley. *Exercise Physiology: Theory and Application to Fitness and Performance,* 4th ed. St. Louis: McGraw-Hill, 2001.

Roitman, J., ed. *ACSM's Resource Manual for Guidelines for Exercise Testing and Prescription*. Philadelphia: Lippincott Williams & Wilkins, 2001.

For links to the Web sites below visit Web Links at www.aw.com/fitness and choose Powers/Dodd Web Links from the drop-down menu.

American Heart Association

Contains latest information about ways to reduce your risk of heart and vascular diseases. Site includes information about exercise, diet, and heart disease.

American College of Sports Medicine

Contains information about exercise, health, and fitness.

Fitness Tests

Describes tests for aerobic power, anaerobic power, flexibility, and body composition.

References

1. American College of Sports Medicine. *Guidelines for Exercise Testing,* 6th ed. Philadelphia: Lea and Febiger, 2000.

2. American College of Sports Medicine. *Resource Manual for Exercise Testing and Prescription*. Philadelphia: Lea and Febiger, 1998.

3. Corbin, C., and R. Lindsey. *Concepts of Physical Fitness.* Dubuque, IA: Wm. C. Brown, 2000.

4. Getchell, B. *Physical Fitness: A Way of Life,* 5th ed. Needham Heights, MA: Allyn and Bacon, 1998.

5. Barrow, M. *Heart Talk: Understanding Cardiovascular Diseases*. Gainesville, FL: Cor-Ed Publishing, 1992.

6. McGlynn, G. *Dynamics of Fitness: A Practical Approach,* 5th ed. Dubuque, IA: Wm. C. Brown, 1998.

7. Pollock, M., and J. Wilmore. *Exercise in Health and Disease,* 3rd ed. Philadelphia: W. B. Saunders, 1990.

8. Pollock, M., J. Wilmore, and S. Fox. *Health and Fitness Through Physical Activity*. New York: John Wiley and Sons, 1978.

9. Powers, S., and E. Howley. *Exercise Physiology: Theory and Application to Fitness and Performance,* 4th ed. St. Louis: McGraw-Hill, 2001.

10. Robergs, R., and S. Roberts. *Fundamental Principles of Exercise Physiology: For Fitness, Performance, and Health*. St. Louis: McGraw-Hill, 2001.

11. Cooper, K. *The Aerobics Program for Total Well-Being.* New York: M. Evans, 1982.

12. Cooper, K. *The Aerobics Way.* New York: Bantam Books, 1977.

13. Fox, E. A simple technique for predicting maximal aerobic power. *Journal of Applied Physiology* 35:914–916, 1973.

14. Rippe, J., A. Ward., J. Porcari, and P. Freedson. Walking for fitness and health. *Journal of the American Medical Association* 259:2720–2724, 1988.

15. Rippe, J. Walking for fitness: A roundtable. *Physician and Sports Medicine* 14:144–159, 1986.

16. Ward, A., and J. Rippe. *Walking for Health and Fitness.* Philadelphia: J. B. Lippincott, 1988.

17. Golding, L., C. Myers, and W. Sinning. *Y's Way to Physical Fitness: The Complete Guide to Fitness Testing and Instruction,* 3rd ed. Champaign, IL: Human Kinetics, 1989.

18. Howley, E., and B. D. Franks. *Health Fitness: Instructors Handbook*. Champaign, IL: Human Kinetics, 1997.

19. Roitman, J., ed. *ACSM's Resource Manual for Guidelines for Exercise Testing and Prescription*. Philadelphia: Lippincott Williams & Wilkins, 2001.

20. Axler, C., and S. McGill. Low back loads over a variety of abdominal exercises: Searching for the safest abdominal challenge. *Medicine and Science in Sports and Exercise* 29:804–810, 1997.

21. Sparling, P. Field testing for abdominal muscular fitness; speed versus cadence sit-ups. *ACSM's Health and Fitness Journal* 1(4):30–33, 1997.

22. Faulkner, R., et al. A partial curl-up protocol for adults based on two procedures. *Canadian Journal of Sports Sciences* 14:135–141, 1989.

23. Lamb, D., and M. Williams. *Ergogenics: Enhancement of Performance in Exercise and Sport.* Vol. 4. Dubuque, IA: Brown and Benchmark, 1991.

24. Lohman, T., et al. Body fat measurement goes high-tech: Not all are created equal. *ACSM's Health and Fitness Journal* 1(1):30–35, 1997.

25. Williams, M. *Lifetime Fitness and Wellness.* Dubuque, IA: Wm. C. Brown, 1996.

26. Jackson, A., and M. Pollock. Practical assessment of body composition. *Physician and Sports Medicine* 13:76–90, 1985.

27. DiGirolamo, M. Body composition—roundtable. *Physician and Sports Medicine* (March):144–162, 1986.

28. Van Itallie, T. Topography of body fat: Relationship to risk of cardiovascular and other diseases. In T. Lohman et al., eds. *Anthropometric Standardization Reference Manual.* Champaign, IL: Human Kinetics, 1988.

29. Lohman, T. The use of skinfold to estimate body fatness in children and youth. *Journal of Alliance for Health, Physical Education, Recreation, and Dance* 58:98–102, 1987.

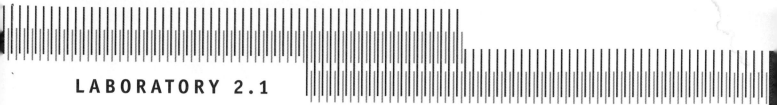
Health Status Questionnaire

NAME _____ DATE _____

The following questions are part of an exercise screening questionnaire originally developed by the Connecticut Mutual Life Insurance Company and modified by the authors. If you answer "yes" to any of the following questions, you should have a thorough medical exam prior to beginning an exercise program.

1. Have you ever had chest pains or a sensation of pressure in your chest that occurred during or immediately following exercise?

2. Do you have chest discomfort when climbing stairs or walking against a cold wind, or during any physical activity?

3. Does your heart ever beat unevenly or irregularly or seem to flutter or skip beats?

4. Do you ever experience sudden bursts of very rapid heart action or periods of slow heart action without apparent cause?

5. Do you take any prescription medicine on a regular basis?

6. Has your doctor ever told you that you have heart problems?

7. Do you have any respiratory problems such as asthma, or do you experience shortness of breath during light physical activity?

8. Do you have arthritis or any condition affecting your joints or back that makes exercise painful?

9. Do you have any of the following risk factors for heart disease: (a) high blood pressure; (b) high blood cholesterol; (c) overweight by more than 30%; (d) smoking; or (e) any close relatives (father, mother, brother, etc.) that have had a history of heart disease prior to age 55?

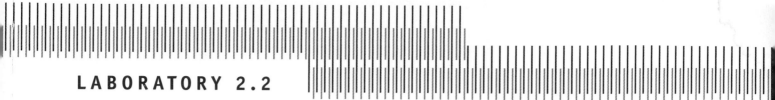

LABORATORY 2.2

Measurement of Cardiorespiratory Fitness:
The 1.5-Mile Run Test

NAME _____ DATE _____

DIRECTIONS

The objective of the test is to complete the 1.5-mile distance as quickly as possible. The run can be completed on an oval track or any properly measured course. You should attempt this test only if you have met the medical clearance criteria discussed in Chapter 2 of this text.

Prior to beginning the test, perform a 5- to 10-minute warm-up. If you become extremely fatigued during the test, slow your pace—do not overstress yourself! If you feel faint or nauseated, or experience any unusual pains in your upper body, stop and notify your instructor!

On completion of the test, cool down and record your time and fitness category (Table 2.1).

TEST 1 DATE: _____

Ambient conditions:

*Temperature: _____ *Relative humidity: _____

Finish time: _____ Fitness category: _____

TEST 2 DATE: _____

Ambient conditions:

*Temperature: _____ *Relative humidity: _____

Finish time: _____ Fitness category: _____

TEST 3 DATE: _____

Ambient conditions:

*Temperature: _____ *Relative humidity: _____

Finish time: _____ Fitness category: _____

*The purpose of recording the temperature and relative humidity is to provide a record of the amount of heat stress during the test. High heat and relative humidity could have a negative impact on your test score.

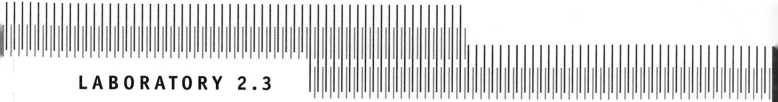

LABORATORY 2.3

Measurement of Cardiorespiratory Fitness: The 1-Mile Walk Test

NAME _____ DATE _____

DIRECTIONS

The objective of the test is to walk the 1-mile distance as quickly as possible. The walk can be completed on an oval track or any properly measured course. You should attempt this test only if you have met the medical clearance criteria discussed in Chapter 2 of this text.

Prior to beginning the test, perform a 5- to 10-minute warm-up. If you become extremely fatigued during the test, slow your pace—do not overstress yourself! If you feel faint or nauseated, or experience any unusual pains in your upper body, stop and notify your instructor!

On completion of the test, cool down and record your time and fitness category (Table 2.2).

TEST 1 DATE: _____

Ambient conditions:

*Temperature: _____ *Relative humidity: _____

Finish time: _____ Fitness category: _____

TEST 2 DATE: _____

Ambient conditions:

*Temperature: _____ *Relative humidity: _____

Finish time: _____ Fitness category: _____

TEST 3 DATE: _____

Ambient conditions:

*Temperature: _____ *Relative humidity: _____

Finish time: _____ Fitness category: _____

*The purpose of recording the temperature and relative humidity is to provide a record of the amount of heat stress during the test. High heat and relative humidity could have a negative impact on your test score.

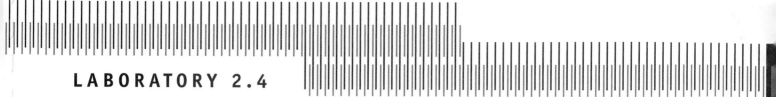

LABORATORY 2.4

Submaximal Cycle Test to Determine Cardiorespiratory Fitness

NAME _____ DATE _____

DIRECTIONS

Warm up for 3 minutes using unloaded pedaling. Set the appropriate load for your age and gender and begin. (See page 21 for load-setting instructions.) Exercise for a 5-minute period. Count your pulse during a 15-second period between minutes 4.5 and 5 of the test.

Cool down for 3 to 5 minutes using unloaded pedaling. Record your heart rate (15-second count) below and compute your relative $\dot{V}O_{2max}$ using Table 2.4. After calculating your relative $\dot{V}O_{2max}$, locate your fitness category in Table 2.5.

TEST 1 DATE: _____

Heart rate (15-second count) during minute 5 of test: _____

Fitness category: _____

TEST 2 DATE: _____

Heart rate (15-second count) during minute 5 of test: _____

Fitness category: _____

TEST 3 DATE: _____

Heart rate (15-second count) during minute 5 of test: _____

Fitness category: _____

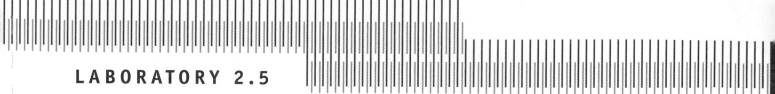

Step Test to Determine Cardiorespiratory Fitness

NAME _____ DATE _____

DIRECTIONS

Perform 30 complete step ups and downs per minute using an 18-inch step over a 3-minute period. On completion of 3 minutes of exercise, sit quietly and count the number of heart beats in 30 seconds during the following time periods: 1 to 1.5 minutes post exercise; 2 to 2.5 minutes post exercise; and 3 to 3.5 minutes post exercise. Record your heart rates below and use Table 2.6 to determine your fitness category.

TEST 1 DATE: _____

Recovery heart rate post exercise (beats)

1–1.5 min: _____

2–2.5 min: _____

3–3.5 min: _____

Total: _____ (recovery index)

Fitness category: _____

TEST 2 DATE: _____

Recovery heart rate post exercise (beats)

1–1.5 min: _____

2–2.5 min: _____

3–3.5 min: _____

Total: _____ (recovery index)

Fitness category: _____

TEST 3 DATE: _____

Recovery heart rate post exercise (beats)

1–1.5 min: _____

2–2.5 min: _____

3–3.5 min: _____

Total: _____ (recovery index)

Fitness category: _____

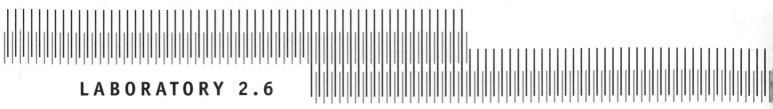

LABORATORY 2.6

Measurement of Muscular Strength: The 1 RM Test

NAME _____ DATE _____

DIRECTIONS

After performance of your 1 RM test, compute your muscular strength scores as follows:

$$\frac{1 \text{ RM weight}}{\text{body weight}} \times 100 = \text{muscle strength score}$$

Record your muscular strength scores below and use Table 2.7 to determine your fitness category.

Age: _____ **Body weight:** _____ **pounds**

TEST 1 DATE: _____

Exercise	1 RM (lbs)	Muscular Strength	Fitness Category
Bench press	_____	_____	_____
Biceps curl	_____	_____	_____
Shoulder press	_____	_____	_____
Leg press	_____	_____	_____

TEST 2 DATE: _____

Exercise	1 RM (lbs)	Muscular Strength	Fitness Category
Bench press	_____	_____	_____
Biceps curl	_____	_____	_____
Shoulder press	_____	_____	_____
Leg press	_____	_____	_____

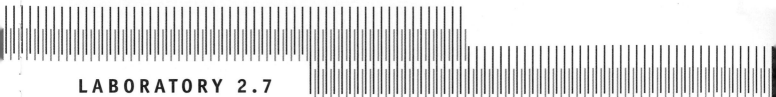

Measurement of Muscular Endurance:
The Push-Up, Sit-Up, and Curl-Up Tests

NAME _____ DATE _____

DIRECTIONS

After completion of the push-up, sit-up, and curl-up tests, record your scores and fitness classifications (Tables 2.9, 2.10, and 2.11).

Age: _____

TEST 1   DATE: _____

Number of push-ups (1 min): _____   Fitness category: _____

Number of sit-ups (1 min): _____   Fitness category: _____

Number of curl-ups: _____   Fitness category: _____

TEST 2   DATE: _____

Number of push-ups (1 min): _____   Fitness category: _____

Number of sit-ups (1 min): _____   Fitness category: _____

Number of curl-ups: _____   Fitness category: _____

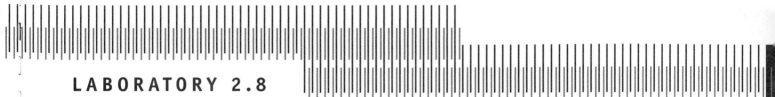

Assessment of Flexibility: Trunk Flexion (Sit and Reach Test) and the Shoulder Flexibility Test

NAME _____ DATE _____

DIRECTIONS

After completion of the sit and reach test and the shoulder flexibility test, record your scores and fitness classifications (Tables 2.10 and 2.11).

TEST 1 DATE: _____

Sit and reach score (inches): _____ Fitness category: _____

Shoulder flexibility (inches): _____ Fitness category: _____

TEST 2 DATE: _____

Sit and reach score (inches): _____ Fitness category: _____

Shoulder flexibility (inches): _____ Fitness category: _____

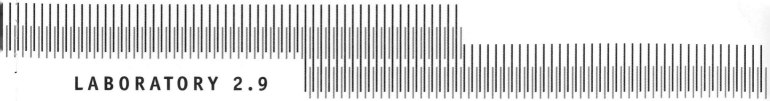

LABORATORY 2.9

Assessment of Body Composition

NAME _____ DATE _____

DIRECTIONS

In the spaces below, record your body composition raw data and fitness categories obtained using the skinfold test, body mass index, and/or the waist-to-hip circumference ratio (Tables 2.14–2.17).

TEST 1   DATE: _____

Skinfold Test

Sum of three skinfolds (mm): _____

Percent body fat: _____

Fitness category: _____

Body Mass Index

Body mass index score: _____

Fitness category: _____

Waist-to-Hip Circumference Ratio

Waist-to-hip circumference ratio: _____

Fitness category: _____

TEST 2   DATE: _____

Skinfold Test

Sum of three skinfolds (mm): _____

Percent body fat: _____

Fitness category: _____

Body Mass Index

Body mass index score: _____

Fitness category: _____

Waist-to-Hip Circumference Ratio

Waist-to-hip circumference ratio: _____

Fitness category: _____

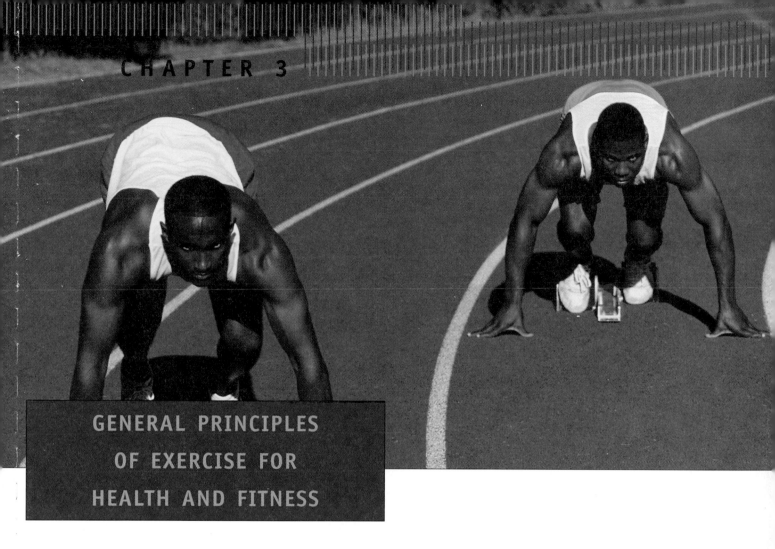

CHAPTER 3

GENERAL PRINCIPLES OF EXERCISE FOR HEALTH AND FITNESS

After studying this chapter, you should be able to:

1. Discuss the following concepts of physical fitness: overload principle; principle of progression; specificity of exercise; principle of recuperation; and reversibility of training effects.

2. Outline the physiological objectives of a warm-up and cool-down.

3. Identify the general principles of exercise prescription.

4. Discuss the concepts of progression and maintenance of exercise training.

5. Explain why individualizing the workout is an important concept for the development of an exercise prescription.

6. Discuss how much exercise is required to reach the "threshold for health benefits."

Research in exercise science has provided guidelines for the development of a safe and efficient program to improve personal fitness (1–9). The purpose of this chapter is to provide you with an overview of general principles for improving your physical fitness. The basic concepts contained within this chapter can be applied to both men and women of all ages and fitness levels. The individual components of health-related physical fitness are covered in Chapters 4, 5, and 6, which detail the development of cardiorespiratory fitness, muscular strength/endurance, and flexibility, respectively.

☀ Principles of Exercise Training to Improve Physical Fitness

Although the specifics of exercise training programs should be tailored to the individual, the general principles of physical fitness are the same for everyone. In the following sections we describe the training concepts of overload, progression, specificity, recuperation, and reversibility.

OVERLOAD PRINCIPLE

The **overload principle** is a key component of all conditioning programs (1–9). In order to improve physical fitness, the body or specific muscles must be stressed. For example, for a skeletal muscle to increase in strength, the muscle must work against a heavier load than normal. In this case we achieve an overload by increasing the intensity of exercise (i.e., by using heavier weights). Note, however, that overload can also be achieved by increasing the duration of exercise. For instance, to increase muscular endurance, a muscle must be worked over a longer duration than normal (by performing a higher number of exercise repetitions). Another practical example of the overload principle applied to health-related physical fitness is the improvement of flexibility. To increase the range of motion at a joint, we must either stretch the muscle to a longer length than normal or hold the stretch for a longer time.

---

overload principle   A basic principle of physical conditioning that states that in order to improve physical fitness, the body or specific muscles must be stressed. For example, for a skeletal muscle to increase in strength, the muscle must work against a heavier load than normal.

principle of progression   A principle of training that dictates that overload should be increased gradually during the course of a physical fitness program.

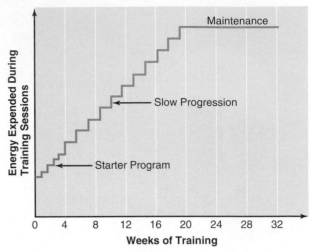

FIGURE 3.1
The progression and maintenance of exercise training during the first several months after beginning an exercise program.
(From Pollock, M. L., Wilmore, J. H., and Fox, S. M., III. *Health and Fitness Through Physical Activity*. New York, Prentice-Hall, 1978. Copyright © 1978. Reprinted by permission of Allyn and Bacon.)

Although improvement in physical fitness requires application of overload, this does not mean that exercise sessions must be exhausting. The often-heard quote, "No pain, no gain," is not completely accurate. In fact, improvement in physical fitness can be achieved without punishing training sessions (5).

PRINCIPLE OF PROGRESSION

The **principle of progression** is an extension of the overload principle. It states that overload should be increased gradually during the course of a physical fitness program. This concept is illustrated in Figure 3.1. Note that the overload of a training program should generally be increased slowly during the first 4 to 6 weeks of the exercise program. After this initial period, the overload can be increased at a steady but progressive rate during the next 18 to 20 weeks of training. It is important that the overload not be increased too slowly or too rapidly if optimum fitness improvement is to result. Progression that is too slow will result in limited improvement in physical fitness. Increasing the exercise overload too rapidly may result in chronic fatigue and injury. Muscle or joint injuries that occur because of too much exercise are called *overuse injuries*. Exercise-induced injuries can come from either short bouts of high-intensity exercise or long bouts of low-intensity exercise.

What is a safe rate of progression during an exercise training program? A definitive answer to this question is not possible because individuals vary in their tolerance for exercise overload. However, a common-sense guideline for improving physical fitness and

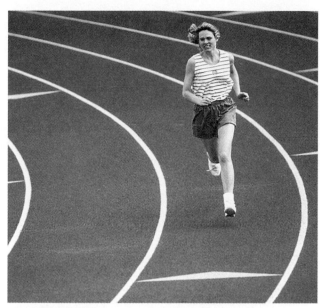

Running illustrates the concept of specificity because it promotes improvements in muscular endurance in the legs.

avoiding overuse injuries is the **ten percent rule** (6). In short, this rule says that the training intensity or duration of exercise should not be increased more than 10% per week. For example, a runner running 20 minutes per day could increase his or her daily exercise duration to 22 minutes per day (10% of 20 = 2) the following week.

When an individual reaches his or her desired level of physical fitness (that is, you have reached your goal as defined by one of the fitness tests described in Chapter 2), it is no longer necessary to increase the training intensity or duration. Indeed, once a desired level of fitness has been achieved, physical fitness can be maintained by regular exercise at a constant level (Figure 3.1). Exercising to sustain a certain level of physical fitness is referred to as a *maintenance program*.

SPECIFICITY OF EXERCISE

Another key concept of training is the **principle of specificity,** which states that the exercise training effect is specific to those muscles involved in the activity (10). You would not expect your arms to become trained following a 10-week jogging program!

Specificity of training also applies to the types of adaptations that occur in the muscle. For example, strength training results in an increase in muscle strength but does not greatly improve the endurance of the muscle. Therefore, strength training is specific to improving muscular strength (11). Similarly, endurance exercise training results in an improvement in muscular endurance without altering muscular strength much (12).

Principle of Recuperation

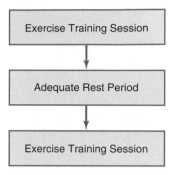

FIGURE 3.2
Principle of recuperation. This principle of training requires that adequate rest periods separate exercise training sessions.

Consider the following simple illustration of exercise specificity. Suppose you want to improve your ability to run a distance of 3 miles. In this case, specific training should include running 3 or more miles several times a week. This type of training would improve muscular endurance in your legs but would not result in large improvements in leg strength (10).

PRINCIPLE OF RECUPERATION

Because the principle of overload requires exercise stress to improve physical fitness, it follows that exercise training places a stress on the body. During the recovery period between exercise training sessions, the body adapts to the exercise stress by increasing endurance or becoming stronger. Therefore, a period of rest is essential for achieving maximal benefit from exercise. This needed rest period between exercise training sessions is called the **principle of recuperation** (Figure 3.2).

How much rest is required between heavy exercise training sessions? One or two days is adequate for most individuals (6). Failure to get enough rest between sessions may result in a fatigue syndrome referred to as

ten percent rule   A rule of training that states that the training intensity or duration of exercise should not be increased more than 10% per week.
principle of specificity   The principle that the effect of exercise training is specific to those muscles involved in the activity.
principle of recuperation   A principle of training that states that the body requires recovery periods between exercise training sessions in order to adapt to the exercise stress. Therefore, a period of rest is essential for achieving maximal benefit from exercise.

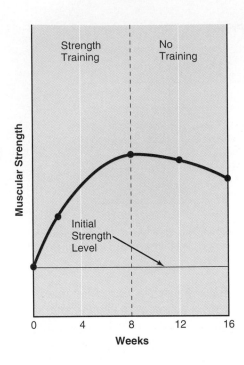

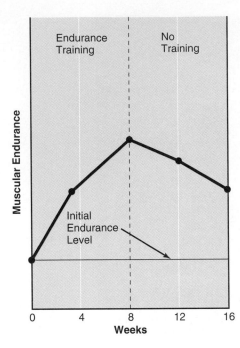

FIGURE 3.3
Retention of muscular strength and muscular endurance after training is stopped.

overtraining. Overtraining may lead to chronic fatigue and/or injuries. A key question is, How do you diagnose overtraining? Sore and stiff muscles or a feeling of general fatigue the morning after an exercise training session, sometimes called a "workout hangover," is a common symptom. The cure is to increase the duration of rest between workouts, reduce the intensity of workouts, or both. Although too much exercise is the primary cause of the overtraining syndrome, failure to consume a well-balanced diet can contribute to the feeling of a workout hangover (Nutritional Links to Health and Fitness).

REVERSIBILITY OF TRAINING EFFECTS

Although rest periods between exercise sessions are essential for maximal benefit from exercise, long intervals between workouts (that is, several days or weeks) can result in a reduction in fitness levels (13). Maintenance of physical fitness requires regular exercise sessions. In other words, physical fitness cannot be stored. The loss of fitness due to inactivity is an example of the **principle of reversibility.** The old adage, "What you don't use, you lose," is true when applied to physical fitness.

How quickly is fitness lost when training is stopped? The answer depends on which component of

physical fitness you are referring to. For example, after cessation of strength training, the loss of muscular strength is relatively slow (11, 14). In contrast, after you stop performing endurance exercise, the loss of muscular endurance is relatively rapid (13). Figure 3.3 illustrates this point. Note that 8 weeks after stopping strength training, only 10% of muscular strength is lost (14). In contrast, 8 weeks after cessation of endurance training, 30% to 40% of muscular endurance is lost (13).

---

overtraining The result of failure to get enough rest between exercise training sessions. Overtraining may lead to chronic fatigue and/or injuries.
principle of reversibility The loss of fitness due to inactivity.

Nutritional Links
TO HEALTH AND FITNESS

Diet and the Workout Hangover

Can a poor diet contribute to fatigue and overtraining? Yes! Failure to consume the recommended amounts of carbohydrates, fats, proteins, vitamins, and minerals can lead to chronic fatigue (15). Of particular importance to people engaged in a regular exercise training program is dietary carbohydrates. Because heavy exercise uses carbohydrates as a primary fuel source (6), diets low in carbohydrates can result in a depletion of muscle carbohydrate stores and can lead to a feeling of chronic fatigue. To maintain muscle carbohydrate stores, these nutrients should make up 60% of the total energy contained in your diet (6, 15). See Chapter 7 for a complete discussion of diet and nutrition for physical fitness.

☀ IN SUMMARY

- Five key principles of exercise training are:
  (1) overload principle; (2) principle of progression;
  (3) specificity of exercise; (4) principle of recuperation; and (5) reversibility of training effects.
- The overload principle refers to the fact that in order to improve physical fitness, the body or the specific muscle group used during exercise must be stressed.
- The principle of progression is an extension of the overload principle and states that overload should be increased gradually over the course of a physical fitness training program.
- The principle of specificity refers to the fact that exercise training is specific to those muscles involved in the activity.
- The requirement for a rest period between training sessions is called "the principle of recuperation."
- Loss of physical fitness due to inactivity is referred to as "the principle of reversibility."

☀ General Principles of Exercise Prescription

Doctors often prescribe medications to treat certain diseases, and for every individual there is an appropriate dosage of medicine to cure an illness. Similarly, for each individual there is a correct "dosage" of exercise to effectively promote physical fitness, called an **exercise prescription** (5, 8). Exercise prescriptions should be tailored to meet the needs of the individual (1–9, 16). They should include fitness goals, mode of exercise, a warm-up, a primary conditioning period, and a cool-down (Figure 3.4). The following sections provide a general introduction to each of these components.

FITNESS GOALS

As mentioned in Chapter 1, establishing short-term and long-term fitness goals is an important part of an exercise prescription. Goals serve as motivation to start an exercise program. Further, attaining your fitness goals improves self-esteem and provides the incentive needed to make a lifetime commitment to regular exercise.

A logical and common type of fitness goal is a performance goal. You can establish performance goals in each component of health-related physical fitness. Table 3.1 on page 68 illustrates a hypothetical example of how Susie Jones might establish short-term and long-term performance goals using fitness testing (Chapter 2) to determine when she has reached her objective. The column labeled "current status" contains

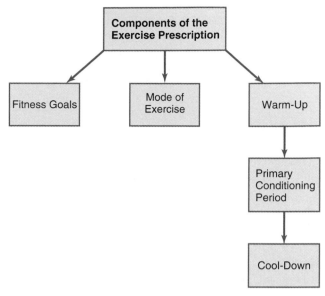

FIGURE 3.4
Components of the exercise prescription.

Susie's fitness ratings based on tests performed prior to starting her exercise program. After consultation with her instructor, Susie has established short-term goals that she hopes to achieve within the first 8 weeks of training. Note that the short-term goals are not "fixed in stone" and can be modified if the need arises. Susie's long-term goals are fitness levels that she hopes to reach within the first 18 months of training. Similar to short-term goals, long-term goals can be modified to meet changing needs or circumstances.

In addition to performance goals, consider establishing exercise adherence goals. That is, set a goal to exercise a specific number of days per week. Exercise adherence goals are important because fitness will improve only if you exercise regularly!

In writing your personal fitness goals, consider the following guidelines:

SET REALISTIC GOALS The most important rule in setting goals is that you must establish realistic ones. After a thorough self-evaluation and consultation with your instructor, set fitness goals that you can reach. Because failure to reach goals is discouraging, establishing realistic short-term goals is critical to the success of your exercise program.

---

exercise prescription The correct dosage of exercise to effectively promote physical fitness. Exercise prescriptions should be tailored to meet the needs of the individual and include fitness goals, mode of exercise, a warm-up, a primary conditioning period, and a cool-down.

TABLE 3.1
Illustration of Short-Term and Long-Term Performance Goals

The fitness categories are the five components of health-related physical fitness. The current status, short-term goals, and long-term goals are the fitness norms presented in Chapter 2.

Fitness Category	Current Status	Short-Term Goal	Long-Term Goal
Cardiorespiratory fitness	Poor	Average	Excellent
Muscular strength	Poor	Average	Excellent
Muscular endurance	Very poor	Average	Good
Flexibility	Poor	Average	Good
Body composition	High fat	Moderately high	Optimal

ESTABLISH SHORT-TERM GOALS FIRST   Reaching short-term fitness goals is a great motivation to continue exercising. Therefore, establishing realistic short-term goals is critical. After reaching a short-term goal, establish a new one.

SET REALISTIC LONG-TERM GOALS   In establishing long-term goals, consider your physical limitations. Heredity plays an important role in determining our fitness limits. Therefore, in establishing long-term goals, set goals that are realistic for you and not based on performance scores of other people.

ESTABLISH LIFETIME MAINTENANCE GOALS   In addition to short-term and long-term goals, consider establishing a fitness maintenance goal. A maintenance goal is established when your fitness goals have been met and your focus becomes remaining physically active and fit.

LIST GOALS IN WRITING   A key to meeting goals is to write them down and put them in a place where you can see them every day. Goals can be forgotten if they are not verifiable in writing. Further, remember that all goals should be periodically reevaluated and modified if necessary. Just because goals are in writing does not mean that they cannot be changed.

RECOGNIZE OBSTACLES TO ACHIEVING GOALS   If you do not make your fitness goals a serious priority, you will keep putting them off until they no longer exist. Once you begin your fitness program, be prepared to make mistakes (such as skipping workouts and losing motivation) and to backslide some (and have your fitness level decline temporarily). This is normal. However, once you realize that you have stopped making progress toward your goals, you must get back on track and start making progress again as soon as you can.

The importance of fitness goals cannot be overemphasized. Goals provide structure and motivation for a personal fitness program. Keys to maintaining a lifelong fitness program are discussed again in Chapter 11.

MODE OF EXERCISE

Every exercise prescription includes at least one **mode of exercise**—that is, a specific type of exercise to be performed. For example, to improve cardiorespiratory fitness, you could select from a wide variety of exercise modes, such as running, swimming, or cycling. Key factors to consider when selecting an exercise mode are enjoyment, availability of the activity, and risk of injury.

Physical activities can be classified as being either high impact or low impact based on the amount of stress placed on joints during the activity. Activities that place a large amount of pressure on joints are called high-impact activities, whereas low-impact activities are less stressful. Because of the strong correlation between high-impact modes of exercise and injuries, many fitness experts recommend low-impact activities for fitness beginners or for those individuals susceptible to injury (such as participants who are older or overweight). Examples of some high-impact activities include running, basketball, and high-impact aerobic dance. Low-impact activities include walking, cycling, swimming, and low-impact aerobic dance.

WARM-UP

A **warm-up** is a brief (5- to 15-minute) period of exercise that precedes a workout. It generally involves light calisthenics or a low-intensity form of the actual mode

mode of exercise   The specific type of exercise to be performed. For example, to improve cardiorespiratory fitness, one could select from a wide variety of exercise modes, including running, swimming, or cycling.
warm-up   A brief (5- to 15-minute) period of exercise that precedes a workout. The purpose of a warm-up is to elevate muscle temperature and increase blood flow to those muscles that will be engaged in the workout.

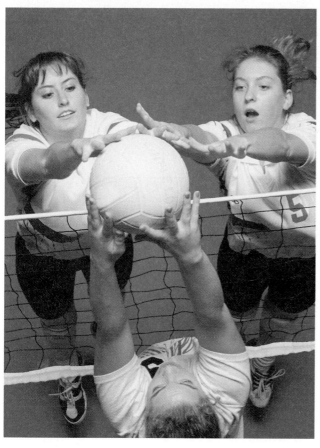

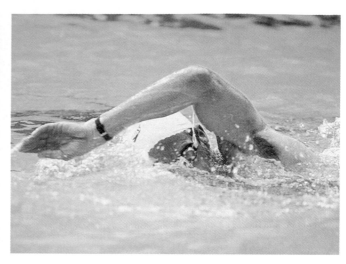

Whereas swimming is considered a low-impact activity, volleyball is considered a high-impact activity.

of exercise and often includes stretching exercises as well (Chapter 6). The purpose of a warm-up is to elevate muscle temperature and increase blood flow to those muscles that will be engaged in the workout (3, 6, 17). A warm-up can also reduce the strain on the heart imposed by rapidly engaging in heavy exercise and may reduce the risk of muscle and tendon injuries (17).

THE WORKOUT

Regardless of the mode of exercise (described earlier), the major components of the exercise prescription that make up the workout (also called the primary conditioning period) are frequency, intensity, and duration of exercise (Figure 3.5). The **frequency of exercise** is the number of times per week that you intend to exercise. In general, the recommended frequency of exercise to improve most components of health-related physical fitness is three to five times per week (5, 18–20).

The **intensity of exercise** is the amount of physiological stress or overload placed on the body during the exercise. The method for determining the intensity of exercise varies with the type of exercise performed. For example, because heart rate increases linearly with energy expenditure (effort) during exercise, measurement of heart rate has become a standard means of determin-

ing exercise intensity during training to improve cardiorespiratory fitness. Although heart rate can also be used to gauge exercise intensity during strength training, the number of exercise repetitions that can be performed before muscular fatigue occurs is more useful for monitoring stress during weight lifting. For instance, a load that can be lifted only five to eight times before complete muscular fatigue is an example of high-intensity weight lifting. In contrast, a load that can be lifted 50 to 60 times without resulting in muscular fatigue is an illustration of low-intensity weight training.

Finally, flexibility is improved by stretching muscles beyond their normal lengths. Intensity of stretching is monitored by the degree of tension or discomfort felt during the stretch. Low-intensity stretching results in only minor tension (or limited discomfort) on the muscles and tendons. In contrast, high-intensity stretching places great tension or moderate discomfort on the muscle groups being stretched.

---

frequency of exercise The number of times per week that one intends to exercise.
intensity of exercise The amount of physiological stress or overload placed on the body during exercise.

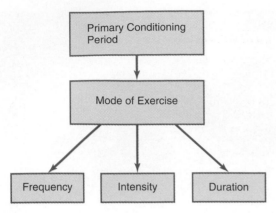

FIGURE 3.5
The components of the primary conditioning period: the frequency, intensity, and duration of exercise.

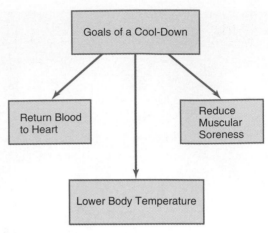

FIGURE 3.6
Purposes of a cool-down.

A key aspect of the primary conditioning period is the **duration of exercise**—that is, the amount of time invested in performing the primary workout. Note that the duration of exercise does not include the warm-up or cool-down. In general, research has shown that 20 to 30 minutes per exercise session (performed at least three times per week) is the minimum amount of time required to significantly improve physical fitness.

COOL-DOWN

The **cool-down** (sometimes called a *warm-down*) is a 5- to 15-minute period of low-intensity exercise that immediately follows the primary conditioning period. For instance, a period of slow walking might be used as a cool-down following a running workout. A cool-down period accomplishes several goals (Figure 3.6). In addition to its goal of lowering body temperature after exercise, one primary purpose of a cool-down is to allow blood to be returned from the muscles back toward the heart (3–6). During exercise, large amounts of blood are pumped to the working muscles. On cessation of exercise, blood tends to remain in large blood vessels located around the exercised muscles (a process called *pooling*). Failure to redistribute pooled blood after exercise could result in your feeling lightheaded or even fainting. Prevention of blood pooling is best accomplished by low-intensity exercise using those muscles utilized during the workout.

Finally, some fitness experts argue that postexercise muscle soreness may be reduced as a result of

a cool-down (21). Although a cool-down period may not eliminate muscular soreness entirely, it seems possible that the severity of exercise-induced muscle soreness may be reduced in people who perform a proper cool-down (21).

INDIVIDUALIZING THE WORKOUT

A key point to remember about exercise prescriptions is that each should be tailored to the needs and objectives of the individual. Although the same general principles of exercise training apply to everyone, no two people are the same. Therefore, the exercise prescription should consider such factors as the individual's general health, age, fitness status, musculoskeletal condition, and body composition. More will be said about individualizing workouts in later chapters.

☀ IN SUMMARY

- The "dosage" of exercise required to effectively promote physical fitness is called the exercise prescription.
- The components of the exercise prescription include fitness goals, mode of exercise, the warm-up, the workout (i.e., the primary conditioning period), and the cool-down.
- Exercise training programs should be individualized by considering such factors as age, health, and fitness status of the individual.

☀ How Much Exercise Is Enough?

Students often ask, "How much exercise is enough to provide health benefits?" Although even low levels of physical activity can provide some health benefits, growing evidence indicates that moderate-to-high

---

duration of exercise The amount of time invested in performing the primary workout.
cool-down A 5- to 15-minute period of low-intensity exercise that immediately follows the primary conditioning period; sometimes called a *warm-down*.

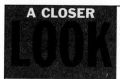

Too Much Exercise Increases Your Risk of Colds

Recent research indicates that intense exercise training (i.e., overtraining) reduces the body's immunity to disease (22). In contrast, light to moderate exercise training boosts the immune system and reduces the risk of infections (23). The relationship between exercise training and the risk of developing on upper respiratory tract infection (i.e., a cold) is shown in the figure in this box. The J-shaped curve in the figure indicates that moderate exercise training reduces the risk of infection, whereas high-intensity and long-duration exercise training increase the risk of infection.

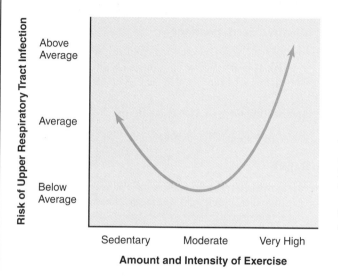

This J-shaped curve illustrates the relationship between physical activity and colds. Note that moderate physical activity reduces your risk of infection, whereas long-duration or high-intensity exercise increases your risk of disease. (Redrawn from Nieman, D., Moderate exercise boosts the immune system: Too much exercise can have the opposite effect. *ACSM's Health and Fitness Journal* 1(5):14–18, 1997.)

levels of physical activity are required to provide major health benefits (18, 20, 24, 25, 26, 27). The theoretical relationship between physical activity and health benefits is illustrated in Figure 3.7. Note that the minimum level of exercise required to achieve some of the health benefits of exercise is called the **threshold for health benefits.** Most experts believe that 20 to 60 minutes of moderate-to-high intensity exercise performed 3 to 5 days per week will surpass the threshold for health benefits and will reduce all causes of death (25, 26, 28). Importantly, any one of many exercise modalities (e.g., running, swimming, cycling) can be used to achieve the exercise threshold for health benefits. Details on how to achieve health-related aspects of physical fitness are discussed in Chapters 4 through 6.

✷ IN SUMMARY

- While low levels of physical activity can provide some health benefits, moderate-to-high levels of physical activity are required to provide major health benefits.
- The minimum level of exercise required to achieve some health benefits of exercise is called the threshold for health benefits.

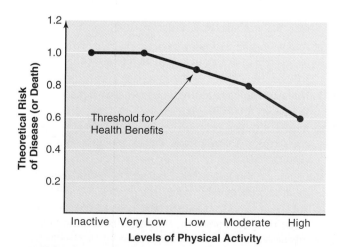

FIGURE 3.7
The relationship between physical activity and improved health benefits. Note that as the level of regular physical activity is increased, the theoretical risk of disease (or death) is decreased. Data are from ref. 25–27.

threshold for health benefits   The minimum level of physical activity required to achieve some of the health benefits of exercise.

Summary

1. The overload principle, which is the most important principle of exercise training, states that in order to improve physical fitness, the body or muscle group used during exercise must be overloaded.

2. The principle of progression states that overload should be increased gradually during the course of a physical fitness program.

3. The need for a rest period between exercise training sessions is called the principle of recuperation.

4. Physical fitness can be lost due to inactivity; this is often called the principle of reversibility.

5. The components of the exercise prescription include fitness goals, mode of exercise, the warm-up, the workout, and the cool-down.

6. All exercise training programs should be tailored to meet the objectives of the individual. Therefore, the exercise prescription should consider the individual's age, health, fitness status, musculoskeletal condition, and body composition.

7. The minimum level of physical activity required to achieve some of the health benefits of exercise is called the threshold for health benefits.

Study Questions

1. Define the following terms: *overtraining* and *principle of recuperation*.

2. What are the general purposes of a cool-down and a warm-up?

3. Describe and discuss the components of the exercise prescription.

4. How does the principle of progression apply to the exercise prescription?

5. Discuss the overload principle.

6. Define the term *threshold for health benefits*.

7. What happens to physical fitness if you stop training?

8. Explain why the exercise prescription should be individualized.

Suggested Reading

Howley, E. T. You asked for it: Is rigorous exercise better than moderate activity in achieving health-related goals? *ACSM's Health and Fitness Journal* 4(2):6, 2000.

Maughan, R., ed. *Basic and Applied Sciences for Sports Medicine.* Oxford, England: Butterworth-Heinemann, 1999.

Powers, S., and E. Howley. *Exercise Physiology: Theory and Application to Fitness and Performance,* 4th ed. St. Louis: McGraw-Hill, 2001.

Roitman, J. *ACSM's Resource Manual for Exercise Testing and Prescription.* Philadelphia: Lippincott Williams & Wilkins, 2001.

For links to the Web sites below visit Web Links at www.aw.com/fitness and choose Powers/Dodd Web Links from the drop-down menu.

American Heart Association

Contains the latest information about ways to reduce your risk of heart and vascular diseases. Site includes information about exercise, diet, and heart disease.

American College of Sports Medicine

Contains information about exercise, health, and fitness.

WebMD

Contains the latest information on a variety of health-related topics, including diet, exercise, and stress. Includes links to nutrition, fitness, and wellness topics.

References

1. Getchell, B. *Physical Fitness: A Way of Life.* Needham Heights, MA: Allyn and Bacon, 1997.

2. Hockey, R. *Physical Fitness: The Pathway to Healthful Living.* St. Louis: Times Mirror/Mosby, 1996.

3. Howley, E., and B. D. Franks. *Health Fitness: Instructors Handbook.* Champaign, IL: Human Kinetics, 1997.

4. Fleck, S. and W. Kraemer. *Designing Resistance Training Programs.* Champaign, Il: Human Kinetics, 1997.

5. Pollock, M., and J. Wilmore. *Exercise in Health and Disease.* Philadelphia: W. B. Saunders, 1990.

6. Powers, S., and E. Howley. *Exercise Physiology: Theory and Application to Fitness and Performance,* 4th ed. St. Louis: McGraw-Hill, 2001.

7. Williams, M. *Lifetime Fitness and Wellness.* Dubuque, IA: Wm. C. Brown, 1996.

8. American College of Sports Medicine. *Guidelines for Exercise Testing and Prescription.* Philadelphia: Lea and Febiger, 1991.

9. Corbin, C., and R. Lindsey. *Concepts of Physical Fitness and Wellness.* Dubuque, IA: Brown and Benchmark, 1997.

10. Roberts, J., and J. Alspaugh. Specificity of training effects resulting from programs of treadmill running and bicycle ergometer riding. *Medicine and Science in Sports* 4:6–10, 1972.

11. Abernethy, P., J. Jurimae, P. Logan, A. Taylor, and R. Thayer. Acute and chronic response of skeletal muscle to resistance exercise. *Sports Medicine* 17:22–28, 1994.

12. Powers, S., D. Criswell, J. Lawler, L. Ji, D. Martin, R. Herb, and G. Dudley. Influence of exercise and fiber type on antioxidant enzyme activity in rat skeletal muscle. *American Journal of Physiology* 266:R375–R380, 1994.

13. Coyle, E., W. Martin, D. Sinacore, M. Joyner, J. Hagberg, and J. Holloszy. Time course of loss of adaptations after stopping prolonged intense endurance training. *Journal of Applied Physiology* 57:1857–1864, 1984.

14. Costill, D., and A. Richardson. *Handbook of Sports Medicine: Swimming*. London: Blackwell Publishing, 1993.

15. Lamb, D., and M. Williams. *Ergogenics: Enhancement of Performance in Exercise and Sport*. Vol. 4. Madison, WI: Brown and Benchmark, 1991.

16. McGlynn, G. *Dynamics of Fitness: A Practical Approach*. Dubuque, IA: Wm. C. Brown, 1996.

17. DeVries, H., and T. Housh. *Exercise Physiology*, 5th ed. Dubuque, IA: Brown and Benchmark, 1994.

18. Bouchard, C., R. Shephard, T. Stephens, J. Sutton, and B. McPherson, eds. *Exercise, Fitness, and Health: A Consensus of Current Knowledge*. Champaign, IL: Human Kinetics, 1990.

19. Barrow, M. *Heart Talk: Understanding Cardiovascular Diseases*. Gainesville, FL: Cor-Ed Publishing, 1992.

20. Morris, J. Exercise in the prevention of coronary heart disease: Today's best buy in public health. *Medicine and Science in Sports and Exercise* 26:807–814, 1994.

21. Robergs, R., and S. Roberts. *Fundamental Principles of Exercise Physiology: For Fitness, Performance, and Health*. St. Louis: McGraw-Hill, 2000.

22. Nieman, D. Immune response to heavy exertion. *Journal of Applied Physiology* 82:1385–1394, 1997.

23. Nieman, D. Moderate exercise boosts the immune system: Too much exercise can have the opposite effect. *ACSM's Health and Fitness Journal* 1(5):14–18, 1997.

24. Paffenbarger, R., J. Kampert, I-Min Lee, R. Hyde, R. Leung, and A. Wing. Changes in physical activity and other lifeway patterns influencing longevity. *Medicine and Science in Sports and Exercise* 26:857–865, 1994.

25. Blair, S., H. W. Kohl, N. Gordon, and R. Paffenbarger. How much physical activity is good for health? *Annual Review of Public Health* 13:99–126, 1992.

26. Lee, I., and R. Paffenbarger. Associations of light, moderate, and vigorous intensity physical activity with longevity. *American Journal of Epidemiology* 151:293–299, 2000.

27. Williams, P. Physical fitness and activity as separate heart disease risk factors: A meta-analysis. *Medicine and Science in Sports and Exercise* 33:754–761, 2001.

28. Pollock, M., G. Gaesser, J. Butcher, J. P. Despres, R. Dishman, B. Franklin, and C. Garber. The recommended quantity and quality of exercise for developing and maintaining cardiorespiratory fitness and muscular fitness, and flexibility in healthy adults. *Medicine and Science in Sports and Exercise* 30:975–991, 1998.

29. Howley, E. T. You asked for it: Is rigorous exercise better than moderate activity in achieving health-related goals? *ACSM's Health and Fitness Journal* 4(2):6, 2000.

30. Roitman, J. *ACSM's Resource Manual for Exercise Testing and Prescription*. Philadelphia: Lippincott Williams & Wilkins, 2001.

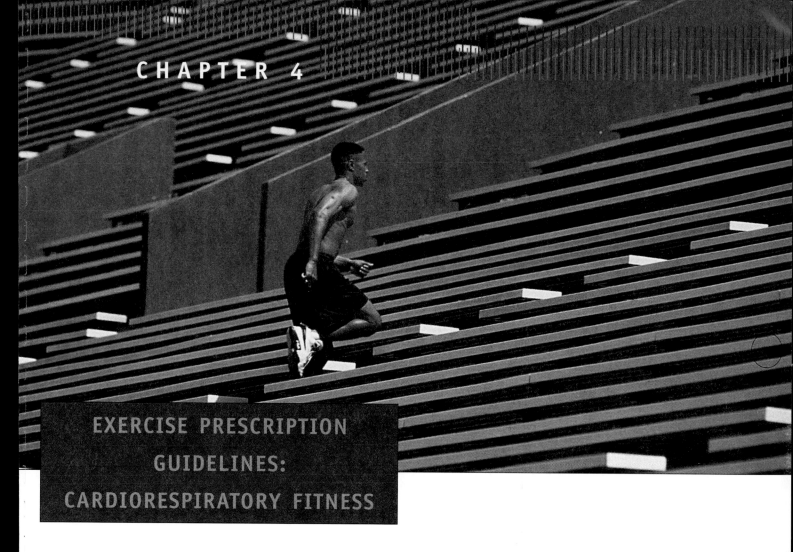

CHAPTER 4

EXERCISE PRESCRIPTION GUIDELINES: CARDIORESPIRATORY FITNESS

After studying this chapter, you should be able to:

1. Explain the benefits of developing cardiorespiratory fitness.

2. Identify the three energy systems involved in the production of adenosine triphosphate for muscular contraction.

3. Discuss the role of the circulatory and respiratory systems during exercise.

4. Define $\dot{V}O_{2max}$.

5. Identify the major changes that occur in skeletal muscles, the circulatory system, and the respiratory system in response to aerobic training.

6. List several modes of training used to improve cardiovascular fitness.

7. Outline the general components of an exercise prescription designed to improve cardiorespiratory fitness.

8. Design an exercise program for improving cardiorespiratory endurance.

Much of the current interest in cardiorespiratory training began in 1968 with the publication of Dr. Kenneth Cooper's best-selling fitness book, *Aerobics* (1). After the book's appearance, the term **aerobics** became commonly used to describe all forms of low-intensity exercise designed to improve cardiorespiratory fitness (such as jogging, walking, cycling, and swimming). Because aerobic exercise has proven effective in promoting weight loss (2) and reducing the risk of cardiovascular disease (3), many exercise scientists consider cardiorespiratory fitness to be one of the most important components of health-related physical fitness.

In the first three chapters of this book we discussed the health benefits of exercise, fitness assessment, and the general principles of exercise training. In the next three chapters we describe how to design a comprehensive, scientifically based exercise program to promote health-related physical fitness. This chapter describes techniques for promoting cardiorespiratory fitness. Before we discuss the exercise prescription for cardiovascular fitness, however, let's review the benefits of cardiorespiratory fitness and some basic concepts concerning how your body works during aerobic exercise.

Benefits of Cardiorespiratory Fitness

The benefits of cardiorespiratory fitness are many. A key advantage is that people with high levels of cardiorespiratory fitness have a lower risk of heart disease and increased longevity. Other health benefits include a reduced risk of type II diabetes, lower blood pressure, and increased bone density in weight-bearing bones (4).

Another positive factor associated with developing cardiorespiratory fitness is that as fitness improves, energy for work and play increases. This translates into your being able to perform more work with less fatigue. Indeed, people with high levels of cardiorespiratory fitness often state that one of the reasons they exercise is because they feel better as a result.

Development of cardiorespiratory fitness through regular exercise has been shown to improve self-esteem (5). This improvement probably comes from several factors. First, starting and maintaining a regular exercise program provides a strong sense of accomplishment. Second, regular exercise improves muscle tone and assists in weight control. Combined, these factors result in an improved appearance and therefore improved self-esteem. Finally, studies have shown that people with high levels of cardiorespiratory fitness sleep better than less fit individuals (6). Fit individuals tend to sleep longer without interruptions (i.e., they enjoy more restful sleep) compared with less fit people. This exercise-related improved sleep results in a better night's rest and a more complete feeling of being mentally restored.

Physiological Basis for Developing Cardiorespiratory Fitness

ENERGY TO PERFORM EXERCISE

The prolonged type of exercise that is necessary to develop cardiovascular fitness requires that an enormous amount of energy be supplied to the exercising muscles. Where do muscles get the energy to contract during exercise? The answer is: from the chemical energy released by the breakdown of food (such as carbohydrates, proteins, and fat). However, food energy cannot be used directly for energy by the muscles. Instead, the energy released from the breakdown of food is used to manufacture another biochemical compound, called **adenosine triphosphate (ATP),** a high-energy compound that is synthesized and stored in small quantities in muscle and other cells. The breakdown of ATP results in the release of energy that can be used to fuel muscular contraction. ATP is the only compound in the body that can provide this immediate source of energy. Therefore, for muscles to contract during exercise, a supply of ATP must be available.

Two "systems" in muscle cells can produce ATP. One system does not require oxygen and is called the **anaerobic** (without oxygen) system. The second system

---

aerobics A common term to describe all forms of low-intensity exercise designed to improve cardiorespiratory fitness (e.g., jogging, walking, cycling, and swimming). Because aerobic exercise has proved effective in promoting weight loss and reducing the risk of cardiovascular disease, many exercise scientists consider cardiorespiratory fitness to be one of the most important components of health-related physical fitness.

adenosine triphosphate (ATP) A high-energy compound that is synthesized and stored in small quantities in muscle and other cells. The breakdown of ATP results in a release of energy that can be used to fuel muscular contraction. ATP is the only compound in the body that can provide this immediate source of energy.

anaerobic Means "without oxygen"; in cells pertains to energy-producing biochemical pathways that do not require oxygen to produce energy.

requires oxygen and is called the **aerobic** (with oxygen) system. Let's discuss the anaerobic system first.

ANAEROBIC ATP PRODUCTION   Most of the anaerobic ATP production in muscle occurs in a metabolic process called *glycolysis,* which breaks down carbohydrates (sugars) in cells. The end result of glycolysis is the anaerobic production of ATP and often the formation of lactic acid. Because lactic acid is often a byproduct of glycolysis, this pathway for ATP production is often called the **lactic acid system.** The lactic acid system can use only carbohydrates as an energy source. Carbohydrates are supplied to muscles from blood sugar (*glucose*) and from muscle stores of glucose (a compound called *glycogen*).

Conceptually, it is convenient to think of the lactic acid system as the energy pathway that produces ATP at the beginning of exercise and during short-term (30–60 seconds) high-intensity exercise. For instance, most of the ATP required to sprint 400 meters (which may require 60–80 seconds) would be derived from the lactic acid system. During this type of intense exercise, muscles produce large amounts of lactic acid because the lactic acid system is operating at high speed. The accumulation of lactic acid in muscles results in fatigue and explains the decline in running speed of a 400-meter runner struggling toward the finish line.

AEROBIC ATP PRODUCTION   Exercise lasting longer than 60 seconds requires ATP production by the aerobic system. Therefore, activities of daily living and many types of exercise depend on aerobic ATP production.

Whereas the anaerobic lactic acid system uses only carbohydrate as a food source, aerobic metabolism can use all three foodstuffs (fats, carbohydrates, and protein) to produce ATP. In a healthy individual consuming a balanced diet, however, proteins play a limited role as an energy source during exercise; therefore, carbohydrates and fats are the primary sources. In general, at the beginning of exercise, carbohydrate is the principal foodstuff broken down during aerobic ATP production. During prolonged exercise (i.e., longer than 20 minutes' duration), there is a gradual shift from carbohydrate to fat as an energy source. This process is illustrated in Figure 4.1.

THE ENERGY CONTINUUM   Although it is common to speak of aerobic versus anaerobic exercise, in reality the energy to perform many types of exercise comes from both sources. Figure 4.2(a) illustrates the anaerobic–aerobic energy continuum as a function of the exercise duration. Anaerobic energy production dominates during short-term exercise, whereas aerobic energy production is greatest during long-term exercise. For example, maximal exercise of 10 seconds' duration uses anaerobic

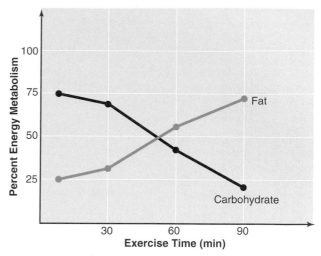

FIGURE 4.1
Changes in carbohydrate and fat use during 90 minutes of aerobic exercise.

energy sources almost exclusively. On the other end of the energy spectrum, notice that aerobic energy production dominates during 2 hours of continuous exercise. Running a maximal-effort 800-meter race (exercise of 2–3 minutes' duration) is an example of an exercise duration that uses almost an equal amount of aerobic and anaerobic energy sources.

Figure 4.2(b) applies the anaerobic–aerobic energy continuum to various sports activities. Weight lifting, gymnastics, and football are examples of sports that use anaerobic energy production almost exclusively. Boxing and skating (1500 meters) are examples of sports that require an equal contribution of anaerobic and aerobic energy production. Finally, cross-country skiing and jogging are examples of activities in which aerobic energy production dominates.

☼ IN SUMMARY

- ATP is required for muscular contraction and can be produced by two energy systems: the anaerobic (without oxygen) system and the aerobic (with oxygen) system.
- In general, anaerobic energy production dominates in short-term exercise, whereas aerobic energy production dominates during prolonged exercise.

---

aerobic   Means "with oxygen"; in cells pertains to energy-producing biochemical pathways that use oxygen to produce energy.
lactic acid   A by-product of glucose metabolism. Produced primarily during intense exercise (i.e., greater than 50–60% of maximal aerobic capacity). Results in inhibition of muscle contraction and, therefore, fatigue.

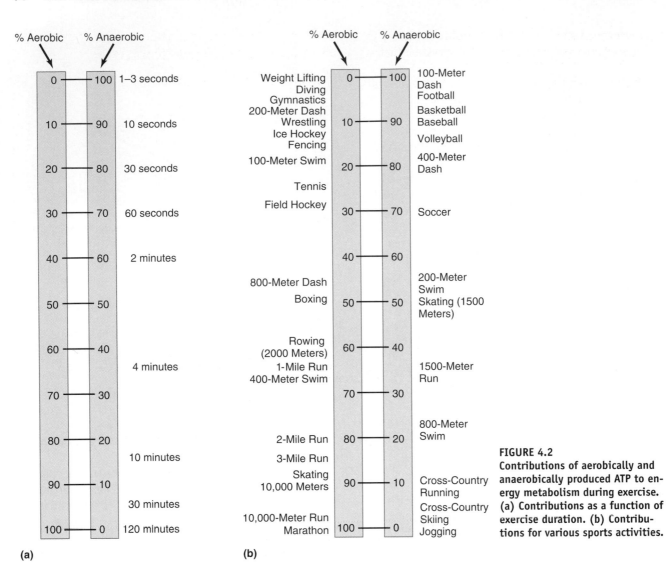

FIGURE 4.2
Contributions of aerobically and anaerobically produced ATP to energy metabolism during exercise. (a) Contributions as a function of exercise duration. (b) Contributions for various sports activities.

Exercise and the Cardiorespiratory System

The term *cardiorespiratory system* refers to the cooperative work of the circulatory and respiratory systems. Together they are responsible for the delivery of oxygen and nutrients as well as for the removal of waste products (e.g., carbon dioxide) from tissues. Exercise poses a major challenge to the cardiorespiratory system by increasing the muscular demand for oxygen and nutrients. The cardiorespiratory system must meet this demand to allow the individual to continue exercising. In the following sections we present a brief overview of cardiorespiratory function during exercise.

THE CIRCULATORY SYSTEM

The circulatory system is a closed loop composed of the heart and blood vessels. The pump in this system is the heart, which, by contracting, generates pressure to move blood through the system. Figure 4.3 illustrates that the heart can be considered two pumps in one. The right side pumps oxygen-depleted (deoxygenated) blood through the lungs (a pathway called the **pulmonary circuit**), while the left side pumps oxygen-rich (oxygenated) blood to tissues throughout the body (a pathway called the **systemic circuit**). Let's consider these two circuits in more detail.

> **pulmonary circuit** The blood vascular system that circulates blood from the right side of the heart, through the lungs, and back to the left side of the heart.
> **systemic circuit** The blood vascular system that circulates blood from the left side of the heart, throughout the body, and back to the right side of the heart.

Nutritional Links
TO HEALTH AND FITNESS

What Nutrients Are Most Important for Endurance Performance?

Whether you're an athlete or fitness enthusiast, nutrition is fundamental to your performance. A balanced eating plan that accounts for the type and level of activity is essential for cardiorespiratory endurance. Your diet should not vary considerably from a normal diet—that is, it should include plenty of fluids and low-fat, high-carbohydrate foods for energy. You should tailor the caloric content of your diet to reflect the amount of energy you expend during workouts. Carbohydrates should constitute at least 60% of the calories you consume, because they are the most critical supply of energy. Since muscles replenish stored carbohydrates most efficiently within the first 2 hours following exercise, you should consume 200–400 calories as soon as possible after exercise. Some good things to eat as a source of complex carbohydrates just after exercising include the following:

Two pieces of fruit

1 cup nonfat yogurt + 1 cup fruit topping

1 oz. cereal + ½ cup skim milk

1 low-fat muffin + ½ cup skim milk

12 oz. fruit juice

1 cup grapes + 1 bagel

1 cup vegetable soup + 1 slice bread

The intake of fluids is critical during exercise. Fluids are necessary to maintain blood volume and to replenish water lost through sweating. Because thirst is not a good regulator of fluid balance over the short run, fluids should be consumed before, during, and after your workout. Consume about 6 oz. of water 30 minutes before the workout, 3–6 oz. every 15 minutes during the workout, and 16 oz. for every pound lost during the workout.

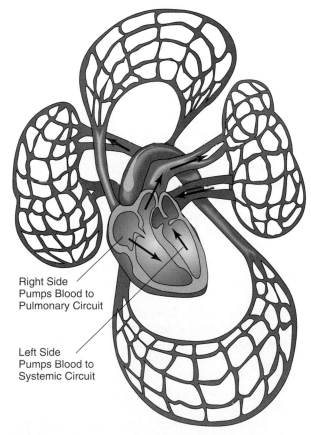

Right Side Pumps Blood to Pulmonary Circuit

Left Side Pumps Blood to Systemic Circuit

FIGURE 4.3
The concept of the heart as "two pumps in one."
(From Wilmore, J. H., and D. L. Costill. *Physiology of Sport and Exercise* (p. 173). Champaign, IL: Human Kinetics. Copyright © 1994 by Jack H. Wilmore and David L. Costill. Reprinted with permission.)

In the systemic circuit, blood carrying oxygen leaves the heart in **arteries,** which branch to form microscopic vessels called *arterioles;* arterioles eventually branch into beds of smaller vessels called *capillaries.* **Capillaries** are thin-walled vessels that permit the exchange of gases (oxygen and carbon dioxide) and nutrients between the blood and tissues. After this exchange, blood passes from the capillaries into microscopic vessels called *venules.* As venules move back toward the heart, they increase in size and form **veins,** which carry oxygen-depleted blood back to the heart.

Venous blood (i.e., blood carried by veins) from all parts of the body returns to the right side of the heart and is pumped through the lungs. In the lungs, oxygen is loaded into the blood, and carbon dioxide is removed from the blood into the lungs. The oxygen-rich blood is then returned to the left side of the heart and pumped to all body tissues by the systemic circuit.

arteries   The blood vessels that transport blood away from the heart.
capillaries   Thin-walled vessels that permit the exchange of gases (oxygen and carbon dioxide) and nutrients between the blood and tissues.
veins   Blood vessels that transport blood toward the heart.

The amount of blood the heart pumps per minute is called **cardiac output.** Cardiac output is the product of the **heart rate** (number of heartbeats per minute) and the **stroke volume** (how much blood is pumped per heartbeat, generally expressed in milliliters). During exercise, cardiac output can be increased by increasing either heart rate or stroke volume or both. Stroke volume does not increase beyond light work rates (i.e., low-intensity exercise). Therefore, the increase in cardiac output needed for moderate work rates and above is achieved by increases in heart rate alone. (Changes in cardiac output in response to exercise are discussed later in this chapter.)

Maximal cardiac output declines in both men and women after approximately 20 years of age, primarily due to a decrease in maximal heart rate. The decrease in maximal heart rate (HR_{max}) with age can be estimated by the formula

$$HR_{max} = 220 - \text{age (in years)}$$

According to this formula, a 20-year-old individual would have maximal HR of 200 beats per minute ($220 - 20 = 200$), whereas a 60-year-old would have a maximal HR of 160 beats per minute ($220 - 60 = 160$).

BLOOD PRESSURE

Blood is moved through the circulatory system by pressure generated by the pumping heart. The pressure that blood exerts against the walls of arteries is called *blood pressure.* Measurement of arterial blood pressure is generally attained by a device called a *sphygmomanometer* (Figure 4.4). During contraction of the heart (called *systole*), arterial blood pressure reaches its highest value. Blood pressure during systole is called **systolic blood pressure;** the normal resting systolic blood pressure for a young male adult is approximately 120 mm Hg (women may register 10–20 mm Hg lower). During the relaxation phase of the heart (called *diastole*),

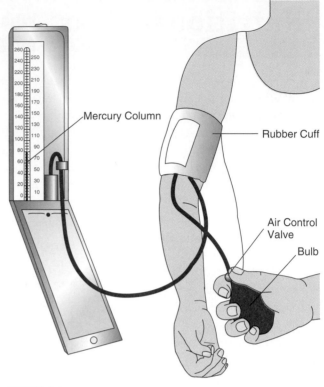

FIGURE 4.4
Measuring blood pressure using a sphygmomanometer.

blood pressure declines and reaches its lowest value. Blood pressure during diastole is called **diastolic blood pressure;** normal diastolic blood pressure for a young male adult is approximately 80 mm Hg (again, women may register 10–20 mm Hg lower). It is important to measure both systolic and diastolic blood pressure because it is the combination of these two pressures that determines your mean (average) arterial pressure.

The walls of arteries are elastic, and they expand during the contraction of the heart. The increase in blood pressure during systole causes a pulsation in the arteries that can be felt by placing your finger (don't use the thumb) on the skin near a major artery. One pulse represents one heartbeat. This technique can be used to count your heart rate during or after exercise (discussed in Chapter 2).

Approximately 20% of all adults living in the United States (7) have abnormally high blood pressure, or **hypertension.** Systolic blood pressure of 140 mm Hg, and diastolic blood pressure of 90 mm Hg, are "threshold" blood pressure values; all higher values indicate hypertension. Hypertension is a serious health problem because it increases the risk of heart attack and stroke (8). As we saw in Chapter 1, regular exercise has been shown to reduce blood pressure in many individuals. Therefore, physicians often prescribe light exercise for hypertensive patients in an effort to lower their blood pressure.

---

cardiac output   The amount of blood the heart pumps per minute.

heart rate   Number of heartbeats per minute.

stroke volume   The amount of blood pumped per heartbeat (generally expressed in milliliters).

systolic blood pressure   The pressure of the blood in the arteries at the level of the heart during the contraction phase of the heart (systole).

diastolic blood pressure   The pressure of the blood in the arteries at the level of the heart during the resting phase of the heart (diastole).

hypertension (high blood pressure)   Usually considered to be a blood pressure of greater than 140 for systolic or 90 for diastolic.

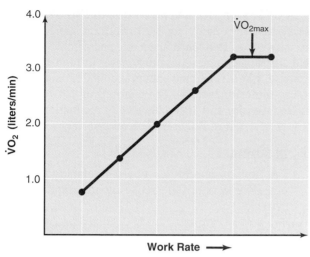

FIGURE 4.5
The relationship between exercise intensity (work rate) and $\dot{V}O_2$. $\dot{V}O_{2max}$ is the highest oxygen uptake that can be obtained during heavy exercise.

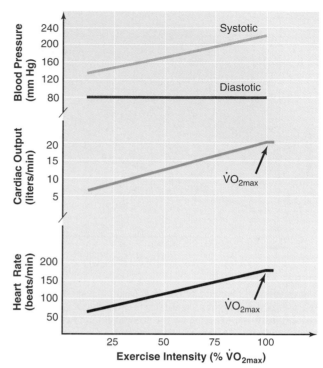

FIGURE 4.6
Changes in blood pressure, cardiac output, and heart rate as a function of exercise intensity.

THE RESPIRATORY SYSTEM

The primary purpose of the respiratory system (also called the *pulmonary system*) is to provide a means of supplying oxygen to the blood and removing carbon dioxide from the blood. This is achieved by bringing oxygen-rich air into the lungs, which we do by breathing. Oxygen then moves from the lungs into the blood, and carbon dioxide moves from the blood into the lungs and is then exhaled.

MAXIMAL CARDIORESPIRATORY FUNCTION: $\dot{V}O_{2max}$

The body's maximum ability to transport and use oxygen during exercise (called $\dot{V}O_{2max}$ or *maximal aerobic capacity*) was introduced in Chapter 2. $\dot{V}O_{2max}$ is considered by many exercise physiologists to be the most valid measurement of cardiorespiratory fitness. Indeed, graded exercise tests designed to measure $\dot{V}O_{2max}$ are often conducted by fitness experts to determine an individual's cardiorespiratory fitness. These tests require expensive equipment to measure oxygen consumption and are usually conducted on a treadmill or stationary exercise cycle. This type of test is often called an incremental exercise test.

Figure 4.5 illustrates the change in oxygen consumption (called *oxygen uptake*) at every exercise intensity (work rate) during a typical incremental exercise test. Note that oxygen uptake increases in a straight line with respect to work rate until $\dot{V}O_{2max}$ is reached; thus, $\dot{V}O_{2max}$ represents a "physiological ceiling" for the ability of the cardiorespiratory system to transport oxygen and for the muscles to use it.

PHYSIOLOGICAL RESPONSES TO EXERCISE

Now that we have an idea how the cardiovascular, respiratory, and energy-producing systems function, let's discuss the specifics of how these systems respond to exercise.

CIRCULATORY RESPONSES Exercise increases the body's need for oxygen. To meet this need, blood flow (and therefore oxygen delivery) to working muscle must increase in proportion to the demand. Increased oxygen transport to skeletal muscle is accomplished by increasing cardiac output and redistributing blood flow toward working muscle. The change in cardiac output, heart rate, and blood pressure in response to exercise of various intensities is illustrated in Figure 4.6. Note that both heart rate and cardiac output increase in a straight line as exercise intensity increases.

The fact that heart rate increases as a function of exercise intensity is useful for monitoring the intensity of exercise or the amount of physiological stress. For

> $\dot{V}O_{2max}$ The highest oxygen consumption achievable during exercise. Practically speaking, $\dot{V}O_{2max}$ is a laboratory measure of the endurance capacity of both the cardiorespiratory system and exercising skeletal muscles.

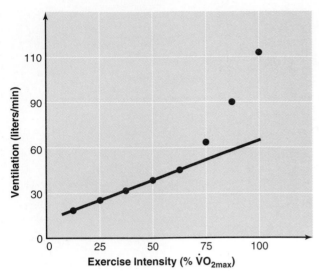

FIGURE 4.7
The ventilatory response to exercise. Each point on the graph represents the amount of ventilation required at a specific exercise intensity. Points lying on the straight line indicate exercise work rates below the anaerobic threshold (A Closer Look).

instance, a person riding a bicycle or running can stop exercising and quickly check heart rate (the pulse) to measure how hard he or she is working. Because it is easy to check heart rate during exercise, this has become the standard means of determining exercise intensity. Also, notice in Figure 4.6 that both heart rate and cardiac output reach a plateau when $\dot{V}O_{2max}$ is achieved. Again, $\dot{V}O_{2max}$ represents a physiological ceiling of the body's ability for delivery and utilization of oxygen in exercising muscles.

Finally, let's consider the changes in blood pressure in response to exercise of varying intensity (Figure 4.6). The key point in Figure 4.6 is that systolic blood pressure increases as the exercise intensity rises; in contrast, note that diastolic blood pressure remains relatively unchanged from the resting state. The rise in systolic blood pressure with higher exercise intensity provides the increased driving pressure to push blood toward the exercising muscles.

RESPIRATORY RESPONSES The responsibility of the respiratory system during exercise is to maintain constant arterial oxygen and carbon dioxide levels. Therefore, because exercise increases oxygen consumption and carbon dioxide production, the breathing rate must increase to bring more oxygen into the body and to remove carbon dioxide. Notice in Figure 4.7 that breathing (called *ventilation*) increases in proportion to exercise intensity up to approximately 65% of $\dot{V}O_{2max}$. At higher work rates, breathing increases rapidly, resulting in increases in delivery of oxygen and removal of carbon dioxide.

RESPONSES OF THE ENERGY-PRODUCING SYSTEMS

Recall that the energy needed to perform many types of exercise comes from both anaerobic and aerobic sources, and that anaerobic exercise dominates in high-intensity exercise, whereas aerobic energy production is greatest in low-intensity exercise. The relationship between exercise intensity and anaerobic energy production is discussed in detail in A Closer Look on page 83.

☀ IN SUMMARY

- The term *cardiorespiratory system* refers to the cooperative work of the circulatory and respiratory systems.
- The primary function of the circulatory system is to transport blood carrying oxygen and nutrients to body tissues.
- The principal function of the respiratory system is to load oxygen into and remove carbon dioxide from the blood.
- The maximum capacity to transport and utilize oxygen during exercise is called $\dot{V}O_{2max}$.
- $\dot{V}O_{2max}$ is considered by many exercise physiologists to be the most valid measure of cardiorespiratory fitness.
- During exercise, cardiac output, systolic blood pressure, heart rate, and breathing rate increase as a function of exercise intensity.

☀ Exercise Prescription for Cardiorespiratory Fitness

After assessing your health status and evaluating your current cardiorespiratory fitness level (Chapter 2), you are ready to develop your exercise prescription to improve your cardiorespiratory fitness. As we have discussed, the exercise training session is composed of three primary elements: warm-up, workout (primary conditioning period), and cool-down.

WARM-UP

Every workout should begin with a warm-up. For an activity such as jogging, the warm-up might consist of the following steps:

1. 1 to 3 minutes of light calisthenics
2. 1 to 3 minutes of walking at a pace that elevates heart rate by 20 to 30 beats/min above rest
3. 2 to 4 minutes of stretching (optional; see Chapter 6 for details)
4. 2 to 5 minutes of jogging at a slow pace to gradually elevate the heart rate toward the desired target heart rate (discussed later in the section on intensity).

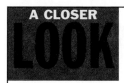

Exercise Intensity and Lactic Acid Production: Concept of the Anaerobic Threshold

High-intensity exercise results in an increased production of lactic acid. The relationship between exercise intensity and blood levels of lactic acid is illustrated in the figure in this box. Note that blood levels of lactic acid during exercise remain low until an exercise intensity of 50–60% of $\dot{V}O_{2max}$ is achieved. However, exercise above 50–60% of $\dot{V}O_{2max}$ results in a rapid accumulation of blood lactic acid. The exercise intensity that results in an increased rate of muscle lactic acid accumulation is called the **anaerobic threshold** (9).

During exercise above the anaerobic threshold, muscles begin to produce large amounts of lactic acid, resulting in muscular fatigue. This explains why exercise below the anaerobic threshold can be tolerated for a long period, whereas exercise above the anaerobic threshold results in rapid fatigue. Those of us who have experimented with finding the maximum speed that we can maintain while running or cycling have had ex-

perience with the anaerobic threshold. We learn that there is some maximal speed we can tolerate for the full duration of the exercise session, and that any attempt to pick up the pace results in muscle fatigue that forces us to slow our pace. This is so because the maximal speed we can

maintain represents an exercise intensity close to but below the anaerobic threshold. Accordingly, prolonged exercise sessions (i.e., 20–60 minutes' duration) aimed at improving cardiorespiratory fitness are generally performed at exercise intensities below the anaerobic threshold.

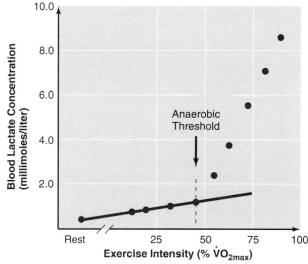

The relationship between blood lactic acid concentration and exercise intensity. Points lying on the straight line indicate exercise work rates below the anaerobic threshold.

If the workout is to consist of exercise modes other than jogging, the same general warm-up routine could be followed by substituting other exercise modes, as in steps 2 and 4. For instance, if cycling is the primary mode of exercise, low-intensity cycling exercise would take the place of walking and jogging in steps 2 and 4.

WORKOUT: PRIMARY CONDITIONING PERIOD

The components of an exercise prescription to improve cardiovascular fitness include the mode, frequency, intensity, and duration of exercise. Let's discuss each of these factors briefly.

MODE Several modes of exercise can be used to improve cardiorespiratory fitness. Some of the most common are walking, jogging, cycling, and swimming. In general, any activity that uses a large muscle mass (e.g., the legs) in a slow, rhythmical pattern can be

used to improve cardiorespiratory fitness. Table 4.1 on page 84 lists several activities that have been shown to improve cardiorespiratory fitness.

There are several key factors to consider when choosing an exercise mode. First, the activity must be fun! Choose an exercise mode that you enjoy. Your chances of sticking with an exercise program are much greater if you choose an activity that you like. A second consideration is that the type of exercise you choose must be convenient and accessible. For example, don't choose swimming if the nearest pool is 50 miles from your home. Similarly, don't choose cycling if you

anaerobic threshold The work intensity during graded, incremental exercise at which there is a rapid accumulation of blood lactic acid. This usually occurs at 50–60% of $\dot{V}O_2$ and contributes to muscle fatigue.

TABLE 4.1
Popular Activities That Promote Cardiorespiratory Fitness

Aerobic dance
Bicycling
Calisthenics (heavy)
Cross-country skiing
Rope skipping
Rowing
Running
Skating (ice or roller)
Stair climber
Swimming
Walking

don't have use of a bicycle. A final factor is the risk of injury. High-impact activities such as running present a greater risk of injury than low-impact activities such as cycling and swimming. A commonsense rule when choosing an exercise mode is that if you tend to be injury prone, choose a low-impact activity. In contrast, if you rarely experience exercise-related injuries, feel free to choose either a high- or low-impact activity mode.

Historically, most exercise prescriptions for improving cardiorespiratory fitness have used only one activity mode. However, there is a current trend toward using **cross training** (i.e., a variety of activity modes) for training the cardiorespiratory system. Many fitness experts feel that participating in only one mode of exercise is boring and leads to more exercise dropouts. Further, cross training may also reduce the frequency of injury. (Cross training is discussed in detail later in this chapter.)

FREQUENCY Although cardiorespiratory fitness gains can be achieved with as few as two exercise sessions per week, the general recommendation for exercise frequency is three to five sessions per week to achieve near-optimal gains in cardiorespiratory fitness with

cross training   The use of a variety of activity modes for training the cardiorespiratory system.
training threshold   The training intensity above which there is an improvement in cardiorespiratory fitness. This intensity is approximately 50% of $\dot{V}O_{2max}$.
target heart rate (THR)   The range of heart rates that corresponds to an exercise intensity of approximately 50–85% $\dot{V}O_{2max}$. This is the range of training heart rates that results in improvements in aerobic capacity.

minimal risk of injury (10). If you remain injury free while training, then if you desire you could increase exercise frequency to 5 days per week. It is, however, unlikely that even greater health or fitness benefits will accrue from exercising more than 5 days per week.

INTENSITY Improvements in cardiorespiratory fitness occur when the training intensity is approximately 50% of $\dot{V}O_{2max}$ (this work rate is often called the **training threshold**). Although improvements in cardiorespiratory fitness can be achieved by exercising at $\dot{V}O_{2max}$, most people could only exercise for 1 to 2 minutes at that intensity. Thus, the recommended range of exercise intensity for improving health-related physical fitness is between 50% and 85% $\dot{V}O_{2max}$.

Recall that training intensity can be monitored indirectly by measurement of heart rate. The range of heart rates that corresponds to an exercise intensity sufficient to improve health-related physical fitness is called the **target heart rate (THR).** The most popular method of determining THR is the percentage of maximal heart rate (HR_{max}) method. This method works on

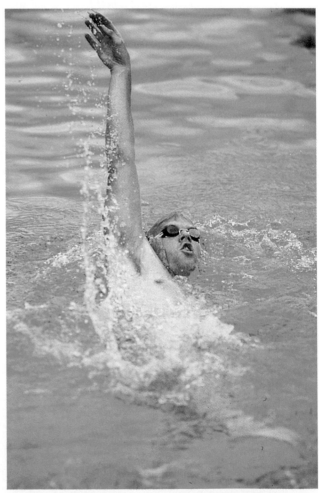

Walking, jogging, cycling, and swimming are popular modes of exercise that can be used to improve cardiorespiratory fitness.

the principle that exercise intensity (i.e., % $\dot{V}O_{2max}$) can be estimated by measuring exercise heart rate. To compute your THR using this method, simply multiply your HR_{max} by both 90% and 70% to arrive at the high and low ends of your THR. For example, the maximal HR of a 20-year-old college student can be estimated by the formula

$$HR_{max} = 220 - 20 = 200 \text{ beats/min}$$

The THR is then computed as

$$200 \text{ beats/min} \times 0.70 = 140 \text{ beats/min}$$

$$200 \text{ beats/min} \times 0.90 = 180 \text{ beats/min}$$

$$THR = 140 \text{ to } 180 \text{ beats/min}$$

In this example, the THR to be maintained during a workout to improve cardiorespiratory fitness is between 140 and 180 beats/min; this range of exercise intensities is sometimes called the *training sensitive zone*.

The reasoning behind using 70% and 90% of your maximal heart rate to compute your target rate is based on the relationship between percent HR_{max} and percent $\dot{V}O_{2max}$ (Table 4.2). Note that 70% of HR_{max} represents the heart rate associated with an exercise intensity that is close to 50% $\dot{V}O_{2max}$ (the lower end of the training sensitive zone), and that 90% of the HR_{max} represents 85% $\dot{V}O_{2max}$ (the upper end of the recommended training sensitive zone).

Finally, it is important to remember that your THR will change as you get older due to the decrease in maximal heart rate. This point is illustrated in Figure 4.8. For instance, while the THR for a 20-year-old college student is between 140 and 180 beats per min, the THR for a 60-year-old is 108 to 139 beats per min.

DURATION Recall that the duration of exercise does not include the warm-up or cool down. In general, exercise durations that have been shown to be most effective in improving cardiorespiratory fitness are between 20 and 60 minutes (10). The reason for this large "window" of duration is that the time required to obtain training benefits depends on both the individual's initial level of fitness and the training intensity. For example, a poorly conditioned individual may only require 20 to 30 minutes of daily exercise at his or her THR to improve cardiorespiratory fitness. In contrast, a highly trained person may require daily exercise sessions of 40 to 60 minutes' duration to improve cardiorespiratory fitness.

Another key point to understand is that improvement of cardiorespiratory fitness by engaging in low-intensity exercise requires a longer daily training duration than high-intensity exercise. For example, an individual training at 50% of $\dot{V}O_{2max}$ may require a daily exercise duration of 40 to 50 minutes to improve cardiorespiratory fitness. In contrast, the same person

TABLE 4.2
The Relationship of Target Heart Rate (THR) to Percent $\dot{V}O_{2max}$ and Percent HR_{max} for a 20-Year-Old Individual

THR (beats/minute*)	% $\dot{V}O_{2max}$	% HR_{max}
186	90	93
180	85	90
173	80	87
166	75	83
160	70	80
153	65	76
146	60	73
140	55	70
134	49	67

*Heart rate based on a HR_{max} of 200 beats/min.

Source: Adapted from Fox, E., R. Bowers, and M. Foss. The Physiological Basis for Exercise and Sport. *Dubuque, IA: Brown and Benchmark, 1989.*

exercising at 70% of $\dot{V}O_{2max}$ may require only 20 to 30 minutes of daily exercise to achieve the same effect. A summary of the guidelines for improving cardiorespiratory fitness is illustrated in Figure 4.9.

SAFETY: IMPROVING CARDIORESPIRATORY FITNESS WITHOUT INJURY

What is the optimal combination of exercise intensity, duration, and frequency to promote cardiorespiratory fitness while minimizing risk of injury? The answer to this question is illustrated in Figure 4.10. The optimal exercise intensity to improve cardiorespiratory fitness without increasing the risk of injury is between 60% and 80% of $\dot{V}O_{2max}$ (73–87% HR_{max}). Further, note that the optimal frequency and duration are 3 to 4 days per week and 20 to 30 minutes per day, respectively.

COOL-DOWN

Every training session should conclude with a cool-down (5–15 minutes of light exercises and stretching). A primary purpose of a cool-down is to promote blood return to the heart, thereby preventing blood from pooling in the arms and legs, which could result in dizziness and/or fainting. A cool-down may also decrease the muscle soreness and cardiac irregularities that sometimes appear after a vigorous workout. Although cardiac irregularities are rare in healthy individuals, it is prudent to cool down and reduce the risk.

A general cool-down of at least 5 minutes (of light exercise such as walking and calisthenics) should be

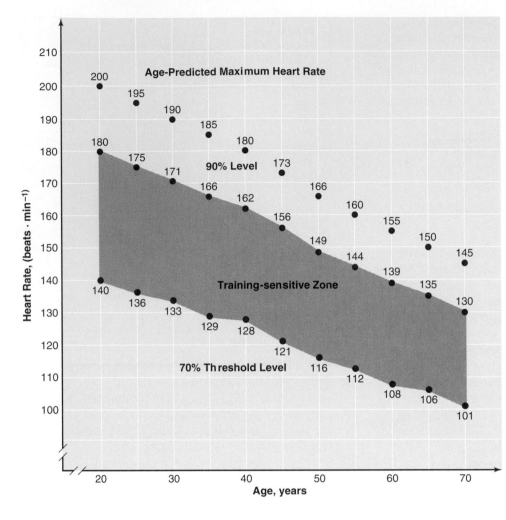

FIGURE 4.8
Target heart rate zones for individuals of ages 20 through 70. The zones cover 70–90% of maximum heart rate, which is indicated above the zones for selected ages.
(Used with permission from *Fitness and Sports Medicine: A Health-Related Approach*, by David C. Nieman. Bull Publishing Co., Palo Alto, CA, 1995.)

Exercise Intensity

70-90% of HR $_{max}$

Exercise Duration

20-60 minutes per session

Exercise Frequency

| S | M | T | W | Th | F | S |

3-5 times per week

FIGURE 4.9
The suggested intensity, duration, and frequency of exercise necessary for improving cardiovascular fitness.

followed by 5 to 30 minutes of flexibility exercises. In general, stretching exercises should focus on the muscles used during training. The type and duration of the stretching session depends on your flexibility goals (Chapter 6).

☀ **IN SUMMARY**

- A key factor in prescribing exercise to improve cardiorespiratory fitness is knowledge of the individual's initial fitness and health status.

- Three primary elements make up the exercise prescription: (1) warm-up; (2) workout, or primary conditioning period; and (3) cool-down.

- The purpose of a warm-up is to slowly elevate heart rate, muscle blood flow, and body temperature.

- The components of the workout are the mode, frequency, intensity, and duration of exercise.

- In general, the best mode of exercise is one that uses a large muscle mass in a slow, rhythmical pattern for 20 to 60 minutes.

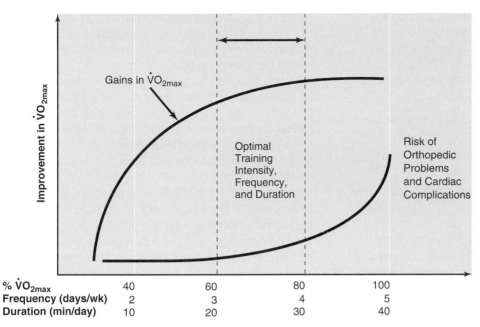

FIGURE 4.10
The effects of increasing intensity, frequency, and duration on the improvements in $\dot{V}O_{2max}$ versus the increased risk of injury.
(Source: Powers, S., and E. Howley. *Exercise Physiology: Theory and Application to Fitness and Performance*. Dubuque, IA: Wm. C. Brown, 2001. Copyright © 2001 Wm. C. Brown Communications, Inc. Reprinted by permission of Times Mirror Higher Education Group, Inc., Dubuque, Iowa. All rights reserved.)

- The intensity of the workout is gauged by the target heart rate, which should be in the range of exercise heart rates that correspond to 50–85% of $\dot{V}O_{2max}$.

- The recommended frequency of exercise to improve cardiorespiratory fitness is three to five times per week.

- The purpose of a cool-down is to slowly decrease the pulse rate and return blood to the heart. To accomplish this, the activity used during the training phase should be continued, but the intensity gradually decreased.

☀ Starting and Maintaining a Cardiorespiratory Fitness Program

Two key elements in any fitness program are the specific short-term and long-term goals. Without these, motivation to continue training is hard to maintain. Many fitness experts agree that the lack of goals is a major contributor to the high dropout rates seen in many organized fitness programs (11). It pays to establish both short-term and long-term fitness goals *before* you start your training program.

If your training plans include running, walking, aerobic dance, or other weight-bearing activities, it is important to exercise in good shoes. Unfortunately, good running, walking, or aerobics shoes are not cheap (costs range from $50–$150). However, investing in good shoes is important for both comfort and injury prevention. Look for a well-cushioned shoe with the following features: soft, comfortable upper material; adequate toe room (as indicated by comfort); well-padded heel and ankle collar; firm arch support; and a heel lift (a wedge that raises the heel about 1/2 inch higher than the sole). Many athletic shoe stores have well-trained sales personnel to assist you in the selection process.

DEVELOPING AN INDIVIDUALIZED EXERCISE PRESCRIPTION

Regardless of your initial fitness level or your choice of exercise mode, the exercise prescription for improving cardiovascular fitness usually has three stages: the starter phase, the slow progression phase, and the maintenance phase. Let's see how each of these training phases can be tailored to an individual's needs.

STARTER PHASE The quickest way to extinguish enthusiasm for an exercise program is to try to accomplish too much too soon. Many people begin an exercise program with great excitement and anticipation of improved fitness levels and weight loss. Unfortunately, this early excitement can lead to exercising too hard during the first training session! This can promote sore muscles and undue fatigue. Therefore, start your fitness program slowly.

The objective of the starter phase is to permit the body to adapt gradually to exercise and to avoid soreness, injury, and personal discouragement. This phase usually lasts 2 to 6 weeks, depending on your initial fitness level. For example, if you are in a poor cardiorespiratory fitness category, you may spend 6 weeks in the starter phase. In contrast, if you have a relatively high initial cardiorespiratory fitness level, you may spend only 2 weeks in the starter phase.

The starter program should include a warm-up, a low-intensity training phase, and then a cool-down. In general, the intensity of exercise during the starter phase should be relatively low (up to 70% of HR_{max}). The following are key points to remember during the starter phase of an exercise program:

1. Start at an exercise intensity that is comfortable for you.
2. Don't increase your training duration or intensity if you are not comfortable.
3. Be aware of new aches or pains. Pain is a symptom of injury and indicates that rest is required to allow the body to repair itself.

SLOW PROGRESSION PHASE The slow progression phase may last 12 to 20 weeks, with exercise progression being more rapid than during the starter phase. The intensity can be gradually elevated, and the frequency and duration of exercise increased, depending on fitness goals and the presence or absence of injuries. In general, this stage should involve an exercise frequency of 3 to 4 times per week and an exercise duration of at least 30 minutes per session. Exercise intensity should range between 70% and 90% HR_{max}, depending on your personal fitness goals.

MAINTENANCE PHASE The average college-age student will generally reach the maintenance phase of the exercise prescription after 16 to 28 weeks of training. At this stage you should have achieved your fitness goal and are no longer interested in increasing your training load. The objective now becomes to maintain this level of fitness. As the old saying goes, "Fitness is not something you can put in the bank." To maintain cardiorespiratory fitness, you must continue to train on a regular basis. The key question now is, How much training is required during the maintenance phase to prevent a decline in cardiorespiratory fitness?

Several studies have shown that the primary factor in maintaining cardiorespiratory fitness is the intensity of exercise (12–14). If the exercise intensity and duration remain the same as during the final weeks of the slow progression phase, frequency can be reduced to as few as 2 days per week without a significant loss in fitness. In addition, if frequency and intensity remain the same as during the final weeks of the slow progression phase, duration can be reduced to as few as 20 to 25 minutes per day. In contrast, when frequency and duration are held constant, a one-third decrease in intensity results in a significant decline in cardiorespiratory fitness. To summarize, if exercise intensity is maintained, the exercise frequency and duration necessary to maintain a given level of cardiorespiratory fitness are substantially less than those required to improve fitness levels.

SAMPLE EXERCISE PRESCRIPTIONS As mentioned, the exercise prescription must be tailored to the individual. The key factor to consider when designing a personal training program is your current fitness level. Programs designed for people with good or excellent cardiorespiratory fitness levels start at a higher level and progress more rapidly, compared with programs designed for people in poor condition. Tables 4.3 through 4.5 illustrate three sample cardiorespiratory training programs designed for college-aged people who are beginning a fitness program. Table 4.3 contains an exercise prescription that might be appropriate for people in very poor or poor cardiorespiratory fitness. Table 4.4 on page 90 illustrates a sample program designed for people in good or average cardiorespiratory fitness, while Table 4.5 on page 91 contains a program aimed at people with a cardiorespiratory rating of excellent or above. Note that these programs are merely sample programs, and each can be modified to meet your individual fitness levels and goals. If you feel that none of these training programs meet your training needs, use Laboratory 4.1 on page 99 to develop your personal exercise prescription. After designing your cardiorespiratory training program, use Laboratory 4.2 on page 101 to keep a record of your exercise training habits. The following is an illustration of a typical training record:

Date	Activity	Duration	Exercise Heart Rate	Comments

☀ IN SUMMARY

- Establishing both short-term and long-term fitness goals is essential before beginning a fitness program.
- Regardless of your initial fitness level, an exercise prescription to improve cardiorespiratory fitness has three phases: (1) the starter phase, (2) the slow progression phase, and (3) the maintenance phase.

☀ Training Techniques

Endurance training is a generic term that refers to any mode of exercise aimed at improving cardiorespiratory fitness. Over the years, numerous endurance training techniques have evolved. In the next section we discuss several common ones.

CROSS TRAINING

As previously mentioned, cross training is a popular form of training that uses several different training modes. It may mean running on one day, swimming on

---

TABLE 4.3
Sample Cardiorespiratory Exercise Program Designed for People in the Very Poor or Poor Fitness Category

General guidelines:
1. *Begin each session with a warm-up.*
2. *Don't progress to the next level until you feel comfortable with your current level of exercise.*
3. *Monitor your heart rate during each training session.*
4. *End each session with a cool-down.*
5. *Be aware of aches and pains. If you are injury prone, choose a low-impact activity mode, and limit your exercise duration to 20 to 30 minutes per day.*

Week No.	Phase	Duration (min/day)	Intensity (% of HR_{max})	Frequency (days/wk)
1	Starter	10	60	3
2	Starter	10	60	3
3	Starter	12	60	3
4	Starter	12	70	3
5	Starter	15	70	3
6	Starter	15	70	3
7	Slow progression	20	70	3
8	Slow progression	20	70	3
9	Slow progression	25	70	3
10	Slow progression	25	70	3
11	Slow progression	30	70	3
12	Slow progression	30	70	3
13	Slow progression	35	70	3
14	Slow progression	35	70	3
15	Slow progression	40	70	3
16	Slow progression	40	70	3
17	Slow progression	40	75	3
18	Slow progression	40	75	3
19	Slow progression	40	75	3
20	Slow progression	40	75	3–4
21	Slow progression	40	75	3–4
22	Slow progression	40	75	3–4
23	Maintenance	30	75	3–4
24	Maintenance	30	75	3–4
25	Maintenance	30	75	3–4
26	Maintenance	30	75	3–4

another day, and cycling on another day. One advantage of cross training is that it reduces the boredom of performing the same kind of exercise day after day. Further, it may reduce the incidence of injuries by avoiding overuse of the same body parts. The disadvantage of cross training is the lack of training specificity. For example, jogging does not improve swimming endurance because the arm muscles are not trained during jogging. Similarly, swimming does not improve jogging endurance. In general, to improve endurance in a particular activity, training should consist of exercises similar to that activity.

LONG, SLOW DISTANCE TRAINING

Long, slow distance training, or continuous training, requires a steady, submaximal exercise intensity (i.e., the intensity is generally around 70% HR_{max}). It is one of the most popular cardiorespiratory training techniques and can be applied to any mode of exercise.

---

long, slow distance training The term used to indicate continuous exercise that requires a steady, submaximal exercise intensity (i.e., the intensity is generally around 70% HR_{max}).

TABLE 4.4
Sample Cardiorespiratory Exercise Program Designed for People in the Average or Good Fitness Category

General guidelines:
1. *Begin each session with a warm-up.*
2. *Don't progress to the next level until you feel comfortable with your current level of exercise.*
3. *Monitor your heart rate during each training session.*
4. *End each session with a cool-down.*
5. *Be aware of aches and pains. If you are injury prone, choose a low-impact activity mode, and limit your exercise duration to 20 to 30 minutes per day.*

Week No.	Phase	Duration (min/day)	Intensity (% of HR_{max})	Frequency (days/wk)
1	Starter	10	70	3
2	Starter	15	70	3
3	Starter	15	70	3
4	Starter	20	70	3
5	Slow progression	25	70	3
6	Slow progression	25	75	3
7	Slow progression	25	75	3
8	Slow progression	30	75	3
9	Slow progression	30	75	3
10	Slow progression	35	75	3
11	Slow progression	35	75	3
12	Slow progression	40	75	3
13	Slow progression	40	75	3
14	Slow progression	40	75	3
15	Slow progression	40	80	3
16	Slow progression	40	80	3–4
17	Slow progression	40	80	3–4
18	Slow progression	40	80	3–4
19	Maintenance	30	80	3–4
20	Maintenance	30	80	3–4
21	Maintenance	30	80	3–4
22	Maintenance	30	80	3–4

During the progression phase of the exercise program, an individual may find this type of training enjoyable because the exercise intensity does not increase. If injuries are not a problem, there is no reason why the duration of the training cannot be extended to 40 to 60 minutes per session. An advantage of continuous training is that risk of injury is lower than in more intensive training.

interval training Repeated sessions or intervals of relatively intense exercise. The duration of the intervals can be varied, but a 1- to 5-minute duration is common. Each interval is followed by a rest period, which should be equal to or slightly longer than the interval duration.

INTERVAL TRAINING

Interval training means undertaking repeated sessions or intervals of relatively intense exercise. The duration of the intervals can be varied, but a 1- to 5-minute duration is common. Each interval is followed by a rest period, which should be equal to, or slightly longer than, the interval duration. For example, if you are running 400-meter intervals on a track, and it takes you approximately 90 seconds to complete each run, your rest period between efforts should be at least 90 seconds.

Interval training is a common training technique among athletes who have already established a base of endurance training and wish to attain much higher fitness levels in order to be more competitive in a particular sport. With correct spacing of exercise and rest periods, more work can be accomplished with interval training than with long, slow distance training. A major

---

TABLE 4.5
Sample Cardiorespiratory Exercise Program Designed for People in the Excellent Fitness Category

General guidelines:
1. *Begin each session with a warm-up.*
2. *Don't progress to the next level until you feel comfortable with your current level of exercise.*
3. *Monitor your heart rate during each training session.*
4. *End each session with a cool-down.*
5. *Be aware of aches and pains. If you are injury prone, choose a low-impact activity mode, and limit your exercise duration to 20 to 30 minutes per day.*

Week No.	Phase	Duration (min/day)	Intensity (% of HR_{max})	Frequency (days/wk)
1	Starter	15	75	3
2	Starter	20	75	3
3	Slow progression	25	75	3
4	Slow progression	30	75	3
5	Slow progression	35	75	3
6	Slow progression	40	75	3
7	Slow progression	40	75	3–4
8	Slow progression	40	75	3–4
9	Slow progression	40	80	3–4
10	Slow progression	40	80	3–4
11	Slow progression	40	80	3–4
12	Slow progression	40	80–85	3–4
13	Slow progression	40	80–85	3–4
14	Slow progression	40	80–85	3–4
15	Maintenance	30	80–85	3–4
16	Maintenance	30	80–85	3–4
17	Maintenance	30	80–85	3–4
18	Maintenance	30	80–85	3–4

advantage of interval training is the variety of workouts it allows, which may reduce the tedium associated with other forms of training.

FARTLEK TRAINING

Fartlek is a Swedish word meaning "speed play," and it refers to a popular form of training for long-distance runners. **Fartlek training** is much like interval training, but it is not as rigid in its work-to-rest interval ratios. It consists of inserting sprints into long, slow running done on trails, roads, golf courses, and the like. An advantage of fartlek training is that these workouts provide variety and reduce the possibility of boredom.

☀ IN SUMMARY

- Common endurance training techniques to improve cardiorespiratory fitness include cross training; long, slow distance training; interval training; and fartlek training.

- Each of these techniques manipulates the frequency, intensity, and duration of training to improve endurance.

☀ Aerobic Exercise Training: How the Body Adapts

How does the body adapt to aerobic exercise training? Endurance exercise training induces changes in the cardiovascular and respiratory systems, skeletal muscles

fartlek training   *Fartlek* is a Swedish word meaning "speed play," and it refers to a popular form of training for long-distance runners. It is much like interval training, but it is not as rigid in its work-to-rest interval ratios. It consists of inserting sprints into long, slow running done on trails, roads, golf courses, and so on.

Frequently Asked Questions About Aerobic Workouts

What is a simple way to judge my workout intensity?

A very simple way to gauge intensity is the talk test. You should be able to talk without gasping for air while exercising. If you cannot, you should slow down. In contrast, if your intensity allows you to laugh and sing, then you need to work harder.

Is it better to exercise for several short sessions, or exercise for one longer period?

Either approach can be beneficial. You do need to warm-up for 5 to 10 minutes and cool-down for 5 to 10 minutes no matter the session length. So if you exercise for one 60-minute period, 40 to 50 minutes of that time should be for aerobic training, with the remainder for warm-up and cool-down. If you exercise for shorter periods, make sure to get at least 15 to 20 minutes of aerobic training.

Should I train my muscles in addition to doing aerobic activity?

Yes. Weight training is an important part of any aerobic program because strength will help protect you from injuries. Moreover, when you are strong it is easier to maintain proper form.

Can steam, the sauna, or a hot tub be helpful after a workout?

After an aerobic workout, blood vessels in the skin are open because blood is sent to the skin to aid in cooling the body. Any form of additional heat tends to open the blood vessels there even more, which diverts blood from critical areas such as the brain, the heart, and muscles. Therefore, heating up the body right after exercise is not the best thing to do. However, if you have thoroughly cooled down and have waited until your heart rate has returned to near its normal resting rate, you might use steam, the sauna, or a hot tub to help relax. If you feel any weakness or dizziness, however, get out immediately.

What is step aerobics?

Step aerobics is a form of aerobic activity performed on a "step" or platform that is approximately 4–10 inches in height. It was developed to provide aerobic training without the high impact of other aerobic exercise such as running or aerobic dance. It is done in a small area, so in a given space more people can do it than aerobic dance.

How good are exercise gadgets?

Trends and fads come and go in the fitness industry. Some gadgets are useful and will help you reach your fitness goals, but some are worthless. Before buying a new gadget, follow the guidelines in this text to determine if the equipment is useful. In general, the best piece of cardiovascular training equipment is the one that you will actually use. If you are simply concerned with which modality burns the most calories, the best piece is the one that you use for the *longest amount of time.*

Is the meal before a workout important, and what should it be?

Most of the energy expended during the workout will come from the meals you ate the previous day. That energy was stored in your muscles and liver. Thus, the pre-workout meal is important in that it (1) should be something easily digestible to keep from upsetting your stomach and thus preventing your workout, and (2) high in complex carbohydrates to replace the energy expended in the workout.

What is the best time of day to exercise?

The same principle that applies to choosing exercise equipment applies here: The best time of day to exercise is the time of day that you are most likely to maintain your workout routine. The best time of day to work out is when you want to exercise, so pick a time of day that works best for you.

Should I train if I'm sick?

Generally, if the sickness is above the neck (sinus, headache, sore throat, etc.), light exercise may not be a problem. Just take it easy, and be sure to respect others who aren't sick by wiping off any equipment that you use when you are finished with it and by washing your hands frequently.

and the energy-producing systems, $\dot{V}O_{2max}$, flexibility, and body composition, in response to regular aerobic training. A brief overview of each of these adaptations follows.

CARDIOVASCULAR SYSTEM

Several adaptations occur in the cardiovascular system as a result of endurance training (15). First, although endurance training does not alter maximal heart rate, this type of training results in a decrease in heart rate during submaximal exercise compared to before training. This reduction in heart rate results because the stroke volume at submaximal loads is increased with training. Further, endurance exercise results in an increase in maximal stroke volume (SV) and a corresponding increase in maximal cardiac output (because maximal cardiac output = maximal HR × maximal SV).

An increased maximal cardiac output results in an increased oxygen delivery to the exercising muscles and improved exercise tolerance.

RESPIRATORY SYSTEM

Some fitness proponents report that exercise improves lung function by expanding the volume of the lungs and increasing the efficiency of oxygen and carbon dioxide exchange. Unfortunately, there is no scientific evidence to support this belief. However, although endurance training does not alter the structure or function of the respiratory system, it does increase respiratory muscle endurance (16, 17). That is, the diaphragm and other key muscles of respiration can work harder and longer without fatigue. This improvement in respiratory muscle endurance may reduce the sensation of breathlessness during exercise and eliminate the pain in the side (often called a *stitch*) that is sometimes associated with exercise.

SKELETAL MUSCLES AND ENERGY-PRODUCING SYSTEMS

Endurance training increases the muscles' capacity for aerobic energy production. The practical result of an improvement in muscle aerobic capacity is an improved ability to use fat as an energy source and an increase in muscular endurance (15). Note that these changes occur only in those muscles used during the training activity. For example, endurance training using a stationary exercise cycle results in an improvement in muscular endurance in leg muscles, but has little effect on arm muscles. Finally, although endurance training improves muscle tone, this type of exercise training does not result in large increases in muscle size or muscular strength.

$\dot{V}O_{2max}$

Recall that $\dot{V}O_{2max}$ is considered by many exercise physiologists to be the best single measure of cardiorespiratory fitness. Therefore, improvement in $\dot{V}O_{2max}$ is an important physiological adaptation that occurs in response to endurance training. In general, 12 to 15 weeks of endurance exercise results in a 10–30% improvement in $\dot{V}O_{2max}$ (15). This improvement is due to a combination of improved aerobic capacity in skeletal muscles and increased maximal cardiac output. The net result is increased oxygen delivery and use by skeletal muscles during exercise. Therefore, an increase in $\dot{V}O_{2max}$ translates to improved muscular endurance and less fatigue during routine daily activities.

How much $\dot{V}O_{2max}$ increases after an endurance training program is dependent on several factors: fit-

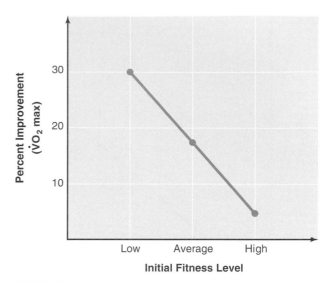

FIGURE 4.11
The relationship between initial fitness levels and improvements in $\dot{V}O_{2max}$ after a 12-week training period.

ness status at the beginning of the training program, intensity of the training program, and nutritional status during the training program. In general, people who start exercise programs with high $\dot{V}O_{2max}$ values improve less than those with low initial $\dot{V}O_{2max}$ values. For example, a person entering an endurance training program with a high $\dot{V}O_{2max}$ may achieve only a 5% improvement over a 12-week period, whereas an individual with a low $\dot{V}O_{2max}$ may improve as much as 30% (Figure 4.11). The explanation for this is that a physiological ceiling or limit for improvement in $\dot{V}O_{2max}$ exists. Those people who enter fitness programs with relatively high $\dot{V}O_{2max}$ values are probably closer to their limits than are people who enter programs with low $\dot{V}O_{2max}$ values.

The magnitude of the exercise-induced increase in $\dot{V}O_{2max}$ is directly related to the intensity of the training program (12). High-intensity training programs result in greater $\dot{V}O_{2max}$ gains than low-intensity and short-duration programs (Figure 4.12). Notice that a plateau exists in the relationship between training intensity and improvement in $\dot{V}O_{2max}$. Therefore, once a high intensity of training is reached, increasing the intensity does not result in further improvement in fitness. In fact, training at extremely high intensities may increase the risk of injury and illness.

Finally, failure to maintain proper nutritional habits during an endurance training program will impair improvements in $\dot{V}O_{2max}$. Proper nutrition means a diet that provides all of the necessary nutrients for good health. In Chapter 7 we discuss how to construct the proper diet for health and fitness.

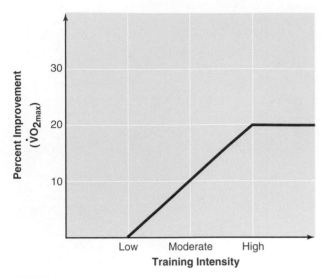

FIGURE 4.12
The relationship between training intensity and improvements in $\dot{V}O_{2max}$ following a 12-week training period.

FLEXIBILITY

Most endurance training programs do not improve flexibility. In fact, several months of endurance training may reduce the range of motion at some joints due to muscle and tendon shortening. Therefore, to prevent a loss of flexibility, stretching exercises should always be a part of an endurance training program (Chapter 6).

BODY COMPOSITION

Endurance training generally results in a reduction in the percent of body fat (15). However, a loss of body

fat in response to endurance training is not guaranteed. Whether or not an individual loses body fat due to exercise training is a result of many factors, including diet and the amount of exercise performed. More is said about this topic in Chapter 8.

☀ IN SUMMARY

- Endurance exercise training results in improvements in maximal cardiac output, endurance of muscles of respiration, skeletal muscle endurance, and $\dot{V}O_{2max}$.
- Endurance exercise can assist in the loss of body fat.
- Endurance training does not improve flexibility and may even reduce flexibility if regular stretching exercises are not performed.

☀ Motivation to Maintain Cardiorespiratory Fitness

Every year, millions of people make the decision to start an exercise routine. Unfortunately, over half those who begin a cardiorespiratory fitness program quit within the first 6 months (11). Although there are many reasons for this high dropout rate, a lack of time is commonly cited as a major one. Although finding time for exercise in a busy schedule is difficult, it is not impossible. The key is to schedule a regular time for exercise and to stick with it. A small investment in time to exercise can reap large improvements in fitness and health. Think about the time required to improve cardiorespiratory fitness in the following way. There are 168 hours in every week. All you need is three, 30-minute workouts

---

FITNESS AND WELLNESS FOR ALL

Wellness Issues Across the Population

DON'T LET A DISABILITY STOP YOU!
Although any type of temporary or permanent disability can certainly be a disincentive to exercise, you can take comfort in knowing that even with most disabilities you can obtain all of the benefits of cardiovascular exercise. Swimming and other water activities are popular ways to take away the burden of supporting your body weight and safely exercise capable muscle

groups. Exercise in water is beneficial for several reasons:

- Exercising in water eliminates the dangers of falling.
- Flexibility exercises are much easier to do in water.
- Water provides resistance that allows capable muscle groups to work at an intensity that provides progressive overload to the cardiorespiratory system.
- A variety of water aids, including hand paddles, pull-buoys, flotation

belts, and kick boards can be used to help maintain buoyancy and balance as well as help you work in the water.

You must take responsibility for knowing about the medical complications associated with your disability, and for knowing how you can prevent and/or control those complications. Finally, remember that the potential for drowning always exists; never swim or work out in the water while alone.

per week to improve cardiorespiratory fitness. Including the associated warm-ups, cool-downs, and showers, this is about 3 hours per week, which is less than 2% of the total week. This leaves you with 165 hours per week to accomplish all of the other things you need to do. The bottom line is, with proper time management, anyone can find time to exercise.

In order for you to keep your commitment to develop cardiorespiratory fitness, exercise must be fun. Therefore, choose a training technique that you enjoy. Further, your chosen exercise mode should be convenient. Failure to meet either of these criteria increases your risk of becoming an exercise dropout.

One of the things that makes exercise enjoyable is the interaction with friends. Therefore, exercising with a partner is an excellent idea because it makes physical activity more fun and helps maintain your sense of commitment to a regular exercise routine. In choosing an exercise partner, choose someone that you enjoy interacting with and someone who is a good exercise role model.

Keeping a record of your training program is helpful in several ways. It assists you in keeping track of your training progress and serves as a motivating factor when you begin to notice improvements in your fitness level.

Finally, it is normal to experience some discomfort and soreness associated with your first several exercise sessions. Don't let this discourage you. In a short time the soreness will fade and the discomfort associated with exercise will begin to disappear. As your fitness level improves, you will start to feel better and look better. Although reaching and maintaining a reasonable level of cardiorespiratory fitness will always require time and effort, the rewards will be well worth the labor.

Summary

1. Benefits of cardiorespiratory fitness include a lower risk of disease, feeling better, increased capacity to perform everyday tasks, and improved self-esteem.

2. Adenosine triphosphate, which is required for muscular contraction, can be produced in muscles by two systems: anaerobic (without oxygen) and aerobic (with oxygen).

3. The energy to perform many types of exercise comes from both anaerobic and aerobic sources. In general, anaerobic energy production dominates in short-term exercise, whereas aerobic energy production dominates during prolonged exercise.

4. The term *cardiorespiratory system* refers to the cooperative work of the circulatory and respiratory systems. The primary function of the circulatory system is to transport blood carrying oxygen and nutrients to body tissues. The principal function of the respiratory system is to load oxygen into and remove carbon dioxide from the blood.

5. The maximum capacity to transport and utilize oxygen during exercise is called $\dot{V}O_{2max}$; many exercise physiologists consider $\dot{V}O_{2max}$ to be the most valid measurement of cardiorespiratory fitness.

6. Cardiac output, systolic blood pressure, and heart rate increase as a function of exercise intensity. Breathing (ventilation) also increases in proportion to exercise intensity.

7. A key factor in prescribing exercise to improve cardiorespiratory fitness is knowledge of the individual's initial fitness and health status.

8. Three primary elements make up the exercise prescription: warm-up, workout (primary conditioning period), and cool-down.

9. The components of the workout are the mode, frequency, intensity, and duration of exercise.

10. In general, the mode of exercise to be used to obtain increased cardiorespiratory endurance is one that uses a large muscle mass in a slow, rhythmical pattern for 20 to 60 minutes.

11. The target heart rate is the range of exercise heart rates that lie between 70% and 90% of maximal heart rate.

12. The recommended frequency of exercise to improve cardiorespiratory fitness is three to five times per week.

13. Establishing both short-term and long-term fitness goals is essential before beginning a fitness program.

14. Regardless of your initial fitness level, an exercise prescription for improving cardiorespiratory fitness has three phases: the starter phase, the slow progression phase, and the maintenance phase.

15. Common endurance training techniques to improve cardiorespiratory fitness include cross training; long, slow distance training; interval training; and fartlek training.

16. Aerobic exercise training results in an improvement in cardiorespiratory fitness ($\dot{V}O_{2max}$) and muscular endurance and can result in a reduction in percent body fat.

17. Maintaining a regular exercise routine requires proper time management and the choice of physical activities that you enjoy.

Study Questions

1. Discuss the two energy pathways used to produce muscle ATP during exercise.

2. Which energy pathway (aerobic or anaerobic) is predominantly responsible for production of ATP during the following activities: 100-meter dash, 800-meter run, 10,000-meter run, tennis, football, and weight lifting?

3. What is meant by the term *cardiorespiratory system*? List the major functions of the circulatory and respiratory systems.

4. Why is the heart considered "two pumps in one"?

5. Define the following terms:
   adenosine triphosphate (ATP)
   cross training
   hypertension
   target heart rate

6. Graph the changes in heart rate, blood pressure, cardiac output, and ventilation as a function of exercise intensity.

7. Define $\dot{V}O_{2max}$.

8. Discuss the relationship between exercise intensity and lactic acid production in muscles. Define the anaerobic threshold. What is the practical significance of the anaerobic threshold for exercise?

9. What physiological changes occur as a result of endurance training?

10. Will endurance training alone result in improvement in all of the components of health-related physical fitness? Why or why not?

11. What information is necessary to develop an individualized exercise prescription?

12. List the criteria that must be met to obtain improvement in aerobic capacity.

13. What effect does mode of training have on obtaining increased aerobic capacity?

14. What range in frequency of exercise is needed to improve aerobic capacity?

15. Define training threshold and give the range of intensities that are considered necessary to elicit an increase in $\dot{V}O_{2max}$.

16. What training techniques are generally used in exercise programs for improving cardiorespiratory fitness?

Suggested Reading

American College of Sports Medicine. American College of Sports Medicine position stand: The recommended quantity and quality of exercise for developing and maintaining cardiorespiratory and muscular fitness and flexibility in healthy adults. *Medicine and Science in Sports and Exercise* 30:975–991, 1998.

Neiman, D. C. *Fitness and Sports Medicine: A Health-Related Approach,* 3rd ed. Palo Alto, CA: Bull Publishing, 1995.

Pollock, M. L., and J. H. Wilmore. *Exercise in Health and Disease,* 3rd ed. Philadelphia: W. B. Saunders, 1998.

Powers, S., and E. Howley. *Exercise Physiology: Theory and Application to Fitness and Performance,* 4th ed. Dubuque, IA: McGraw-Hill, 2001.

Warburton, D. E., N. Gledhill, and A. Quinney. Musculoskeletal fitness and health. *Canadian Journal of Applied Physiology* 26(2):217–237, 2001.

For links to the Web sites below visit Web Links at www.aw.com/fitness and choose Powers/Dodd Web Links from the drop-down menu.

FitnessOnline

Provides information, tools, and support to achieve health and fitness goals. Online home of *Shape, Men's Fitness, Muscle & Fitness, Flex, Natural Health,* and *Fit Pregnancy* magazines.

Sympatico: Health

Includes numerous articles, book reviews, and links to nutrition, fitness, and wellness topics.

Gatorade Sports Science Institute

Presents many articles relating to fluid replacement during exercise. Enables registration to be on a mailing list to receive new articles.

Marathoning Start to Finish

Provides guides to exercise in heat and cold, and presents information on training for racing, ergogenic aids, and sports nutrition.

The Running Page

Contains information about racing, running clubs, places to run, running-related products, magazines, and treating running injuries.

Meriter Fitness

Contains information on injury prevention and treatment, weight training, flexibility, exercise prescriptions, and more.

References

1. Cooper, K. H. *Aerobics.* New York: Bantam Books, 1968.

2. Ross, R., and I. Janssen. Physical activity, total and regional obesity: Dose-response considerations. *Medicine and Science in Sports and Exercise* 33(6):S345–S641, 2001.

3. Kohl, H. W. Physical activity and cardiovascular disease: Evidence for a dose response. *Medicine and Science in Sports and Exercise* 33(6):S472–S483, 2001.

4. Kesaniemi. Y. A., E. Danforth, M. D. Jensen, P. G. Kopelman, P. Lefebvre, and B. A. Reeder. Dose-response issues

concerning physical activity and health: An evidence-based symposium. *Medicine and Science in Sports and Exercise* 33(6):S351–S358, 2001.

5. Dunn, A. L., M. H. Trivedi, and H. A. O'Neal. Physical activity dose-response effects on outcomes of depression and anxiety. *Medicine and Science in Sports and Exercise* 33(6):S587–S597, 2001.

6. Gambelunghe, C., R. Rossi, G. Mariucci, M. Tantucci, and M. V. Ambrosini. Effects of light physical exercise on sleep regulation in rats. *Medicine and Science in Sports and Exercise* 33(1):57–60, 2001.

7. American Heart Association. *Are You at Risk of Heart Attack or Stroke?* Dallas: American Heart Association, 1999.

8. American Heart Association. *2001 Heart and Stroke Statistical Update.* Dallas: American Heart Association, 2000.

9. Brooks, G. Anaerobic threshold: Review of the concept and directions for future research. *Medicine and Science in Sports and Exercise* 17:22–23, 1985.

10. *ACSM's Resource Manual for Guidelines for Exercise Testing and Prescription,* 4th ed. Philadelphia: Lippincot Williams, & Wilkins 2001.

11. Mullineaux, D. R., C. A. Barnes, and E. F. Barnes. Factors affecting the likelihood to engage in adequate physical activity to promote health. *Journal of Sports Sciences* 19(4):279–288, 2001.

12. Hickson, R. C., et al. Reduced training intensities and loss of aerobic power, endurance, and cardiac growth. *Journal of Applied Physiology* 58:492, 1985.

13. Hickson, R. C., et al. Reduced training duration effects on aerobic power, endurance, and cardiac growth. *Journal of Applied Physiology* 53:255, 1982.

14. Hickson, R. C., and M. A. Rosenkoetter. Reduced training frequencies and maintenance of aerobic power. *Medicine and Science in Sports and Exercise* 13:13, 1982.

15. Powers, S., and E. Howley. *Exercise Physiology: Theory and Application to Fitness and Performance,* 4th ed. Dubuque, IA: McGraw-Hill, 2001.

16. Powers, S., D. Criswell, F.-K. Lieu, S. Dodd, and II. Silverman. Exercise-induced cellular alterations in the diaphragm. *American Journal of Physiology* 263:R1093–R1098, 1992.

17. Powers, S., S. Grinton, J. Lawler, D. Criswell, and S. Dodd. High intensity exercise training–induced metabolic alterations in respiratory muscles. *Respiration Physiology* 89:169–177, 1992.

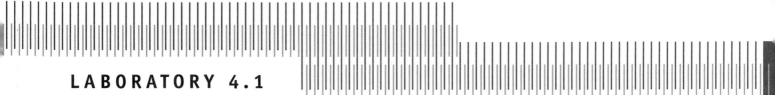

LABORATORY 4.1

Developing Your Personal Exercise Prescription

NAME _____ DATE _____

Using Tables 4.3 through 4.5 as models, develop your personal exercise prescription based on your current fitness level and goals. Record the appropriate information in the spaces provided below. Monitor your fitness levels periodically and adjust your prescription accordingly.

Week No.	Phase	Duration (min/day)	Intensity (% of HR_{max})	Frequency (days/wk)	Exercise Mode	Comments
1						
2						
3						
4						
5						
6						
7						
8						
9						
10						
11						
12						
13						
14						
15						
16						

Cardiorespiratory Training Log

(Note: Make additional copies as needed)

NAME _____ DATE _____

In the spaces below keep a record of your exercise training program. Exercise heart rate can be recorded as the range of heart rates measured at various times during the training session. Use the comments section to record any useful information concerning your exercise session, such as weather conditions, time of day, how you felt, and so on.

Date	Activity	Warm-Up Duration	Exercise Duration	Cool-Down Duration	Exercise Heart Rate	Comments

(continued on next page)

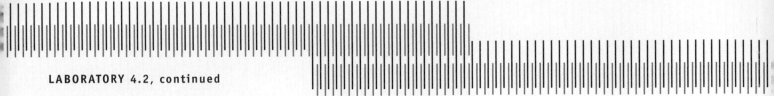

Date	Activity	Warm-Up Duration	Exercise Duration	Cool-Down Duration	Exercise Heart Rate	Comments

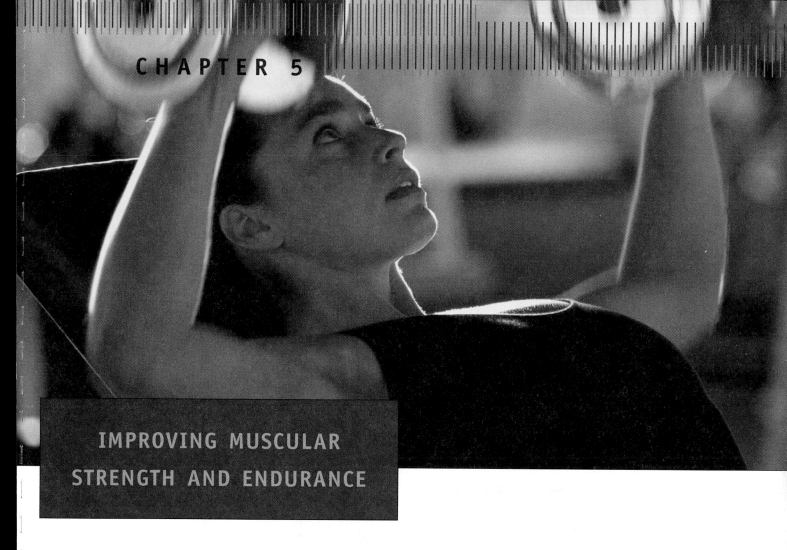

CHAPTER 5

IMPROVING MUSCULAR STRENGTH AND ENDURANCE

After studying this chapter, you should be able to:

1. Explain the benefits of developing muscular strength and endurance.

2. Describe how muscles contract.

3. Distinguish among the various types of muscle fibers.

4. Classify the types of muscular contractions.

5. Identify the major changes that occur in skeletal muscles in response to strength training.

6. List the factors that determine muscle strength and endurance.

7. Outline the general principles used in designing a strength and endurance program.

8. Distinguish among the various types of training programs for improving strength and endurance.

9. Design a program for improving strength and endurance.

Lifting weights or performing other types of resistance exercises to build muscular strength and endurance is commonly referred to as weight training or strength training. This chapter discusses the principles and techniques employed in strength training programs. We begin with a brief overview of the benefits associated with developing muscular strength and endurance.

☀ Benefits of Muscular Strength and Endurance

Regular strength training promotes numerous health benefits. For example, we know that the incidence of low back pain, a common problem in both men and women, can be reduced with the appropriate strengthening exercises for the lower back and abdominal muscles (1). Further, recent studies demonstrate that muscle-strengthening exercises may reduce the occurrence of joint and/or muscle injuries that may occur during physical activity (2, 3). In addition, strength training can postpone the decreases in muscle strength experienced by sedentary older individuals (4), as well as contribute to the prevention of the bone-wasting disease called osteoporosis (5).

Another positive aspect of strength training is the improvement in personal appearance and self-esteem associated with increased muscular tone and strength (6). Also, increased muscular strength has many practical benefits in daily activities, such as an improved ability to carry heavy boxes, perform routine yard work, or do housework.

One of the most important benefits of strength training is that increasing muscle size results in an elevation in resting energy expenditure. Resting energy expenditure (called *resting metabolic rate*) is the total amount of energy that the body requires to perform all of the necessary functions associated with maintaining life. For example, resting metabolic rate includes the energy required to drive the heart and respiratory muscles and to build and maintain body tissues.

How does strength training influence resting metabolic rate? One of the primary results of strength training is an increase in muscle mass. Because muscle tissue requires energy even at rest, muscular enlargement promotes an increase in resting energy expenditure. An increase of 1 pound of muscle elevates resting metabolism by approximately 2–3%. Further, this increase can be magnified with larger gains in muscle. For instance, a 5-pound increase in muscle mass would result in a 10–15% increase in resting metabolic rate. Changes in resting metabolic rate of this magnitude can play an important role in assisting in weight loss or maintaining desirable body composition throughout life. There-

fore, strength training is a key component of any physical fitness program.

☀ Physiological Basis for Developing Strength and Endurance

The human body contains approximately 600 skeletal muscles, the primary function of which is to provide force for bodily movement. The body and its parts move when the appropriate muscles shorten and apply force to the bones. Skeletal muscles also assist in maintaining posture and regulating body temperature during cold exposure (for example, by causing heat production through the mechanism of shivering in cold weather). Because all fitness activities require the use of skeletal muscles, some appreciation of their structure and function is essential for anyone entering a physical fitness program.

Before we discuss how muscles work, let's revisit the definitions of muscular strength and endurance. Muscular strength and endurance are related, but they

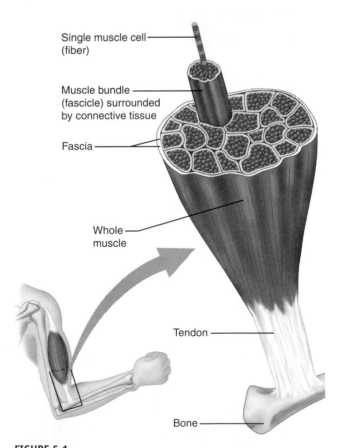

FIGURE 5.1
Muscle structure.
(*Source:* Johnson, Michael, *Human Biology.* Benjamin Cummings, San Francisco, 2001.)

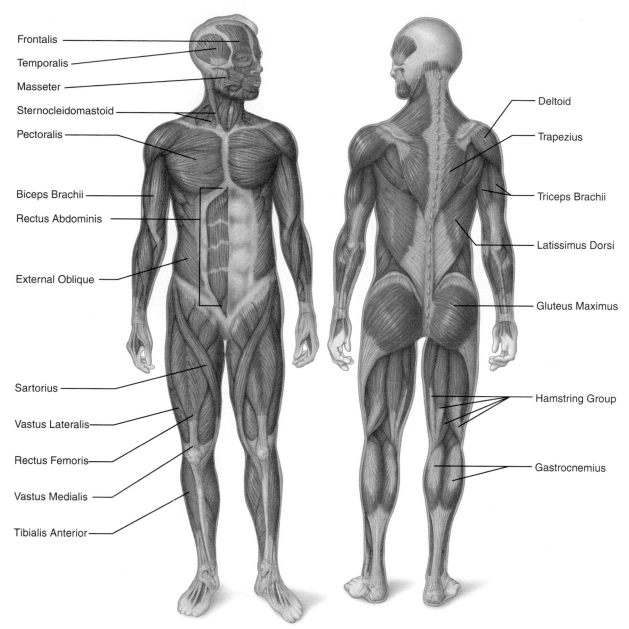

FIGURE 5.2
Major muscles of the human body.
(*Source:* Johnson, Michael. *Human Biology.* Benjamin Cummings, San Francisco, 2001.)

are not the same thing. Recall that muscular strength is defined as the ability of a muscle to generate maximal force (Chapter 1). In simple terms, muscular strength is the amount of weight that an individual can lift during one maximal effort. In contrast, muscular endurance is defined as the ability to generate force over and over again. In general, increasing muscular strength by exercise training will increase muscular endurance as well. However, training aimed at improving muscular endurance does not always result in significant improvements in muscular strength. Techniques to improve both muscular strength and muscular endurance are discussed later in this chapter.

MUSCLE STRUCTURE AND CONTRACTION

MUSCLE STRUCTURE   Skeletal muscle is a collection of long thin cells called *fibers*. These fibers are surrounded by a dense layer of connective tissue called *fascia* that holds the individual fibers together and separates muscle from surrounding tissues (Figure 5.1).

Muscles are attached to bone by connective tissues known as *tendons*. Muscular contraction causes the tendons to pull on the bones, thereby causing movement. Most of the muscles involved in movement are illustrated in Figure 5.2.

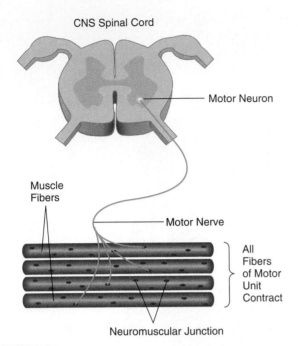

CNS Spinal Cord

Motor Neuron

Muscle
Fibers

Motor Nerve

All
Fibers
of Motor
Unit
Contract

Neuromuscular Junction

FIGURE 5.3
The concept of a motor unit. A motor nerve from the central nervous system is shown innervating several muscle fibers. With one impulse from the motor nerve, all fibers contract.
(*Source:* Fox, E., R. Bowers, and M. Foss. *The Physiological Basis of Physical Education and Athletics.* Madison, WI: Brown and Benchmark, 1997.)

MUSCLE CONTRACTION Muscle contraction is regulated by signals coming from motor nerves. Motor nerves originate in the spinal cord and send nerve fibers to individual muscles throughout the body. A motor nerve and an individual muscle fiber meet and make contact at a neuromuscular junction. The relationship between a motor nerve and skeletal muscle fibers is illustrated in Figure 5.3. Note that each motor nerve branches and then connects with numerous individual muscle fibers. The motor nerve and all of the muscle fibers it controls is called a **motor unit.**

motor unit A motor nerve and each of the muscle fibers it innervates.
isotonic Refers to muscle contractions in which there is movement of a body part. Most exercise or sports skills use isotonic contractions.
dynamic Means "movement"; in reference to muscle contractions, dynamic contraction is synonymous with isotonic contraction.
isometric Refers to muscle contractions in which muscular tension is developed but no movement of body parts takes place.
static Stationary; in reference to muscle contractions, static contraction is synonymous with isometric contraction.

Isometric vs. Isotonic Contraction

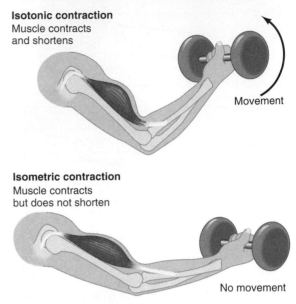

Isotonic contraction
Muscle contracts
and shortens

Movement

Isometric contraction
Muscle contracts
but does not shorten

No movement

FIGURE 5.4
Illustration of isotonic (also called *dynamic*) and isometric contractions.
(*Source:* Powers, S., and E. Howley. *Exercise Physiology: Theory and Application to Fitness and Performance.* Dubuque, IA: McGraw-Hill, 2001.)

A muscle contraction begins when a message to contract (called a *nerve impulse*) reaches the neuromuscular junction (Figure 5.3). The arrival of the nerve impulse triggers the contraction process by permitting the interaction of contractile proteins in muscle.

Because the nerve impulse initiates the contractile process, it is logical that the removal of the nerve signal from the muscle would "turn off" the contractile process. Indeed, when a motor nerve ceases to send signals to a muscle, the contraction stops. Occasionally, however, an uncontrolled muscular contraction occurs, resulting in a muscle cramp.

TYPES OF MUSCLE CONTRACTIONS

Muscle contractions are classified into two major categories: isotonic and isometric. **Isotonic** (also called **dynamic**) contractions are those that result in movement of a body part. Most exercise or sports skills utilize isotonic contractions. For example, lifting a dumbbell (Figure 5.4, top) involves movement of a body part and is therefore classified as an isotonic contraction. An **isometric** (also called **static**) contraction requires the development of muscular tension but results in no movement of body parts (Figure 5.4, bottom). A classic example of isometric contraction involves an individual exerting force against an iron bar mounted on the wall of a building; the muscle is developing tension but the

Concentric contraction

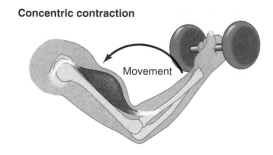

Eccentric contraction

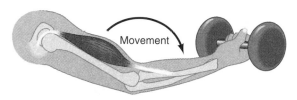

FIGURE 5.5
Illustration of concentric and eccentric contractions.
(*Source:* Adapted from Powers, S., and E. Howley. *Exercise Physiology: Theory and Application to Fitness and Performance.* Dubuque, IA: McGraw-Hill, 2001.)

wall is not moving, and therefore neither is the body part. Isometric contractions occur commonly in the postural muscles of the body during sitting or standing; for instance, isometric contractions are responsible for holding the head upright.

Note that isotonic contractions can be further subdivided into concentric, eccentric, and isokinetic contractions. **Concentric contractions** are isotonic muscle contractions that result in muscle shortening. The upward movement of the arm in Figure 5.5 is an example of a concentric contraction. In contrast, **eccentric contractions** (also called *negative contractions*) are defined as contractions in which the muscle exerts force while it lengthens. An eccentric contraction occurs when, for example, an individual resists the pull of a weight during the lowering phase of weight lifting (Figure 5.5). Here, the muscle is developing tension, but the force developed is not great enough to prevent the weight from being lowered.

Isokinetic contractions are concentric or eccentric contractions performed at a constant speed. That is, the speed of muscle shortening or lengthening is regulated at a fixed, controlled rate. This is generally accomplished by a weight-lifting machine that controls the rate of muscle shortening.

MUSCLE FIBER TYPES

There are three types of skeletal muscle fibers: slow twitch, fast twitch, and intermediate. These fiber types differ in their speeds of contraction and in fatigue resistance (7). Because most human muscles contain a

Nutritional Links
TO HEALTH AND FITNESS

Do Weight Lifters Need Large Amounts of Protein in Their Diets?

Many of the companies that manufacture nutritional supplements claim that weight lifters require large amounts of protein in their diets to ensure maximal strength gains during training. However, there is no evidence to support this claim. Although a well-balanced diet is essential for anyone engaging in regular weight lifting, research shows that the recommended daily allowance of protein (about one-third gram of protein per pound of body weight per day) is adequate to ensure maximal strength gains (8). Thus, for people eating balanced diets, a protein supplement during weight training is not recommended. See Chapter 7 for a complete discussion of nutrition and exercise.

mixture of all three fiber types, it is helpful to have an understanding of each before beginning a strength-training process.

SLOW-TWITCH FIBERS   As the name implies, **slow-twitch fibers** contract slowly and produce small amounts of force; however, these fibers are highly resistant to fatigue. Slow-twitch fibers, which are red in appearance, have the capacity to produce large quantities of ATP aerobically, making them ideally suited for a low-intensity prolonged exercise like walking or slow jogging. Further, because of their resistance to fatigue, most postural muscles are composed primarily of slow-twitch fibers.

concentric contractions   Isotonic muscle contractions that result in muscle shortening.
eccentric contractions   Isotonic contractions in which the muscle exerts force while the muscle lengthens (also called *negative contractions*).
isokinetic contractions   Concentric or eccentric isotonic contractions performed at a constant speed.
slow-twitch fibers   Muscle fibers that contract slowly and are highly resistant to fatigue. Red in appearance, they have the capacity to produce large quantities of ATP aerobically, making them ideally suited for low-intensity, prolonged exercise like walking or slow jogging.

TABLE 5.1
Properties of Human Skeletal Muscle Fiber Types

Property	Fiber Type		
	Slow-twitch	Intermediate	Fast-twitch
Contraction speed	Slow	Intermediate	Fast
Resistance to fatigue	High	Intermediate	Low
Predominant energy system	Aerobic	Combination aerobic and anaerobic	Anaerobic
Force generation	Low	Intermediate	High

FAST-TWITCH FIBERS   **Fast-twitch fibers** contract rapidly and generate great amounts of force but fatigue quickly. These fibers are white and have a low aerobic capacity, but they are well equipped to produce ATP anaerobically. With their ability to shorten rapidly and produce large amounts of force, fast-twitch fibers are used during activities requiring rapid or forceful movement, such as jumping, sprinting, and weight lifting.

INTERMEDIATE FIBERS   **Intermediate fibers,** although more red in color, possess a combination of the characteristics of fast- and slow-twitch fibers. They contract rapidly, produce great force, and are fatigue resistant due to a well-developed aerobic capacity. Intermediate fibers contract more quickly and produce more force than slow-twitch fibers but contract more slowly and produce less force than fast-twitch fibers. They are more fatigue resistant than fast-twitch fibers but less fatigue resistant than slow-twitch fibers. Table 5.1 summarizes the properties of all three fiber types.

RECRUITMENT OF MUSCLE FIBERS DURING EXERCISE

Many types of exercise use only a small fraction of the muscle fibers available in a muscle group. For example, walking at a slow speed may use fewer than 30% of the muscle fibers in the legs. More intense types of exer-

cise, however, require more force. In order for a muscle group to generate more force, a greater number of muscle fibers must be called into play. The process of involving more muscle fibers to produce increased muscular force is called fiber **recruitment.** Figure 5.6 illustrates the order of recruitment of muscle fibers as the intensity of exercise increases. Note that during low-intensity exercise, only slow-twitch fibers are used. As the exercise intensity increases, progressive recruitment of fibers occurs, from slow-twitch to intermediate fibers and finally to fast-twitch fibers. High-intensity activities like weight training recruit large numbers of fast-twitch fibers.

fast-twitch fibers   Muscle fibers that contract rapidly but fatigue quickly. These fibers are white and have a low aerobic capacity, but they are well equipped to produce ATP anaerobically.
intermediate fibers   Muscle fibers that possess a combination of the characteristics of fast- and slow-twitch fibers. They contract rapidly and are fatigue resistant due to a well-developed aerobic capacity.
recruitment   The process of involving more muscle fibers to increase muscular force.

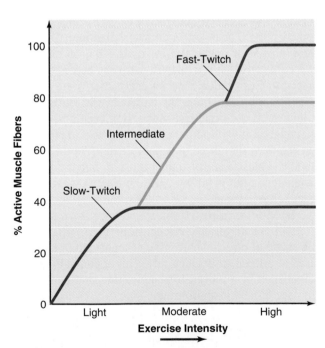

FIGURE 5.6
The relationship between exercise intensity and recruitment of muscle–fiber type.
(*Source:* Adapted from Powers, S., and E. Howley. *Exercise Physiology: Theory and Application to Fitness and Performance.* Dubuque, IA: McGraw-Hill, 2001.)

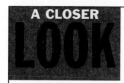

Anabolic Steroid Use Increases Muscle Size but Has Serious Side Effects

The abuse of **anabolic steroids** (primarily the hormone testosterone, which is important in muscle growth) has mushroomed over the past several decades. The fierce competition in body building and sports in which strength and power are necessary for success has driven both men and women to risk serious health consequences in order to develop large muscles.

The large doses of steroids needed to increase muscle mass produce several health risks. A partial list of the side effects caused by abusing steroids includes liver cancer, increased blood pressure, increased levels of "bad" cholesterol, and prostate cancer. Prolonged use and high doses of steroids can be lethal.

GENETICS AND FIBER TYPE

People vary in the percentage of slow-twitch, intermediate, and fast-twitch fibers their muscles contain. Research by exercise scientists has shown that a relationship exists between muscle fiber type and success in athletics. For example, champion endurance athletes, such as marathon runners, have a predominance of slow-twitch fibers. This is logical, because endurance sports require muscles with high fatigue resistance. In contrast, elite sprinters, such as 100-meter dash runners, possess a predominance of fast-twitch fibers. The average non-athlete generally has equal numbers of all three fiber types.

Although endurance exercise training has been shown to cause some fiber type conversion, the number and percentage of skeletal muscle fiber types is primarily determined by genetics. Because of the interrelationship among genetics, fiber type, and athletic success, some researchers have jokingly suggested that if you want to be a champion athlete, you must pick your parents wisely!

FACTORS THAT DETERMINE MUSCULAR STRENGTH

Two primary physiological factors determine the amount of force that a muscle can generate: the size of the muscle and the number of fibers recruited during the contraction.

MUSCLE SIZE The primary determinant of how much force a muscle can generate is its size. The larger the muscle, the greater the force it can produce. Although there is no difference in the chemical makeup of muscle in men and women, men are generally stronger than women because men have more muscle mass (i.e., larger muscles). The larger muscle mass in men is due to hormonal differences between the sexes; men have higher levels of the male sex hormone testosterone. The fact that testosterone promotes an increase in muscle size has led some athletes to attempt to improve muscular strength with drugs (A Closer Look).

MUSCLE FIBER RECRUITMENT We have seen that muscle fiber recruitment influences the production of muscle force. The more muscle fibers that are stimulated to shorten, the greater the muscle force generation, because the force generated by individual fibers is additive (Figure 5.7).

Muscle fiber recruitment is regulated voluntarily through the nervous system. That is, we determine how many muscle fibers to recruit by voluntarily making a decision about how much effort to put into a particular movement. For instance, when we choose to make a minimal effort in lifting an object, we recruit only a few motor units, and the muscle develops limited force. However, if we make a decision to exert our maximal effort in lifting a heavy object, many muscle fibers are recruited and great force is generated (Figure 5.7).

❖ IN SUMMARY

- Strength training can reduce low back pain, reduce the incidence of exercise-related injuries, decrease the incidence of osteoporosis, and aid in maintenance of functional capacity that normally decreases with age.
- Muscular strength is the ability to generate maximal force, whereas muscular endurance is the ability to generate force over and over again.
- Skeletal muscle is composed of fibers that are attached to bone by tendons.

anabolic steroids Hormones produced by the body that enhance muscle growth. Usually refers to the synthetic form of the hormone testosterone.

- Muscle contraction is regulated by signals coming from motor nerves. A motor unit comprises a motor nerve and all the muscle fibers it controls.
- Isotonic, or dynamic, muscle contractions result in movement of a body part, whereas isometric contractions result in no movement.
- Slow-twitch muscle fibers shorten slowly but are fatigue resistant. Fast-twitch fibers shorten rapidly but fatigue rapidly. Intermediate fibers shorten quickly but fatigue slowly.
- The process of involving more muscle fibers to produce increased muscular force is called *fiber recruitment.*
- The percentages of slow-twitch, intermediate, and fast-twitch fibers vary among individuals and play a major role in determining success in athletics.
- Two factors that determine muscle force are the size of the muscle and the number of fibers recruited.

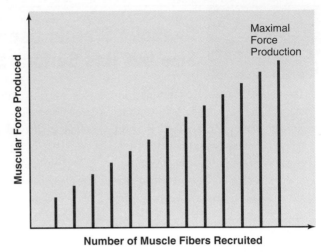

FIGURE 5.7
The relationship between motor unit recruitment and muscular force production.

☀ Guiding Principles for Designing a Strength and Endurance Program

In Chapter 3 we discussed the general principles for developing training programs to improve physical fitness. Before we discuss the specifics of how to develop a strength training program, let's discuss several principles that should be considered in developing a muscular strength and endurance training program.

☀ Progressive Resistance Exercise

The concept of **progressive resistance exercise (PRE)** is an application of the overload principle applied to strength and endurance exercise programs. Even though the two terms can be used interchangeably, PRE is preferred when discussing weight training. Progressive resistance exercise means that as strength and endurance are increased, the load against which the muscle works

must be periodically elevated if strength and endurance gains are to be realized.

PRINCIPLE OF SPECIFICITY OF TRAINING

The principle of **specificity of training** means that development of muscular strength and endurance is specific to both the muscle group that is exercised and the training intensity. First, only those muscles that are trained will improve in strength and endurance. For example, if an individual has low back pain and wishes to improve the strength of the supporting musculature of the lower back, it would be of no benefit to strengthen the arm muscles. The specific muscles involved with movement of the lower back should be the ones trained. Second, the training intensity determines whether the muscular adaptation is primarily an increase in strength or endurance. High-intensity training (i.e., lifting heavy weights four to six times) results in an increase in both muscular strength and size with only limited improvements in muscular endurance. Conversely, high-repetition, low-intensity training (i.e., lifting light weights 15 times or more) promotes an increase in muscular endurance, with only limited improvements in muscular size and strength.

☀ Designing a Training Program for Increasing Muscle Strength

There are numerous approaches to the design of weight-training programs. Any program that adheres to the basic principles described earlier will result in an improvement in strength and endurance. However, the type of weight-training program that you develop for yourself

---

progressive resistance exercise (PRE)   The application of the overload principle applied to strength and endurance exercise programs. Even though the overload principle and PRE can be used interchangeably, PRE is preferred when discussing weight training.
specificity of training   The concept that the development of muscular strength and endurance, as well as cardiorespiratory endurance, is specific to both the muscle group exercised and the training intensity.

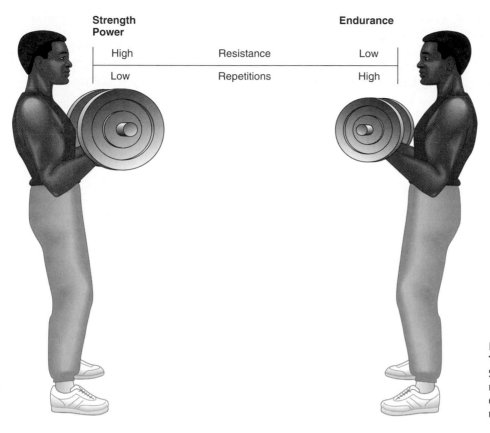

Strength Power		Endurance
High	Resistance	Low
Low	Repetitions	High

FIGURE 5.8
The strength–endurance continuum. Strength is achieved by using low repetitions/high weight, and endurance is achieved by using high repetitions/low weight.

depends on your goals and the types of equipment available to you. Next, we discuss several other considerations in the development of a weight-training program.

SAFETY CONCERNS

Before we discuss the specifics of how to develop a weight-training program, the need for safety should be emphasized. Although weight training can be performed safely, some important guidelines should be followed:

1. When using free weights (like barbells), have spotters (helpers) assist you in the performance of exercises. They can help you if you are unable to complete a lift. Many weight machines reduce the need for spotters.

2. Be sure that the collars on the end of the bars of free weights are tightly secured to prevent the weights from falling off. Dropping weight plates on toes and feet can result in serious injuries. Again, many weight machines reduce the potential risk of dropping weights.

3. Warm up properly before doing any weight-lifting exercise.

4. Do not hold your breath during weight lifting. A recommended breathing pattern to prevent breath holding during weight lifting is to exhale while lifting the weight and inhale while lowering. Also, breathe through both your nose and mouth.

5. Although debate continues as to whether high-speed weight lifting is superior to slow-speed lifting in terms of strength gains, slow movements may reduce the risk of injury. Therefore, because slow movement during weight lifting certainly results in an increase in both muscle size and strength, it would be wise to take this approach.

6. Use light weights in the beginning so that the proper maneuver can be achieved in each exercise. This is particularly true when lifting free weights.

TRAINING TO IMPROVE STRENGTH VERSUS TRAINING TO IMPROVE ENDURANCE

Weight-training programs specifically designed to improve strength and programs designed to improve muscular endurance differ mainly in the number of repetitions (i.e., the number of lifts performed) and the amount of resistance (9). Note in Figure 5.8 that a weight-training program using low repetitions and high resistance results in the greatest strength gains, whereas a weight-training program using high repetitions and low resistance results in the greatest improvement in muscular endurance. However, it is important to appreciate that while low-repetition/high-resistance training appears to be the optimal training method to increase strength, this type of training improves muscular endurance as well. In contrast, although weight training using high

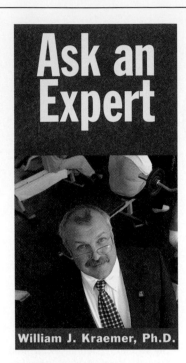

Ask an Expert

William J. Kraemer, Ph.D.

Resistance Training

Dr. Kraemer is Director of Research in the Human Performance Lab at the University of Connecticut. He is an internationally known expert on the adaptation of muscle to resistance training programs. He has published many scientific papers, books, and book chapters related to the acute and chronic adaptations to resistance exercise. In the following interview, Dr. Kraemer addresses several questions related to resistance training.

Q: **I am beginning to work out with weights and want to improve my strength and understand that there is controversy over how many sets are best—one set or three sets. What is your advice?**

A: When starting a program you should use the principle of "progressive resistance training" in your program. How many sets you should do depends on your training goals. Start out with one set to allow your body to develop toleration to the stress of resistance exercise. If your goal is to see continued improvement beyond a base level of fitness, progress to a multiple set program. Understand that not all exercises in a program need to be performed with the same number of sets. The number of sets are part of a volume of exercise equation (sets × reps × resistance = exercise volume). The volume of exercise can also be manipulated over time with the concept of periodization, where you may have training days or training cycles with very low, low-moderate, high, or very high training volumes for the entire body or a particular body part. Most advanced programs utilize multiple sets to expose the body to more total work, and such programs have been found to be significantly better than single set programs in producing strength, power, local muscular endurance, and muscle size gains.

Q: **After starting a weight training program several months ago, my strength gains have plateaued. What can I do to further my strength gains?**

A: Studies overwhelmingly show that gains in strength are highest early in training and that the rate of improvement decreases as higher levels of strength are achieved. To surpass a plateau, adhere to three basic principles of progression: 1) progressive overload; 2) specificity; and 3) variation (periodization).

Progressive overload entails that the program gradually become more difficult. Overload may be introduced for improved strength, hypertrophy, endurance, and power in several ways:

1) Increase load;

2) Add repetitions;

3) Alter repetition speed with submaximal loads;

4) shortened rest periods for endurance improvements or lengthened for strength and power;

5) increase volume within reasonable limits; and/or

6) any combination of the above.

Specificity refers to training that targets one particular (specific) group of muscles. The adaptation of this group of muscles will be specific to the particular muscle action, speed of movement, range of motion, muscle group, energy system, and intensity and volume of training.

Variation (or periodization) refers to systematic alteration in the volume and intensity of work. The technique of variation optimizes the development of strength by increasing the intensity while decreasing volume.

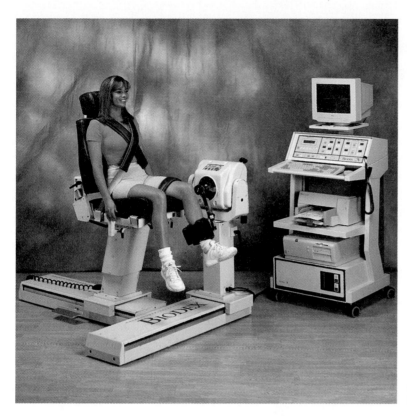

A commercially available isokinetic weight-training device.

repetition and low resistance improves endurance, this training method results in only small strength increases, particularly in less fit individuals.

TYPES OF WEIGHT-TRAINING PROGRAMS

Weight-training programs can be divided into three general categories classified by the type of muscle contraction involved: isotonic, isometric, and isokinetic.

ISOTONIC PROGRAMS Isotonic programs, like isotonic contractions, involve the concept of contracting a muscle against a movable load (usually a free weight or weights mounted by cables or chains to form a weight machine). Isotonic programs are very popular and are the most common type of weight-training program in use today.

ISOMETRIC PROGRAMS An isometric strength-training program is based on the concept of contracting a muscle at a fixed angle against an immovable object, using an isometric or static contraction. Interest in strength training increased dramatically during the 1950s with the finding that maximal strength could be increased by contracting a muscle for 6 seconds at two-thirds of maximal tension once per day for 5 days per week! Although subsequent studies suggested that these claims were exaggerated (8), it is generally agreed that isometric training can increase muscular strength and endurance.

Two important aspects of isometric training make it different from isotonic training. First, in isometric training, the development of strength and endurance is specific to the joint angle at which the muscle group is trained (10). Therefore, if isometric techniques are used, isometric contractions at several different joint angles are needed to gain strength and endurance throughout a full range of motion. In contrast, because isotonic contractions generally involve the full range of joint motion, strength is developed over the full movement pattern. Second, the static nature of isometric muscle contractions can lead to breath holding (called a **valsalva maneuver**), which can reduce blood flow to the brain and cause dizziness and fainting. In an individual at high risk for coronary disease, the maneuver could be extremely dangerous and should always be avoided. Remember: Continue to breathe during any type of isometric or isotonic contraction!

ISOKINETIC PROGRAMS Recall that isokinetic contractions are isotonic contractions performed at a constant speed (*isokinetic* refers to constant speed of movement). Isokinetic training is a relatively new strength training method, so limited research exists to describe

---

valsalva maneuver Breath holding during an intense muscle contraction; can reduce blood flow to the brain and cause dizziness and fainting.

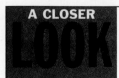

Plyometric Training Is Not for Everyone

You may have heard the term *plyometrics* used in reference to training for athletes. Athletes use this technique to develop explosive power. Plyometric training is performed by quickly stretching a muscle prior to initiating a maximal contraction. A common example is a simple vertical jump. You may have noticed that when you attempt to jump as high as possible, you almost always bend your knees quickly and "rebound" in order to maximize your jump height. You can certainly jump higher by using this "rebound" than by starting the jump with your knees already bent.

Plyometric training is based on the principle that stretching a muscle prior to contraction enables a greater force to be generated by the muscle. The most common method of plyometric training is called "drop jump-

ing"—dropping from a height and rebounding. (See the box figure below.) This exercise requires the athlete to drop (not jump) to the ground from a platform or box, and then immediately jump. The drop prestretches the muscles, and the jump overloads the muscles with the ensuing concentric contraction. The exercise is more effective the shorter the time the feet are in contact with the ground. The amount of load placed on the muscles is determined in part by the height of the drop, which should be in the

range of 12–30 in. Drop jumping is a relatively high-impact form of training and should not be introduced until after an athlete has used lower-impact alternatives, such as two-footed jumping on the ground.

Because of the dynamic nature of plyometric training, there is great potential for injury to both muscles and joints. For a basic fitness program, there is no need to include a high-risk type of training when a low-risk activity will accomplish the same goal. This training technique is best reserved for athletes looking for a competitive edge and for rehabilitation programs that are closely supervised.

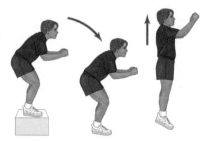

A drop jump.

its strength benefits compared with those of isometric and isotonic programs. Isokinetic exercises require the use of machines that govern the speed of movement during muscle contraction. The first isokinetic machines available were very expensive and were used primarily in clinical settings for injury rehabilitation. Recently, less expensive machines use a piston device (much like a shock absorber on a car) to limit the speed of movement throughout the range of the exercise. Today, these machines are found in fitness centers across the United States.

☼ IN SUMMARY

- The overload principle states that a muscle will adapt only when it works against a workload that is greater than normal. The application of the overload principle to weight training is called progressive resistance exercise (PRE).

- The greatest strength gains are made with a training program using low repetitions and high resistance, whereas the greatest improvement in endurance is made using high repetitions and low resistance.

- Isotonic programs include exercises with moveable loads. Isometric training includes exercises in which a muscle contracts at a fixed angle against an immovable object. Isokinetic exercises involve machines that govern speed of movement during muscle contraction.

☼ Exercise Prescription for Weight Training: An Overview

We introduced the general concepts of the intensity, duration, and frequency of exercise required to improve physical fitness in Chapter 3. Although these same concepts apply to improving muscular strength and endurance via weight training, the terminology used to monitor the intensity and duration of weight training is unique. For example, the intensity of weight training is measured not by heart rate but by the number of "repetition maximums." Similarly, the duration of weight training is monitored not by time but by the number of sets performed. Let's discuss these two concepts briefly.

The intensity of exercise in both isotonic and isokinetic weight-training programs is measured by the concept of the **repetition maximum (RM).** The RM is the maximal load that a muscle group can lift a specified number of times before tiring. For example, 6 RM is the maximal load that can be lifted six times. Therefore, the amount of weight lifted is greater when performing a low number of RMs than a high number of RMs; that is, the weight lifted while performing 4 RMs is greater than the weight lifted while performing 15 RMs.

The number of repetitions (reps) performed consecutively without resting is called a **set.** In the example of 6 RM, 1 set = 6 reps. Because the amount of rest required between sets will vary among individuals depending on how fit they are, the duration of weight training is measured by the number of sets performed, not by time.

Although disagreement exists as to the optimum number of reps and sets required to improve strength and endurance, some general guidelines can be provided. To improve strength, 3 sets of 6 reps for each exercise are generally recommended. The concept of progressive resistance applied to a strength-training program involves increasing the amount of weight to be lifted a specific number of reps. For example, suppose that 3 sets of 6 RMs were selected as your exercise prescription for increasing strength. As the training progresses and you become stronger, the amount of weight lifted must be increased. A good rule of thumb is that once 8 reps can be performed, the load should be increased to a level at which 6 reps are again maximal. Figure 5.9 illustrates the relationship between strength improvement and various combinations of reps and sets. Note that in each strength-training program, 6 reps result in the greatest strength improvement. A key point in Figure 5.9 is that programs involving 3 sets result in the greatest strength gains. This is because the third set requires the greatest effort and thus is the greatest overload for the muscle. Although it may seem that adding a fourth set would elicit even greater gains, most studies suggest 4 or more sets results in overtraining and decreased benefits.

To improve muscular endurance, 4 to 6 sets of 18 to 20 reps for each exercise are recommended. Note that endurance could be improved by either increasing the number of reps progressively while maintaining the same load, or increasing the amount of weight while maintaining the same number of reps. The advantage of the latter program is that it would also improve muscular strength.

What role does training frequency play in the development of strength? Most research suggests that 2 to 3 days of exercise per week is optimal for strength gains (11). However, studies have shown that once the desired level of strength has been achieved, one high-intensity training session per week is sufficient to maintain the new level of strength. Finally, although

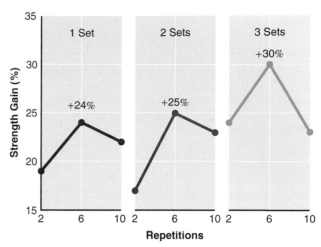

FIGURE 5.9
Strength gains from a resistance training program consisting of various sets and repetitions. All programs were performed 3 days per week for 12 weeks. Note that the greatest strength gains (+30% improvement) were obtained using 3 sets of 6 reps per set.
(*Source:* Adapted from Fox, E., R. Bowers, and M. Foss. *Fox's Physiological Basis of Exercise and Sports.* Boston: WCB-McGraw-Hill, 1998.)

limited research exists regarding the optimal frequency of training to improve muscular endurance, 3 to 5 days per week seem adequate (12).

☀ Starting and Maintaining a Weight-Training Program

You should begin your weight-training program with both short- and long-term goals. Identifying goals is an important means of maintaining interest and enthusiasm for weight training. A key point is to establish realistic short-term goals that can be reached in the first several weeks of training. Reaching these goals provides the motivation needed to continue training.

DEVELOPING AN INDIVIDUALIZED EXERCISE PRESCRIPTION

An exercise prescription for strength training has three stages: the starter phase, the slow progression phase, and the maintenance phase.

---

repetition maximum (RM)   The measure of the intensity of exercise in both isotonic and isokinetic weight-training programs. The RM is the maximal load that a muscle group can lift a specified number of times before tiring. For example, 6 RM is the maximal load that can be lifted six times.
set   The number of repetitions performed consecutively without resting.

TABLE 5.2
Guidelines and Precautions to Follow Prior to Beginning a Strength-Training Program

Warm up before beginning a workout. This involves 5 to 10 minutes of movement (calisthenics) using all major muscle groups.

Start slowly. The first several training sessions should involve limited exercises and light weight!

Use the proper lifting technique, as shown in the Isotonic Strength-Training Exercises in this chapter. Improper technique can lead to injury.

Follow all safety rules (see the section on safety concerns on page 111).

Always lift through the full range of motion. This not only develops strength throughout the full range of motion but also assists in maintaining flexibility.

TABLE 5.3
Suggested Isotonic Strength-Training Routine to Be Included in a Basic Fitness Program

The durations of the starter and slow progression phases will depend on your initial strength level.

Week No.	Phase	Frequency	Sets	Reps	Weight
1–3	Starter	2/week	2	15	15 RM
4–20	Slow progression	2–3/week	3	6	6 RM
20+	Maintenance	1–2/week	3	6	6 RM

STARTER PHASE   The primary objective of the starter phase is to build strength gradually without developing undue muscular soreness or injury. This can be accomplished by starting your weight-training program slowly—beginning with light weights, a high number of repetitions, and only 2 sets per exercise. The recommended frequency of training during this phase is twice per week. The duration of this phase varies from 1 to 3 weeks, depending on your initial strength fitness level. A sedentary person might spend 3 weeks in the starter phase, whereas a relatively well-trained person may only spend 1 to 2 weeks.

SLOW PROGRESSION PHASE   This phase may last 4 to 20 weeks depending on your initial strength level and your long-term strength goal. The transition from the starter phase to the slow progression phase involves three changes in the exercise prescription: increasing the frequency of training from 2 to 3 days per week; increasing the amount of weight lifted and decreasing the number of repetitions; and increasing the number of sets performed from 2 to 3 sets.

The objective of the slow progression phase is to gradually increase muscular strength until you reach your desired level. After reaching your strength goal, your long-term objective becomes to maintain this level of strength by entering the maintenance phase of the strength-training exercise prescription.

MAINTENANCE PHASE   After reaching your strength goals, the problem now becomes, How do I maintain this strength level? The bad news is that maintaining strength will require a lifelong weight-training effort. Strength is lost if you do not continue to exercise. The good news is that the effort required to maintain muscular strength is less than the initial effort needed to gain strength. Research has shown that as little as one workout per week is required to maintain strength. A sample exercise prescription incorporating all three training phases follows.

SAMPLE EXERCISE PRESCRIPTION FOR WEIGHT TRAINING

GETTING STARTED   Similar to training to improve cardiorespiratory fitness, the exercise prescription for improving muscular strength must be tailored to the individual. Before starting a program, keep in mind the guidelines and precautions presented in Table 5.2.

DETAILS OF THE PRESCRIPTION   Table 5.3 illustrates the stages of a suggested strength-training exercise prescription. As mentioned earlier, the durations of both the starter and slow progression phases will vary depending on your initial strength fitness level. When

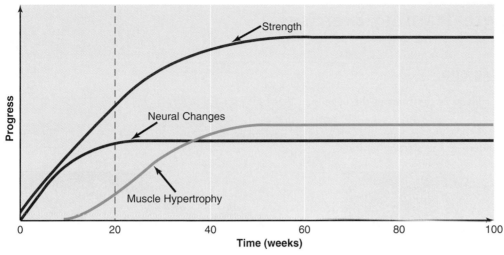

FIGURE 5.10
The relative roles of the nervous system and muscular adaptation in strength development. Strength training increases muscular strength first through changes in the nervous system and then by increasing muscle size.
(*Source:* Wilmore, J. H., and D. L. Costill. *Physiology of Sport and Exercise.* Champaign, IL: Human Kinetics, 1994.)

the strength goals of the program are reached, the maintenance phase begins. This period utilizes the same routine as used during the progression phase but may be done only once per week.

SAMPLE STRENGTH-TRAINING EXERCISES The isotonic strength-training program contains 12 exercises that are designed to provide a whole body workout. Although specific machines are used in the following examples, barbells may be used for performing similar exercises. However, it is important to remember that safety and proper lifting technique are especially important when using barbells. Before beginning a program using barbells, it is a good idea to get advice from someone experienced with their use.

Follow the exercise routines described and illustrated in Exercises 5.1 through 5.12, and develop your program using the guidelines provided in Table 5.3. This selection of exercises is designed to provide a comprehensive strength-training program that focuses on the major muscle groups. Although many more exercises exist, some of them use the same muscle groups as those covered here. Be aware of which muscle groups are involved in an exercise in order to avoid overtraining any one muscle group (Figure 5.2). Note that it is not necessary to perform all 12 exercises in one workout session; you can perform half of the exercises on one day and the remaining exercises on an alternate day.

Use Laboratory 5.1 on page 129 to keep a record of your training progress. Remember: Maintenance and review of your training progress will help motivate you to continue your strength-training program!

☀ IN SUMMARY

- In developing a strength-training program, divide it into three phases: a starter phase, a slow progression phase, and a maintenance phase.

☀ Strength Training: How the Body Adapts

What physiological changes occur as a result of strength training? How quickly can muscular strength be gained? Do men and women differ in their responses to weight-training programs? Let's address each of these questions separately.

PHYSIOLOGICAL CHANGES DUE TO WEIGHT TRAINING

It should now be clear that programs designed to improve muscular strength can do so only by increasing muscular size and/or by increasing the number of muscle fibers recruited. In fact, both these factors are altered by strength training (9). Research has shown that strength-training programs increase muscular strength by first altering fiber recruitment patterns due to changes in the nervous system and then by increasing muscle size (Figure 5.10).

How do muscles increase in size? Muscle size is increased primarily through an increase in fiber size, called **hypertrophy** (9). However, recent research has shown that strength training can also promote the formation of new muscle fibers, a process called **hyperplasia.** To date, the role that hyperplasia plays in the increase in muscle size due to strength training remains controversial. Regardless, the increase in muscle size due to strength training depends on diet, the muscle fiber type (fast fibers may hypertrophy more than slow

---

hypertrophy An increase in muscle fiber size.
hyperplasia An increase in the number of muscle fibers.

Text continues on page 124.

Isotonic Strength-Training Exercises

EXERCISE 5.1   BICEPS CURL

Purpose: To strengthen the muscles in the front of the upper arm that cause flexion at the elbow.

Movement: Holding the grips with palms up and arms extended (a), curl up as far as possible (b) and slowly return to the starting position.

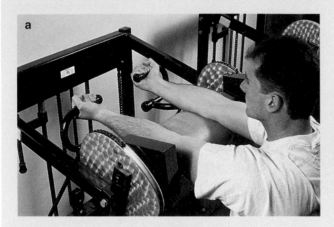
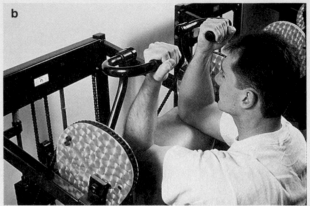

EXERCISE 5.2   ABDOMINAL CURL

Purpose: To strengthen the abdominal muscles.

Movement: Place hands on the abdomen (a) and curl forward, bringing the chest toward the knees (b). Slowly return to the upright position.

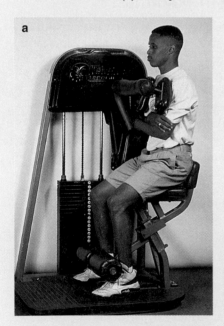
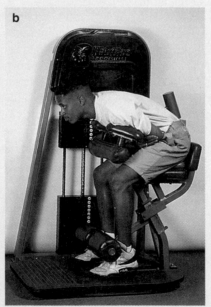

Isotonic Strength-Training Exercises

EXERCISE 5.3 LEG EXTENSION

Purpose: To strengthen the muscles in the front of the upper leg.

Movement: Sitting in a nearly upright position, grasp the handles on the side of the machine (a). Extend the legs until they are completely straight (b) and then slowly return to the starting position.

a
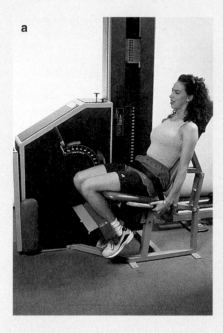

b
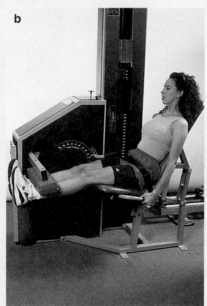

EXERCISE 5.4 BENCH PRESS

Purpose: To strengthen the muscles in the chest, the front of the shoulders, and the back of the upper arm.

Movement: Lie on the bench with the bench press bar above the chest and the feet flat on the foot rest (a). Grasp the bar handles and press upward until the arms are completely extended (b). Return slowly to the original position. **Caution:** Do not arch the back while performing this exercise.

a
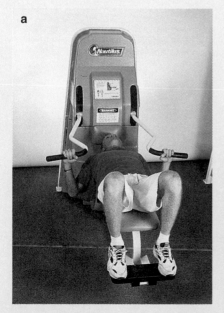

b
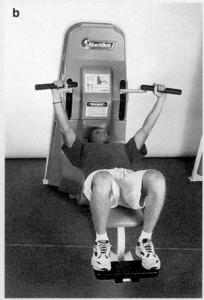

Isotonic Strength-Training Exercises

EXERCISE 5.5   LEG CURL

Purpose: To strengthen the muscles on the back of the upper leg and buttocks.

Movement: Lying on the left side, place the back of the feet over the padded bar (a). Curl the legs to at least a 90° angle (b) and then slowly return to the original position.

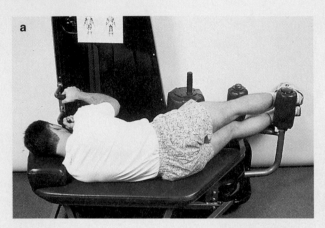
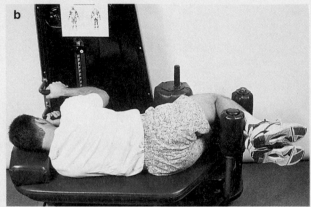

EXERCISE 5.6   LOWER BACK EXTENSION

Purpose: To strengthen the muscles of the lower back and buttocks.

Movement: Position the thighs and upper back against the padded bars (a). Buckle the strap around the thighs. Slowly press backward against the padded bar until the back is fully extended (b). Slowly return to the original position.

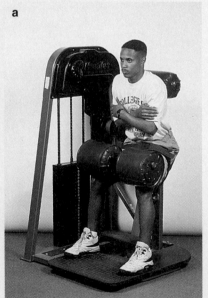
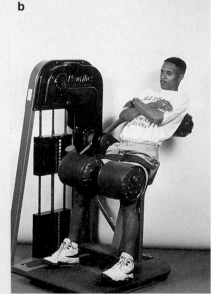

Isotonic Strength-Training Exercises

EXERCISE 5.7   UPPER BACK

Purpose: To strengthen the muscles of the upper back.

Movement: Sit in the machine with elbows bent and the backs of the arms resting against the padded bars (a). Press the arms back as far as possible, drawing the shoulder blades together (b). Slowly return to the original position.

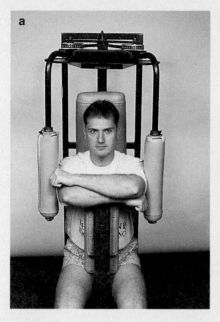

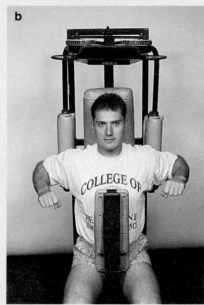

EXERCISE 5.8   HIP AND BACK

Purpose: To strengthen the muscles of the hip and lower back.

Movement: Lying on the left side, grasp the handles at both sides for stability. Place the back of the knees against the padded bars (a). Press the legs back until fully extended (b). Slowly return to the original position.

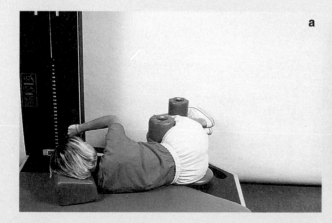

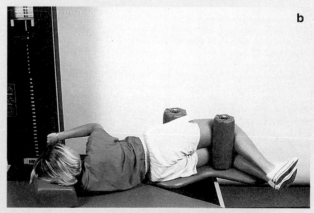

Isotonic Strength-Training Exercises

EXERCISE 5.9   PULLOVER

Purpose: To strengthen the muscles of the chest, shoulder, and side of the trunk.

Movement: Sit with elbows against the padded end of the movement arm and grasp the bar behind your head (a). Press forward and down with the arms, pulling the bar overhead and down to the abdomen (b). Slowly return to the original position.

a

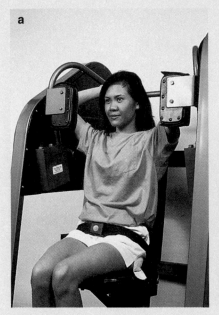

b

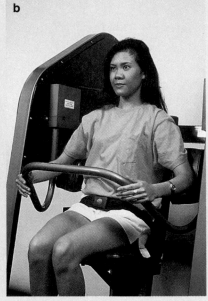

EXERCISE 5.10   TORSO TWIST

Purpose: To strengthen the muscles on the sides of the abdomen.

Movement: Sitting upright with the elbows behind the padded bars, twist the torso as far as possible to one side (a). Slowly return to the original position and repeat to the other side (b).

a

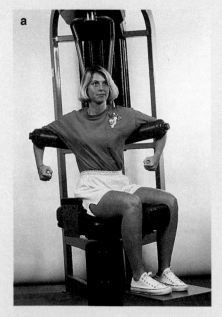

b

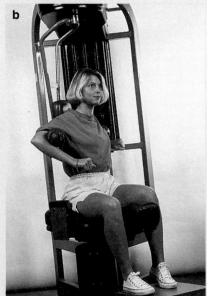

Isotonic Strength-Training Exercises

EXERCISE 5.11   TRICEPS EXTENSION

Purpose: To strengthen the muscles on the back of the upper arm.

Movement: Sit upright with elbows bent (a). With the little-finger side of the hand against the pad, fully extend the arms (b) and then slowly return to the original position.

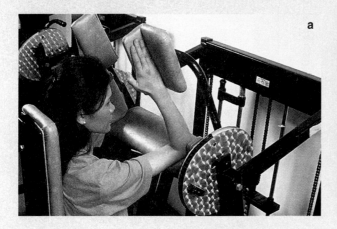
a

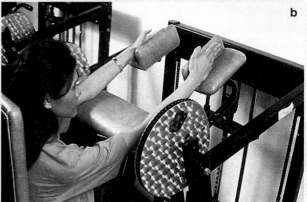
b

EXERCISE 5.12   CHEST PRESS

Purpose: To strengthen the muscles of the chest and shoulder.

Movement: With the elbows bent at a 90° angle and the forearms against the pads (a), press the arms forward as far as possible, leading with the elbows (b). Slowly return to the original position.

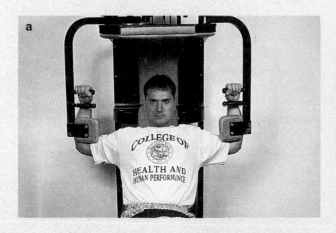
a

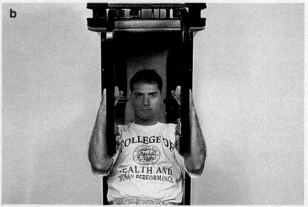
b

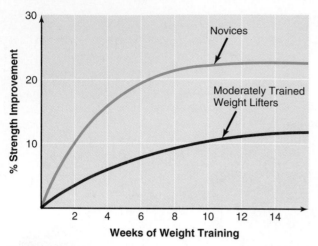

FIGURE 5.11
Time course of strength improvement in novice weight lifters versus moderately well-trained weight lifters. The rate of improvement and the total percent strength improvement is greater in novices compared with moderately trained weight lifters. This occurs because moderately trained weight lifters began the weight-training program with higher initial strength levels.

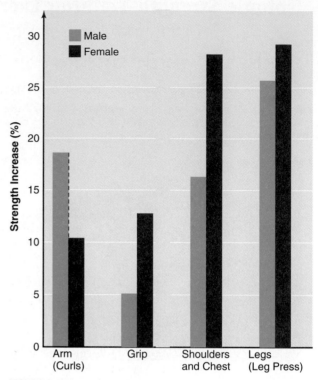

FIGURE 5.12
A comparison of strength gains for men and women. In relation to beginning strength levels, the increase in strength for women over the first 12 weeks of training is equal to or greater than that seen in men for most muscle groups.
(Adapted from Wilmore, J. Body composition and strength development. *Journal of Physical Education Research* 46(1):38–40, 1975.)

fibers), blood levels of testosterone, and the type of training program.

Although strength training does not result in significant improvements in cardiorespiratory fitness (12), a regular weight-training program can provide positive changes in both body composition and flexibility. For most men and women, rigorous weight training results in an increase in muscle mass and a loss of body fat, the end result being a decrease in the percent of body fat.

If weight-training exercises are performed over the full range of motion possible at a joint, flexibility can be improved (8). In fact, many diligent weight lifters have excellent flexibility. Therefore, the notion of weight lifters becoming muscle-bound and losing flexibility is generally incorrect.

RATE OF STRENGTH IMPROVEMENT WITH WEIGHT TRAINING

How rapidly does strength improvement occur? The answer depends on your initial strength level. Strength gains occur rapidly in untrained people, whereas gains are more gradual in individuals with relatively higher strength levels (Figure 5.11). Indeed, an exciting point about weight training for a novice lifter is that strength gains occur very quickly (13). These rapid strength gains provide motivation to continue a regular weight-training program.

GENDER DIFFERENCES IN RESPONSE TO WEIGHT TRAINING

In terms of absolute strength, men tend to be stronger than women because men generally have a greater mus-

cle mass. The difference is greater in the upper body, where men are approximately 50% stronger than women; men are only 30% stronger than women in the lower body.

Do men and women differ in their responses to weight-training programs? The answer is "no" (14). On a percentage basis, women gain strength as rapidly as men during the first 12 weeks of a strength-training program (Figure 5.12). However, as a result of long-term weight training, men generally exhibit a greater increase in muscle size than do women. This occurs because men have 20 to 30 times more testosterone (a male sex hormone that builds muscles) than do women.

IN SUMMARY

- Muscle size increases primarily because of hypertrophy (increase in size) of muscle fibers. Strength training can also promote the formation of new muscle fibers (hyperplasia).

- Strength training promotes positive changes in both body composition and flexibility.

- The rate of improvement in weight training depends on initial strength level.

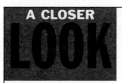

Frequently Asked Questions About Weight Training

How much rest is necessary between training sessions?

Getting the correct amount of rest is as important as doing the proper exercises! Weight training depletes energy stores and damages muscle fibers. With the proper rest, water intake, and nutrition, the muscles grow stronger by replenishing and repairing themselves. If you do not get the proper rest, your muscles will not reach their potential. Depending on the muscle groups used and the intensity and volume of training, you may need 24 to 72 hours to recover and allow muscles to repair themselves. Also, you should try to get 6 to 8 hours of sleep per night.

What is the best kind of equipment for weight training?

No particular kind of resistance-training equipment is "better" than any other. All exercise accessories have their advantages and disadvantages. As discussed in this chapter, equipment should be safe and provide the ability to overload the muscle groups you want to train. Remember, the best equipment is the one that you use regularly!

Should I train a muscle if it's sore?

No. If your legs are sore from squatting and you want to work an upper-body muscle group, that's okay. But if your legs are still sore from the last leg workout, take at least another day off before working the same muscle group again.

Will doing aerobics retard muscle growth?

If you're training for maximum muscle mass, aerobics will slow down muscle growth. However, if you are developing an all-purpose fitness program, both aerobics and resistance training are necessary.

Should I use a lifting belt?

Most people don't need to use a lifting belt. Using a belt all the time actually weakens the abdominals and the lower back by making them work less. Weight belts are recommended for max squats or heavy lifting above the head.

I have reached a plateau in strength gains. What can I do?

First, you could be overtraining. Try taking a week off, and when you come back take it easy for a few weeks while reevaluating your workout. Second, make sure your caloric intake is adequate and rich in nutrients. Don't overeat—doing so will not build muscle. Third, if you have been using the same routine/exercise for every workout, change your routine and use different muscle groups. Remember, the muscles will only respond if overloaded. Finally, you may be hitting your genetic limits. Taking a break, eating more, and changing your workout should help when you hit a strength plateau.

Should I use free weights or machines?

This argument has been ongoing for years. Free weights indirectly work more muscles (those needed for stability and balance), and they allow a larger range of motion. Machines isolate muscles better and are safer since you don't need a spotter. Most people who train use both, and many others use whatever type is available. But realize that a lot can be accomplished by doing exercises with neither, such as push-ups, pull-ups, one-legged squats, lunges, and so on. Each exercise or piece of equipment works the muscles at a slightly different angle. Experiment to find what works for you. For most people, en-

suring that the workout is safe should be the prime concern.

What exercises should I avoid?

Any exercise can cause an injury when done improperly. Again, safety is a primary concern, so go slow, don't bounce, and don't cheat. If you feel any pain during any exercise, STOP!

What is periodization?

Periodization, or cycling, is a training method in which you cycle your routine to keep muscles growing and getting stronger. It is commonly performed by varying the intensity and volume of lifting. It is a valuable training method for athletes. For example, as an athlete's off-season training program progresses, the intensity of the workout is increased and repetitions are reduced. However, for most fitness programs periodization is unnecessary.

Will unexercised muscle turn into fat?

No! Muscle and fat are different types of tissue. In any given area of the body, both muscle mass and fat stores can get either smaller or larger. However, neither one is converted to the other. Fat is gained with increases in caloric intake and/or a reduction in caloric expenditure. Muscle mass can be increased with resistance training.

I don't want to look like a bodybuilder. Should I still lift weights?

YES! For most people, adding muscle is very difficult. Hard work, eating right, and having the right genetics are all needed to get the bodybuilder look. It also takes years, and most often a lot of steroids, to put on the kind of mass that you see in magazines. If you find yourself getting larger muscles than you'd like, you can stop training and they will shrink due to lack of work.

- Men tend to be stronger than women because of their greater muscle mass. Testosterone, a predominantly male hormone, is responsible for this difference.
- Women gain strength as fast as men early in a weight-training program.

☀ Motivation to Maintain Strength Fitness

The problems associated with starting and maintaining a weight-training program are similar to those associated with cardiorespiratory training. You must find time to train regularly, so good time management is critical.

Another key feature of any successful exercise program is that training must be fun. Making weight training fun involves several elements. First, find an enjoyable place to work out. Locate a facility that contains the type of weights that you want to use and also provides a pleasant and motivating environment. Second, develop an enjoyable weight-training routine (exercise prescription). Designing a training routine that is too hard may be good for improving strength but does not increase your desire to train. Therefore, design a program that is challenging, but fun. Further, weight training is more enjoyable if you have a regular training partner. Select a friend who is highly motivated to exercise and has strength abilities similar to yours.

Although the benefits of weight training are numerous, recent studies have shown that improved appearance, elevated self-esteem, and the overall feeling of well-being that result from regular weight training are the most important factors in motivating people to continue to train regularly. Looking your best and feeling good about yourself are excellent reasons to maintain a regular weight-training program.

Summary

1. The importance of training to improve strength and endurance is evident from the fact that strength training can reduce low back pain, reduce the incidence of exercise-related injuries, decrease the incidence of osteoporosis, and aid in maintenance of functional capacity, which normally decreases with age.

2. Muscular strength is defined as the ability of a muscle to generate maximal force (Chapter 1). In simple terms, this refers to the amount of weight that an individual can lift during one maximal effort. In contrast, muscular endurance is defined as the ability of a muscle to generate force over and over again. In general, increasing muscular strength by exercise training will increase muscular endurance as well. In contrast, training aimed at improving muscular endurance does not always result in significant improvements in muscular strength.

3. Skeletal muscle is composed of a collection of long thin cells (fibers). Muscles are attached to bone by thick connective tissue (tendons). Therefore, muscle contraction results in the tendons pulling on bone, thereby causing movement.

4. Muscle contraction is regulated by signals coming from motor nerves. Motor nerves originate in the spinal cord and send nerve fibers to individual muscles throughout the body. The motor nerve and all of the muscle fibers it controls is called a *motor unit*.

5. Isotonic or dynamic contractions are contractions that result in movement of a body part. Isometric contractions involve the development of force but result in no movement of body parts. Concentric contractions are isotonic muscle contractions involving muscle shortening. In contrast, eccentric contractions (negative contractions) are defined as isotonic contractions in which the muscle exerts force while the muscle lengthens.

6. Human skeletal muscle can be classified into three major fiber types: slow-twitch, fast-twitch, and intermediate fibers. Slow-twitch fibers shorten slowly but are highly fatigue resistant. Fast-twitch fibers shorten rapidly but fatigue rapidly. Intermediate fibers possess a combination of the characteristics of fast- and slow-twitch fibers.

7. The process of involving more muscle fibers to produce increased muscular force is called fiber recruitment.

8. The percentages of slow-, intermediate-, and fast-twitch fibers vary among individuals. Research by sports scientists has shown that a relationship exists between muscle fiber type and success in athletics. For example, champion endurance athletes (e.g., marathon runners) have a high percentage of slow-twitch fibers.

9. Two primary physiological factors determine the amount of force that can be generated by a muscle: the size of the muscle and the neural influences (i.e., number of fibers recruited).

10. Muscle size is increased primarily because of an increase in fiber size (hypertrophy). Further, recent

research has shown that strength training can also promote the formation of new muscle fibers (hyperplasia).

11. The overload principle states that a muscle will increase in strength and/or endurance only when it works against a workload that is greater than normal.

12. The concept of progressive resistance exercise (PRE) is the application of the overload principle to strength and endurance exercise programs.

13. A weight-training program using low repetitions/high resistance results in the greatest strength gains, whereas a weight-training program using high repetitions/low resistance results in the greatest improvement in muscular endurance.

14. Isotonic programs, like an isotonic contraction, involve the concept of contracting a muscle against a movable load (usually a free weight or weights mounted by cables or chains to form a weight machine). An isometric strength-training program is based on the concept of contracting a muscle(s) at a fixed angle against an immovable object (isometric or static contraction). Isokinetic exercises require the use of machines that govern the speed of movement during muscle contraction throughout the range of motion.

15. To begin a strength-training program, divide the program into three phases: starter phase—2 to 3 weeks with 2 workouts per week using 2 sets at 15 RM; slow progression phase—20 weeks with 2 to 3 workouts per week using 3 sets at 6 RM; and maintenance phase—continues for life with 1 workout per week using 3 sets at 6 RM.

Study Questions

1. Define the following terms:
   anabolic steroid
   hyperplasia
   hypertrophy
   motor unit
   progressive resistance exercise
   static contraction
   valsalva maneuver

2. List at least three reasons why training for strength and endurance is important.

3. List and discuss the characteristics of slow-twitch, fast-twitch, and intermediate skeletal muscle fibers.

4. Discuss the pattern of muscle fiber recruitment with increasing intensities of contraction.

5. Discuss the relationship of muscle fiber type to success in various types of athletic events.

6. What factors determine muscle strength?

7. What are some of the consequences of steroid abuse?

8. What physiological changes occur as a result of strength training?

9. Compare and contrast the overload principle and progressive resistance exercise.

10. Discuss the concept of specificity of training.

11. Compare and contrast the differences in training to increase strength versus training to increase endurance.

12. Define the concept of repetition maximum.

13. List the phases of a strength and endurance training program and discuss how they differ.

14. Distinguish between *concentric* and *eccentric* contractions.

15. Describe each of the following types of muscle contraction: isokinetic, isometric, and isotonic.

Suggested Reading

American College of Sports Medicine. The recommended quantity and quality of exercise for developing and maintaining cardiorespiratory and muscular fitness, and flexibility in healthy adults. *Medicine and Science in Sports and Exercise* 30:975–991, 1998.

Blair, S. N., and J. C. Connelly. How much physical activity should we do: The case for moderate amounts and intensities of physical activity. *Research Quarterly for Exercise and Sport* 67: 193–205, 1996.

Fleck, S. J., and W. J. Kraemer. *Designing Resistance Training Programs.* Champaign, IL: Human Kinetics, 1997.

Haskell, W. L. Physical activity, sport and health: Toward the next century. *Research Quarterly for Exercise and Sport* 67: S37–S47, 1996.

Howley, E. Type of activity: Resistance, aerobic and leisure versus occupational physical activity. *Medicine and Science in Sports and Exercise* 33(6):S364–S369, 2001.

Komi, P. *Strength and Power in Sport.* Oxford: Blackwell Publishers, 1992.

Powers, S., and E. Howley. *Exercise Physiology: Theory and Application to Fitness and Performance,* 4th ed. Dubuque, IA: McGraw-Hill, 2001.

For links to the Web sites below visit Web Links at www.aw.com/fitness and choose Powers/Dodd from the drop-down menu.

Simpatico: Health

Contains numerous articles, book reviews, and links to nutrition, fitness, and wellness topics.

Fitness Files

Describes fitness fundamentals and flexibility and contraindicated exercises, and discusses exercise nutrition and the treatment of exercise injuries.

Meriter Fitness

Discusses injury prevention and treatment, weight training, flexibility, exercise prescriptions, and more.

Muscle Physiology

Includes in-depth discussions of how muscle works as well as recent research articles from a world-renowned muscle physiology lab.

References

1. Mannion, A. F., A. Junge, S. Taimela, M. Muntener, K. Lorenzo, and J. Dvorak. Active therapy for chronic low back pain, Part 3. Factors influencing self-rated disability and its change following therapy. *Spine* 26(8):920–929, 2001.

2. Stone, M. H. Muscle conditioning and muscle injuries. *Medicine and Science in Sports and Exercise.* 22:457–462, 1990.

3. Kibler, W. B., T. J. Chandler, and E. S. Stracener. Musculoskeletal adaptations and injuries due to overtraining. In *Exercise and Sports Sciences Reviews,* Vol. 20, J. O. Holloszy, ed. Baltimore: Williams and Wilkins, 1992.

4. Spirduso, W. W., and D. L. Cronin. Exercise dose-response effects on quality of life and independent living in older adults. *Medicine and Science in Sports and Exercise* 33(6): S598–S608, 2001.

5. Snow-Harter, C., and R. Marcus. Exercise, bone mineral density, and osteoporosis. In *Exercise and Sports Sciences Reviews,* Vol. 19, J. O. Holloszy, ed. Baltimore: Williams and Wilkins, 1991.

6. Dunn, A. L., M. H. Trivedi, and H. A. O'Neal. Physical activity dose-response effects on outcomes of depression and anxiety. *Medicine and Science in Sports and Exercise* 33(6):S587–S597, 2001.

7. Pette, D. Perspectives: Plasticity of mammalian skeletal muscle. *Journal of Applied Physiology* 90(3):1119–1124, 2001.

8. Kraemer, W. L., N. D. Duncan, and J. S. Volek. Resistance training and elite athletes: Adaptations and program considerations. *Journal of Orthopedic Sports and Physical Therapy* 28(2):110–119, 1998.

9. Fleck, S. J., and W. J. Kraemer. *Designing Resistance Training Programs.* Champaign, IL: Human Kinetics, 1997.

10. Kitai, T. A. Specificity of joint angle in isometric training. *European Journal of Applied Physiology* 58:744, 1989.

11. Powers, S., and E. Howley. *Exercise Physiology: Theory and Application to Fitness and Performance,* 4th ed. Dubuque, IA: McGraw-Hill, 2001.

12. Leveritt, M., P. J. Abernethy, B. K. Barry, and P. A. Logan. Concurrent strength and endurance training: A review. *Sports Medicine* 28(6):413–427, 1999.

13. Enoka, R. M. Neural adaptations with chronic physical activity. *Journal of Biomechanics* 30(5):447–455, 1997.

14. Shephard, R. J. Exercise and training in women, Part 1: Influence of gender on exercise and training responses. *Canadian Journal of Applied Physiology* 25(1):19–34, 2000.

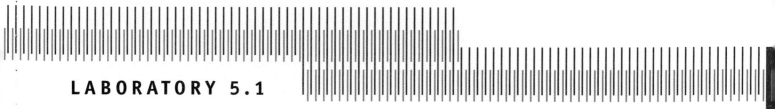

Strength-Training Log

NAME _____ DATE _____

The purpose of this log is to provide a record of progress in building strength in the upper and lower body.

DIRECTIONS

Record the date, number of sets, reps, and the weight for each of the exercises listed in the left column.

St/RP/Wt = Sets/Reps/Weights

Example: 2/6/80 = 2 sets of 6 reps each with 80 lbs.

DATE							
Exercise	St/Rp/Wt	St/Rp/Wt	St/Rp/Wt	St/Rp/Wt	St/Rp/Wt	St/Rp/Wt	St/Rp/Wt
Biceps curl							
Abdominal curl							
Leg extension							
Bench press							
Leg curl							
Lower back extension							
Upper back							
Hip and back							
Pullover							
Torso twist							
Triceps extension							
Chest press							

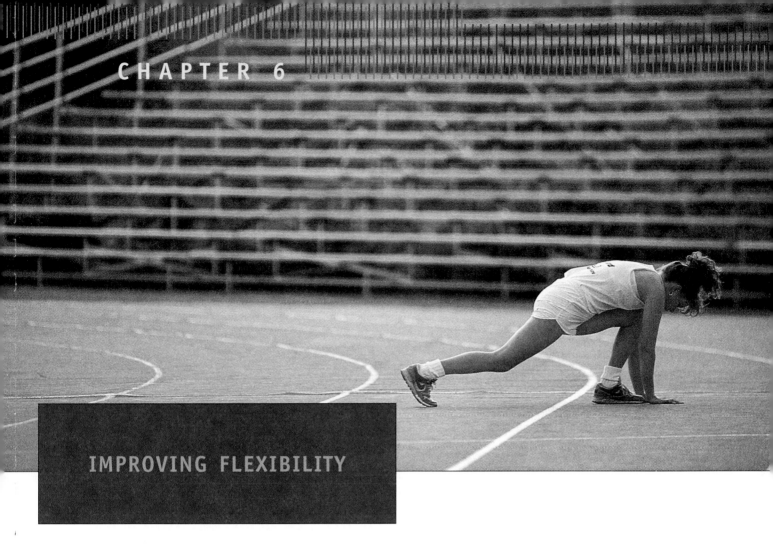

CHAPTER 6

IMPROVING FLEXIBILITY

After studying this chapter, you should be able to:

1. Discuss the value of flexibility.

2. Identify the structural and physiological limits to flexibility.

3. Discuss the stretch reflex.

4. Describe the three categories of stretching techniques.

5. Design a flexibility exercise program.

Flexibility is defined as the ability to move joints freely through their full range of motion. The full range of motion is determined in part by the shapes and positions of the bones that make up the joint, and in part by the composition and arrangement of muscles and tendons around the joint. For example, movement of the elbow (a hinge-type joint) is not limited solely by the arrangement of the bones themselves, because the soft connective tissues surrounding the joint also impose major limitations on the range of movement (1, 2).

Although flexibility varies among individuals because of differences in body structure, it is important to appreciate that flexibility is not a fixed property. The range of motion of most joints can be increased with proper training techniques or can decline with disuse. This chapter introduces exercises designed to improve flexibility.

☀ Benefits of Flexibility

The many benefits of increased flexibility include increased joint mobility, efficient body movement, and good posture (1, 2, 3, 4). Although it is commonly believed that stretching before exercise reduces the incidence of muscle injury during exercise, data from most research studies indicate that this is not the case. A recent critical review article concludes that there is no good evidence that stretching reduces muscle injury and, in fact, cites evidence suggesting that stretching may contribute to injury (5). The only studies suggesting that stretching offers protection from muscle injury combined the stretching with a general warm-up.

While all of these flexibility benefits are important, a key reason to improve flexibility is its role in the prevention of low back problems. For example, most low back pain is due to misalignment of the vertebral column and pelvic girdle caused by a lack of flexibility and/or weak muscles. Low back pain is a significant problem—more than one billion dollars is lost by U.S. business yearly due to reduced productivity by workers suffering from low back problems (3).

☀ Physiological Basis for Developing Flexibility

We have already noted that the limits to flexibility are determined by the way the joint is constructed as well as by the associated muscles and tendons. Let's discuss these factors in more detail.

STRUCTURAL LIMITATIONS TO MOVEMENT

Five primary factors contribute to the limits of movement: bone; muscle; connective tissue within the joint capsule (the joint capsule is composed of **ligaments,** which hold bones together, and **cartilage,** which cushions the ends of bones); **tendons,** which connect muscle to bones and to connective tissue surrounding joints; and skin. Exercise aimed at improving flexibility does not change the structure of bone, but it alters the soft tissues (i.e., muscle, joint connective tissue, and tendons) that contribute to flexibility. Table 6.1 lists the contribution of the various soft tissues to total joint flexibility. Note that the structures associated with the joint capsule, muscles, and tendons provide most of the body's resistance to movement. Therefore, exercises aimed at improving flexibility must alter one of these three factors in order to increase the range of motion around a joint. Stretching the ligaments in the joint capsule may lead to a loose joint that would be highly susceptible to injury. However, muscle and tendon are soft tissues that can lengthen over time with stretching exercises. Stretching exercises increase the range of motion in the joint by reducing the resistance to movement offered by tight muscles and tendons.

STRETCHING AND THE STRETCH REFLEX

Before we examine specific exercises for improving flexibility, it is useful to discuss a key physiological response to stretching exercises. Muscles contain special receptors, called *muscle spindles,* that are sensitive to stretch. When a doctor taps you on the knee with a

---

ligaments Connective tissue within the joint capsule that holds bones together.

cartilage A tough, connective tissue that forms a pad on the end of bones in certain joints, such as the elbow, knee, and ankle. Cartilage acts as a shock absorber to cushion the weight of one bone on another and to provide protection from the friction due to joint movement.

tendons Connective tissue that connects muscles to bones.

TABLE 6.1
Contribution of Soft-Tissue Structures to Limiting Joint Movement

Structure	Resistance to Flexibility (% of total)
Joint capsule	47
Muscle	41
Tendon	10
Skin	2

Nutritional Links

Can Diet Supplements Improve Joint Health?

The ends of the bones in joints are covered by a firm, resilient type of connective tissue called *cartilage,* which absorbs shock and provides smooth surfaces that aid joint movement. Cartilage mostly consists of a gel-like matrix of water, collagen fibers, and chains of sugar-based molecules (glycans) produced by cartilage cells. Joint injury, arthritis, and the natural process of aging can cause deterioration of cartilage in joints, which can lead to pain and reduced flexibility. As a result, preventing joint deterioration and stimulating the re-

generation of cartilage is important to joint health.

Several recent studies have investigated the effects of dietary supplements containing two key substances the body uses to produce cartilage. One substance, chondroitin, is thought to be important in reducing joint wear by combining with other molecules to increase the strength and resiliency of cartilage. The other substance, glucosamine, promotes regeneration of damaged cartilage matrix. Several of these studies have shown that individuals with cartilage deterio-

ration who take glucosamine and chondroitin have thicker joint cartilage compared to controls (5).

Although these results and the apparent lack of side effects of taking these supplements are encouraging, it is not yet known whether taking chondroitin and glucosamine provides long-term improvements in joint health. If you have joint pain or other joint problems, consult your physician to determine whether supplementation with these products might be beneficial for you.

rubber hammer, for example, the rapid stretching of muscle spindles results in a "reflex" contraction of the muscle to prevent it from stretching too far too fast. This reflex contraction, called **stretch reflex,** is counterproductive to stretching exercises because the muscle is shortening instead of lengthening. Fortunately, the stretch reflex can be avoided when muscles and tendons are stretched very slowly. In fact, if a muscle stretch is held for several seconds, the muscle spindles allow the muscle being stretched to further relax and permit an even greater stretch (2, 3). Therefore, stretching exercises are most effective when they avoid promoting a stretch reflex.

IN SUMMARY

- Flexibility is defined as the range of motion of a joint.
- Improved flexibility results in the following benefits: increased joint mobility, resistance to muscle injury, prevention of low back problems, efficient body movement, and improved posture and personal appearance.
- The structural and physiological limits to flexibility are (1) bone, (2) muscle, (3) structures within the joint capsule, (4) the tendons which connect muscle to bones and to connective tissue surrounding joints, and (5) skin.
- If muscle spindles are stretched suddenly, they respond by initiating a stretch reflex that causes the muscle to contract and shorten. However, if the

muscles and tendons are stretched slowly, the stretch reflex can be avoided.

Designing a Flexibility Training Program

Three kinds of stretching techniques are commonly used to increase flexibility: ballistic stretching, static stretching, and proprioceptive neuromuscular facilitation (2, 7). However, because ballistic stretching (quick, bouncing movements that briefly stretch muscles) promotes the stretch reflex and increases the risk of injury to muscles and tendons, only the static and proprioceptive neuromuscular facilitation methods are recommended. For this reason, we do not discuss ballistic stretching techniques. A brief discussion of static and proprioceptive neuromuscular facilitation techniques follows.

STATIC STRETCHING

Static stretching is extremely effective for improving flexibility and has gained popularity over the last decade (2, 4). Static stretching slowly lengthens a

stretch reflex Involuntary contraction of a muscle that occurs due to rapid stretching of that muscle.
static stretching Stretching that slowly lengthens a muscle to a point where further movement is limited.

muscle to a point at which further movement is limited (slight discomfort is felt) and requires holding this position for a fixed period of time. The optimal amount of time to hold the stretch for maximal improvement in flexibility is unknown. However, most investigators agree that holding the stretch position for 20 to 30 seconds (repeated three to four times) results in an improvement in flexibility. Compared with ballistic stretching, the risk of injury associated with static stretching is minimal. Another benefit of static stretching is that, when performed during the cool-down period, it may reduce the muscle stiffness associated with some exercise routines (2, 4).

PROPRIOCEPTIVE NEUROMUSCULAR FACILITATION

A relatively new technique for improving flexibility, **proprioceptive neuromuscular facilitation (PNF),** combines stretching with alternating contraction and relaxation of muscles. There are two common types of PNF stretching: contract-relax (CR) stretching and contract-relax/antagonist contract (CRAC) stretching. The CR stretch technique calls for first contracting the muscle to be stretched. Then, after relaxing the muscle, the muscle is slowly stretched. The CRAC method calls for the same contract-relax routine but adds to this the contraction of the **antagonist** muscle, the muscle on the opposite side of the joint. The purpose of contracting the antagonist muscle is to promote a reflex relaxation of the muscle to be stretched.

How do PNF techniques compare with ballistic and static stretching? First, PNF has been shown to be safer and more effective in promoting flexibility than ballistic stretching (7). Further, studies have shown PNF programs to be equal to, or in some cases superior to, static stretching for improving flexibility (8). However, one disadvantage of PNF stretching is that some stretches require a partner.

---

proprioceptive neuromuscular facilitation (PNF)
A technique that combines stretching with alternating contraction and relaxation of muscles to improve flexibility. There are two common types of PNF stretching: contract-relax (CR) stretching and contract-relax/antagonist contract (CRAC) stretching.
antagonist The muscle on the opposite side of the joint.

The following steps illustrate how a CRAC procedure can be done with a partner (Figure 6.1):

1. After the assistant moves the limb in the direction necessary to stretch the desired muscles to the point of tightness (mild discomfort is felt), the subject isometrically contracts the muscle being stretched for 3 to 5 seconds and then relaxes them.

2. The subject then moves the limb in the opposite direction of the stretch by isometrically contracting the antagonist muscles. The subject holds this isometric contraction for approximately 5 seconds, during which time the muscles to be stretched relax. While the desired muscles are relaxed, the assistant may increase the stretch of the desired muscles.

3. The subject then isometrically contracts the antagonist muscles for another 5 seconds, which relaxes the desired muscles, and then the assistant again stretches the desired muscles to the point of mild discomfort.

This cycle of three steps is repeated three to five times. Figure 6.1 illustrates a partner-assisted CRAC procedure for stretching the calf muscles.

Figure 6.2 shows how some PNF stretches can be done without a partner.

☀ IN SUMMARY

- Static stretches involve stretching a muscle to the limit of movement and holding the stretch for an extended period of time.
- Proprioceptive neuromuscular facilitation (PNF) combines stretching with alternating contraction and relaxation of muscles to improve flexibility.

☀ Exercise Prescription for Improving Flexibility

For safety reasons, all flexibility programs should consist of either PNF or static stretching exercises. The frequency and duration of a stretching exercise prescription should be 2 to 5 days per week for 10 to 30 minutes each day. The first week of a stretching regimen is considered the starter phase. The first week should consist of one stretching session, and one session should be added per week during the first 4 weeks of the slow progression phase of the program. Initially, the duration of each training session should be approximately 5 minutes and should increase gradually to approximately 20 to 30 minutes following 6 to 12 weeks of stretching during the slow progression phase.

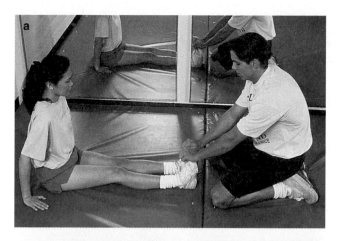

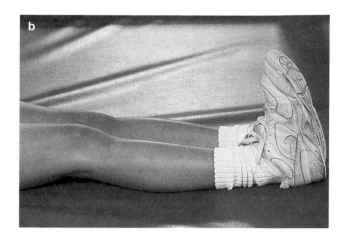

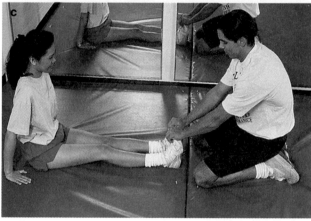

FIGURE 6.1
An example of a partner-assisted CRAC procedure for stretching the calf muscles. The subject contracts the calf muscles against resistance provided by the assistant (a). Unassisted, the subject contracts the shin (antagonist) muscles, which relaxes the calf muscles (b). While the subject continues the contraction of the shin muscles, the assistant stretches the calf muscles (c).

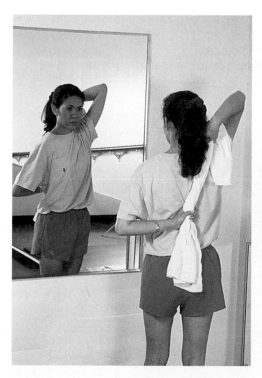

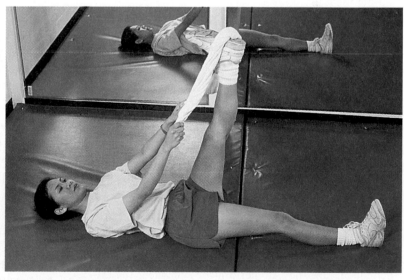

FIGURE 6.2
Examples of how PNF stretches may be done without a partner. What other creative ways to self-assist with PNF stretches can you devise?

TABLE 6.2
Sample Flexibility Program with Considerations for Duration of Stretch Hold, Number of Repetitions, and Frequency of Training

Week No.	Phase	Duration of Stretch Hold	Repetitions	Frequency (times/wk)
1	Starter	15 sec	1	1
2	Slow progression	20 sec	2	2
3	Slow progression	25 sec	3	3
4	Slow progression	30 sec	4	3
5	Slow progression	30 sec	4	3–4
6	Slow progression	30 sec	4	4–5
7+	Maintenance	30 sec	4	4–5

The physiological rationale for increasing the duration of stretching is that each stretch position is held for progressively longer durations as the program continues. For example, begin by holding each stretched position for 15 seconds, then add 5 seconds each week up to 30 seconds. Start by performing each of the exercises once (1 rep) and progress to 4 reps. Table 6.2 illustrates a sample exercise prescription for a flexibility program.

What about the intensity of stretching? In general, a limb should not be stretched beyond a position of mild discomfort. The intensity of stretching is increased simply by extending the stretch nearer to the limits of your range of motion. Your range of motion will gradually increase as your flexibility improves during the training program.

To improve overall flexibility, all major muscle groups should be stretched. Exercises 6.1 through 6.12 illustrate the proper methods of performing 12 different stretching exercises. Integrate these exercises into the program outlined in Table 6.2.

These exercises are designed to be used in a regular program of stretching to increase flexibility. The exercises presented involve the joints and major muscle groups for which range of motion tends to decrease with age and disuse. The exercises include both static and PNF movements and may require a partner.

HOW TO AVOID HAZARDOUS EXERCISES

Many exercises are potentially harmful to the musculoskeletal system. Which exercises actually cause injury depends on how they are performed. Remember the following key points during an exercise session to help prevent injury:

- Avoid breathholding. Try to breath as normally as possible during the exercise.
- Avoid full flexion of the knee or neck.
- Avoid full extension of the knee, neck, or back.
- Do not stretch muscles that are already stretched, such as the abdominal muscles.
- Do not stretch to the point that joint pain occurs.
- Use extreme caution when using an assistant to help with passive stretches.
- Avoid forceful extension and flexion of the spine.

Many commonly practiced exercises may cause injuries and are therefore contraindicated. The illustrations starting on page 141 show some of these exercises (contraindicated exercises) and provide alternatives (substitute exercises) to accomplish the same goals.

IN SUMMARY

- Stretching exercises should be performed 2 to 5 days per week for 10 to 30 minutes each day.
- Week one, the "starter" phase, consists of one stretching session lasting approximately 5 minutes.
- Weeks 2 through 4 are "progression" weeks during which one session should be added each week.
- The duration of stretching exercise sessions should be increased gradually up to 20–30 minutes over 10 to 12 weeks.
- The intensity of a stretch is considered to be maximal where "mild discomfort" is felt.

Sample Flexibility Exercises

EXERCISE 6.1   LOWER LEG STRETCH

Purpose: To stretch the calf muscles and the Achilles' tendon.

Position: Stand on the edge of a surface that is high enough to allow the heel to be lower than the toes. Have a support nearby to hold for balance.

Movement: Rise on the toes as far as possible for several seconds (a), then lower the heels as far as possible (b). Shift your body weight from one leg to the other for added stretch of the muscles.

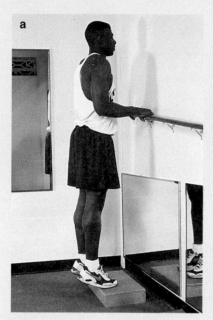

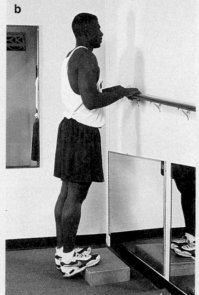

EXERCISE 6.2   INSIDE LEG STRETCH

Purpose: To stretch the muscle on the inside of the thighs.

Position: Sit with bottoms of the feet together and the hands placed just below the knees.

Movement: Using the hands and forearms to resist an effort to raise the knees. Then relax and, using your hands, press the knees toward the floor and hold for several seconds.

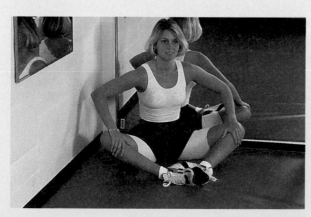

Sample Flexibility Exercises

EXERCISE 6.3   ONE-LEG STRETCH

Purpose: To stretch the lower back muscles and muscles in the back of the thigh.

Position: Stand with the heel of one foot on a support approximately knee-to-waist high. Keep both legs straight.

Movement: Press the heel down on the support for several seconds (a); then relax and bend forward at the waist and attempt to touch your head to your knee, and hold for several seconds (b). Return to the upright position and alternate legs.

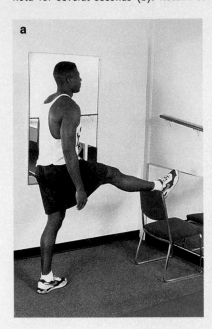
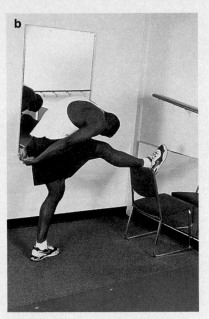

EXERCISE 6.4   LOWER BACK STRETCH

Purpose: To stretch the lower back and buttocks muscles.

Position: Lying on your back with the feet flat on the floor.

Movement: First, arch your back and lift the hips off the floor, and hold for several seconds (a). Relax and place your hands behind the knees. Pull the knees to the chest and hold for several seconds (b). Repeat the sequence for the desired number of repetitions.

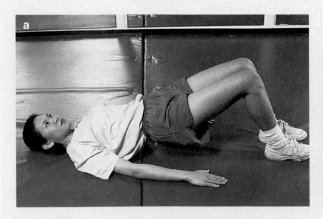
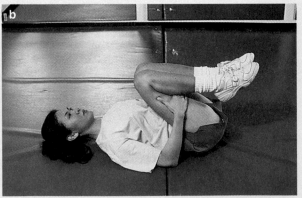

Sample Flexibility Exercises

EXERCISE 6.5
CHEST STRETCH

Purpose: To stretch the muscles across the chest.

Position: Stand in a doorway and grasp the frame of the doorway at shoulder height.

Movement: Press forward on the frame for ~5 seconds. Then, relax and shift your weight forward until you feel the stretch of muscles across the chest, and hold for several seconds.

EXERCISE 6.6
SIDE STRETCH

Purpose: To stretch the muscles of the upper arm and side of the trunk.

Position: Sitting on the floor with legs crossed.

Movement: Stretch one arm over the head while bending at the waist in the same direction. With the opposite arm, reach across the chest as far as possible. Hold for several seconds. Do not rotate the trunk; try to stretch the muscle on the same side of the trunk as the overhead arm. Alternate arms to stretch the other side of the trunk.

EXERCISE 6.7
THIGH STRETCH

Purpose: To stretch the muscles in the front of the thigh of the extended (rear) leg.

Position: Kneel on one knee, resting the rear foot on the ball of the foot and placing the forward foot flat on the floor.

Movement: Lean forward and place your hands on the floor on either side of the forward foot. Lift the knee off the floor and slide the rear leg backward so that the knee is slightly behind the hips; then press the hips forward and down, and hold for several seconds. While stretching, maintain approximately a 90° angle at the knee of the front leg. Switch the positions of the legs to stretch the other thigh.

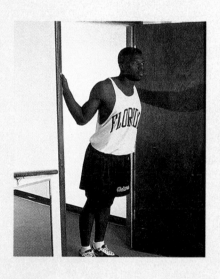 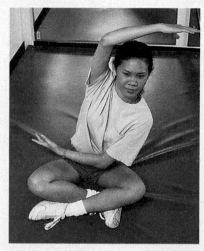 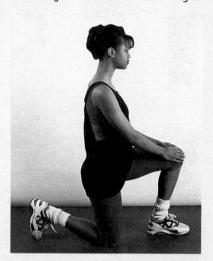

EXERCISE 6.8   SPINE TWISTER

Purpose: To stretch the muscles that rotate the trunk and thighs.

Position: Lie on your back, with one leg crossed over the other and both shoulders and both arms on the floor (a).

Movement: Rotate the trunk such that the crossed-over leg stays on top and both knees approach or touch the floor (b); hold for several seconds. The shoulders and arms should remain on the floor all during the stretch. Reverse the positions of the legs and repeat the stretch.

a

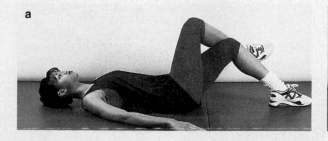

b

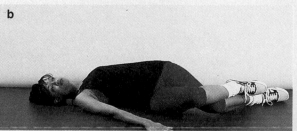

Sample Flexibility Exercises

EXERCISE 6.9   NECK STRETCH

Purpose: To stretch the muscles that rotate the neck.

Position: After turning the head to one side, place the hand against the cheek with fingers toward the ear and elbow forward.

Movement: Try to turn the head and neck against the resistance of the hand; hold for a few seconds. Remove the hand and relax, and then turn the head as far as possible in the same direction as before. Hold this position for several seconds. Then repeat the stretch, this time turning in the other direction.

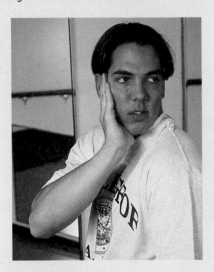

EXERCISE 6.10   SHIN STRETCH

Purpose: To stretch the muscles of the shin.

Position: Kneel on both knees, with the trunk rotated to one side and the hand on that side pressing down on the ankle.

Movement: While pressing down on the ankle, move the pelvis forward; hold for several seconds. Repeat on the other side.

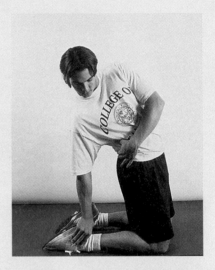

EXERCISE 6.11   LEG STRETCH

Purpose: To stretch the muscles on the back of the hip, the back of the thigh, and the calf.

Position: Lying on your back, bring one knee toward the chest and grasp the toes with the hand on the same side. Place the opposite hand on the back of the leg just below the knee.

Movement: Pull the knee toward the chest while pushing the heel toward the ceiling and pulling the toes toward the shin. Straighten the knee until you feel sufficient stretch in the muscles of the back of the leg, and hold for several seconds. Repeat for the other leg.

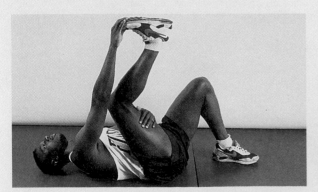

EXERCISE 6.12   TRUNK TWISTER

Purpose: To stretch the trunk muscles and the muscles of the hip.

Position: Sit with the left leg extended, the right leg bent and crossed over the left knee, and the right foot on the floor. Place the right hand on the floor behind the buttocks.

Movement: Placing the left arm on the right side of the right thigh and the left hand on the floor, use the left arm to push against the right leg while twisting the trunk to the right. Hold for several seconds. Then assume the starting position with the right leg extended and so forth, and stretch the opposite side of the body.

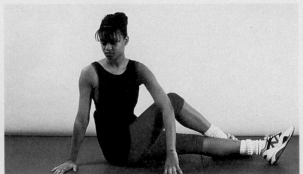

Contraindicated Exercise

Substitute Exercise

ARM CIRCLES (PALMS DOWN)

Purpose: To strengthen the muscles of the shoulder and upper back.

Problem: May result in irritation of the shoulder joint and, if circled forward and down, results in the use of the chest muscles instead of back muscles.

ARM CIRCLES (PALMS UP)

In a sitting position, turn the palms up and circle the arms backward and up.

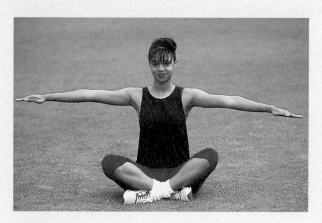

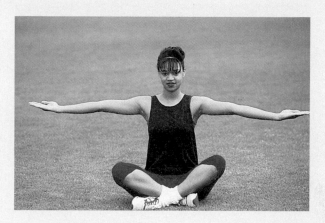

KNEE PULL

Purpose: To stretch the lower back and buttocks.

Problem: Places undue stress on the knee joint.

LEG PULL

Lying on your back, pull the knee toward the chest by pulling on the back of the leg just below the knee. Then, extend the knee joint and point the sole of the foot straight up. Continue to pull the leg toward your chest. Repeat several times with each leg.

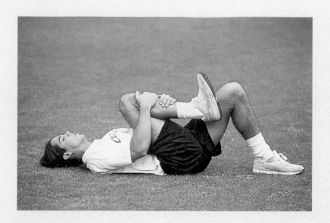

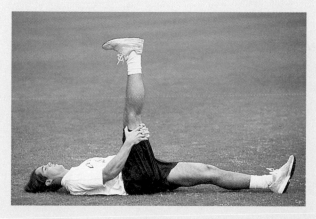

Contraindicated Exercise

Substitute Exercise

DEEP KNEE BENDS

Purpose: To strengthen the upper leg and stretch the lower leg.

Problem: This movement hyperflexes the knee and "opens" the joint while stretching the ligaments.

LUNGES

While standing, step forward with either foot and touch the opposite knee to the ground. Repeat with the opposite leg.

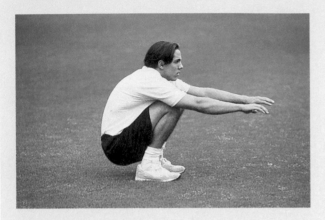

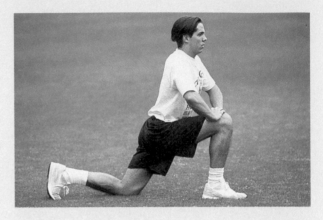

LEG LIFTS

Purpose: To strengthen the abdominal muscles.

Problem: This exercise primarily recruits the hip flexor muscles and thus does not accomplish the intended purpose. These muscles are likely strong enough and do not need strengthening. In addition, this exercise produces excess compression on the vertebral disks.

REVERSE CURL

Lie on your back with the knees bent and the arms and feet flat on the ground. Maintaining about the same degree of bend at the knee joint, pull the knees up toward the chest so that the hips leave the ground. Do not allow the knees to go past the shoulders. Lower the legs back to the ground and repeat.

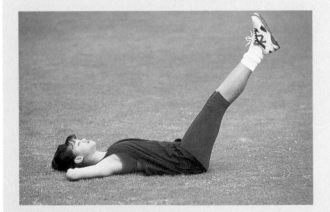

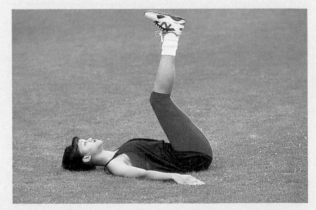

Contraindicated Exercise

STANDING TOE TOUCH

Purpose: To stretch the lower back, buttocks, and hamstrings.

Problems: First, hyperflexion of the knee could cause damage to ligaments and, second, if performed with the back flat, damage could occur to the lower back.

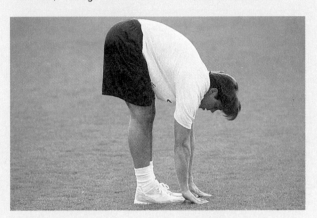

SIT-UP (HANDS BEHIND HEAD)

Purpose: To strengthen the abdominal muscles.

Problem: With hands behind the head, there is a tendency to jerk on the head and neck to "throw" yourself up. This could cause hyperflexion of the neck. In addition, sitting up with the back straight places undue strain on the lower back.

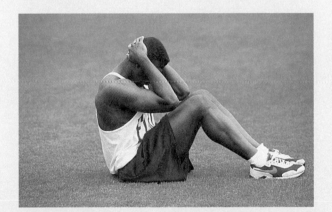

Substitute Exercise

SITTING HAMSTRING STRETCH

Sit at leg-length from a wall. With your foot on the wall and the other knee bent with the foot between the wall and buttocks, bend forward keeping the lower back straight. The bent knee can fall to the side.

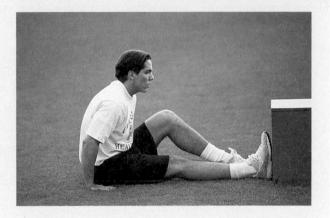

CURL UP

Keeping the knees bent while lying on your back, cross your arms over your chest so that your fingers rest on your shoulders. Using the abdominal muscles, curl up until the upper half of the back is off the floor and then return to the starting position.

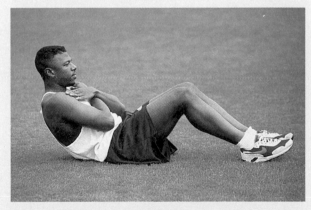

Contraindicated Exercise

NECK CIRCLES

Purpose: To stretch the neck muscles.

Problem: Hyperextension of the neck should always be avoided. This can pinch arteries and nerves, as well as damage disks in the spine.

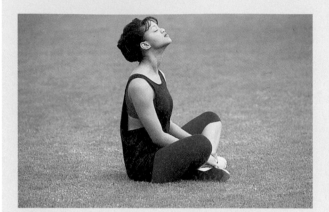

DONKEY KICK

Purpose: To stretch and strengthen the buttocks.

Problem: When kicking the leg back, most people hyperextend the neck and/or back.

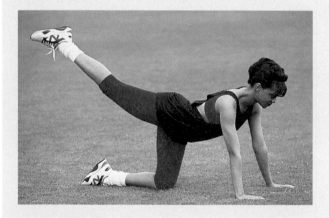

Substitute Exercise

NECK STRETCHES

In a sitting position, with your head and neck straight, move your head down to flex the neck, and return the head upright. Then, slowly turn your head from side to side as far as possible; attempt to point your chin at each shoulder.

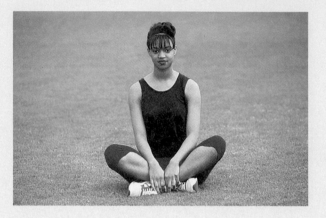

KNEE-TO-NOSE TOUCH

While on your hands and knees, lift one knee toward your nose and then extend that leg to horizontal. Alternate legs. Remember: Your leg should not go higher than your hips, and your neck should remain in line with your back.

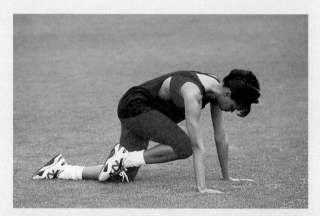

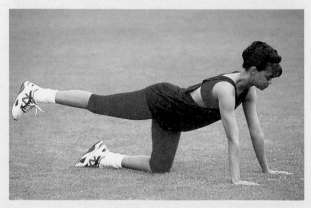

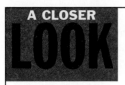

A CLOSER LOOK

When Muscles Cramp

Muscle cramps are one of the most common problems encountered in sports and exercise. For many years the primary causes of muscle cramps were thought to be dehydration and/or electrolyte imbalances. Accordingly, drinking enough fluids and ensuring that the diet contains sufficient amounts of sodium (from table salt, for example) and potassium (from bananas, for example) have long been encouraged as preventive measures. Whenever muscles cramp, stretching and/or massage have been used to relieve the cramping until electrolyte balance can be restored.

More recent research, however, suggests that cramping may be due to abnormal spinal control of motor neuron activity, especially when a muscle contracts while shortened (9). Thus, for example, the cramping that often occurs in the calf muscles of recreational swimmers when their toes are pointed may occur because those calf muscles are contracting while they are shortened.

The most prevalent risk factors for cramps during exercise are muscle fatigue and poor stretching habits (failure to stretch regularly and long enough during each session). Other risk factors include older age, higher body mass index, and a family history of muscle cramps.

If cramping occurs, you should:

• Passively stretch the muscle. Such stretching induces receptors that sense the stretch to initiate nerve impulses that inhibit muscle stimulation.

• Drink plenty of water to avoid dehydration or electrolyte imbalances. Sports drinks can help replenish glucose and electrolytes, but do *not* use salt tablets.

• Seek medical attention if multiple muscle groups are involved, because this could be a sign of more serious problems.

Although no strategies for preventing muscle cramping during exercise have been proven effective, regular stretching using PNF techniques, correction of muscle balance and posture, and proper training for the exercise activity involved may be beneficial.

☀ Motivation to Maintain Flexibility

Maintaining flexibility requires a lifetime commitment to performing regular stretching. Just as in other types of fitness training, good time management is critical if you are going to succeed. Set aside time for 3 to 5 stretching periods per week, and stick to your schedule. A key point to remember is that stretching can be performed almost anywhere because it does not require special equipment. So take advantage of "windows" of free time in your day and plan stretching workouts.

You are not likely to maintain a lifetime stretching program if you do not enjoy your workouts. One suggestion for making stretching more fun is to perform stretching workouts while listening to music or during a television program you enjoy. This will allow time to pass more rapidly and will make your stretching workout more pleasant.

As in other aspects of physical fitness, establishing short-term and long-term flexibility goals is important in maintaining the motivation to stretch. Further, keeping a record of your workouts and improvements allows you to follow your flexibility progress and plan your future training schedule (Laboratory 6.1, page 147). So, establish your stretching goals today and get started toward a lifetime of flexibility.

Summary

1. *Flexibility* is defined as the range of motion of a joint.

2. Improved flexibility results in the following benefits: increased joint mobility, prevention of low back problems, efficient body movement, and improved posture and personal appearance.

3. The five structural and physiological limits to flexibility are bone, muscle, structures within the joint capsule, the tendons that connect muscle to bones and connective tissue that surrounds joints, and skin.

4. If muscle spindles are suddenly stretched, they respond by initiating a stretch reflex that causes the muscle to contract. However, if the muscles and tendons are stretched slowly, the stretch reflex can be avoided.

5. Static stretches involve stretching a muscle to the limit of movement and holding the stretch for an extended period of time.

6. Proprioceptive neuromuscular facilitation combines stretching with alternating contraction and relaxation of muscles to improve flexibility.

Study Questions

1. Define the following terms:
   antagonist
   cartilage
   flexibility
   proprioceptive neuromuscular facilitation
2. Describe the difference in function between ligaments and tendons.
3. Compare static and ballistic stretching.
4. List three primary reasons why maintaining flexibility is important.
5. List all of the factors that limit flexibility. Which factors place the greatest limitations on flexibility?
6. Compare and contrast the two recommended methods of stretching.
7. Briefly outline the exercise prescription for improvement of flexibility.
8. Describe why the stretch reflex is counterproductive to stretching, and explain how this reflex can be avoided.

Suggested Reading

DeVries, H., and T. Housh. *Physiology of Exercise,* 5th ed. Dubuque, IA: Brown and Benchmark, 1994.

Fox, E., R. Bowers, and M. Foss. *The Physiological Basis for Exercise and Sports,* 6th ed. Dubuque, IA: Brown and Benchmark, 1997.

Golding, L. A. Flexibility, stretching, and flexibility testing. *ACSM's Health and Fitness Journal* 1(2):17–20, 1997.

Hutton, R. S. Neuromuscular basis of stretching exercises. In *Strength and Power in Sport,* P. V. Komi, ed. Oxford: Blackwell Scientific, 1992.

Powers, S., and E. Howley. *Exercise Physiology: Theory Application to Fitness and Performance,* 3rd ed. Dubuque, IA: Brown and Benchmark, 1997.

For links to the Web sites below visit Web Links at www.aw.com/fitness and choose Powers/Dodd Web Links from the drop-down menu.

Sports Medicine

Presents detailed information on all aspects of sports medicine.

Fitness Tests

Describes tests for aerobic power, anaerobic power, flexibility, and body composition.

Fitness Files

Covers fitness fundamentals, flexibility and contraindicated exercises, exercise nutrition, and treating exercise injuries.

Meriter Fitness

Discusses injury prevention and treatment, weight training, flexibility, exercise prescriptions, and more.

References

1. Kubo, K., H. Kanehisa, Y. Kawakami, and T. Fukunaga. Influence of static stretching on viscoelastic properties of human tendon structures in vivo. *Journal of Applied Physiology* 90(2):520–526, 2001.
2. Hutton, R. S. Neuromuscular basis of stretching exercises. In *Strength and Power in Sport,* P. V. Komi, ed. Oxford: Blackwell Scientific, 1992.
3. McGill, S. M. Low back stability: From formal description to issues for performance and rehabilitation. *Exercise and Sport Sciences Review* 29(1):26–31, 2001.
4. American College of Sports Medicine. The recommended quantity and quality of exercise for developing and maintaining cardiorespiratory and muscular fitness, and flexibility in healthy adults. *Medicine and Science in Sports and Exercise* 30(6):975–991, 1998.
5. Shrier, I. Stretching before exercise does not reduce the risk of local muscle injury: A critical review of the clinical and basic science literature. *Clinical Journal of Sport Medicine* 9(4):221–227, 1999.
6. Deal, C. L., and R. W. Moskowitz. Neutraceuticals as therapeutic agents in osteoarthritis. The role of glucosamine, chondroitin sulfate, and collagen hydrolysate. *Rheumatic Disease Clinics of North America* 25(2):379–395, 1999.
7. McAtee, Robert. *Facilitated Stretching,* 2nd ed. Champaign, IL: Human Kinetics, 1999.
8. Etnyre, B. R., and E. J. Lee. Comments on proprioceptive neuromuscular facilitation stretching techniques. *Research Quarterly for Exercise and Sport* 58:184–188, 1987.
9. Bentley, S. Exercise-induced muscle cramp. Proposed mechanisms and management. *Sports Medicine* 21(6): 409–420, 1996.

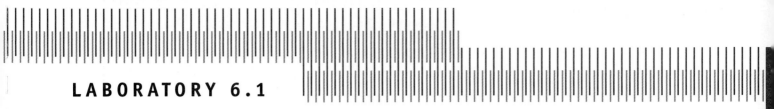

LABORATORY 6.1

Flexibility Progression Log

NAME _____ **DATE** _____

The purpose of this log is to provide a record of progress in increasing flexibility in selected joints.

DIRECTIONS

Record the date, sets and hold time for each of the exercises listed in the left column.

St/Hold = Sets and hold time

Example: 2/30 = 2 sets held for 30 seconds each.

DATE _____

Exercise	St/Hold	St/Hold	St/Hold	St/Hold	St/Hold	St/Hold	St/Hold
Lower leg stretch							
Inside leg stretch							
One-leg stretch							
Lower back stretch							
Chest stretch							
Side stretch							
Thigh stretch							
Spine twister							
Neck stretch							
Shin stretch							
Leg stretch							
Trunk twister							

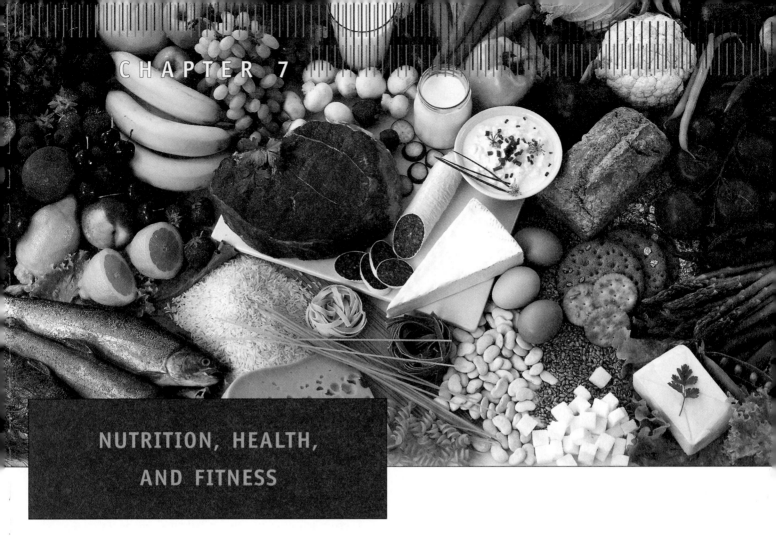

CHAPTER 7

NUTRITION, HEALTH, AND FITNESS

After studying this chapter, you should be able to:

1. Define macro- and micronutrients.

2. Describe the macronutrients and the primary functions of each.

3. Discuss the energy content of fats, carbohydrates, and proteins in the body.

4. Describe the micronutrients and the primary functions of each.

5. Discuss the value of water in the diet.

6. List the dietary guidelines for a well-balanced diet.

7. Define the term *calorie*.

8. Describe the need for protein, carbohydrate, and vitamins for physically active individuals.

9. Define the term *dietary supplement,* and discuss governmental regulations for marketing such supplements.

10. Discuss the benefits of irradiation of foods.

Nutrition can be broadly defined as the study of food and the way the body uses it to produce energy and build or repair body tissues. Good nutrition means that an individual's diet supplies all of the essential foodstuffs required to maintain a healthy body. Although dietary deficiencies were once a problem in many industrialized countries, a primary danger associated with nutrition today is overeating.

Many diets are high in calories (A Closer Look), sugar, fats, and sodium, and diseases linked to these dietary excesses, such as cardiovascular disease, cancer, obesity, and diabetes, are the leading killers in the United States today (1). According to the U.S. Department of Health and Human Services, over one-half of all deaths in the United States are associated with health problems linked to poor nutrition (2). Nevertheless, through diet analysis and modification, it is possible to prevent many of these nutrition-related diseases. An elementary understanding of nutrition is therefore important for everyone. This chapter outlines the fundamental concepts of good nutrition and provides guidelines for developing a healthy diet. We also discuss how exercise training can modify nutritional requirements.

☀ Basic Nutrition

Substances in food that are necessary for good health are called **nutrients.** They can be divided into two categories: macronutrients and micronutrients. **Macronutrients,** which consist of carbohydrates, fats, and proteins, are necessary for building and maintaining body tissues and providing energy for daily activities. **Micronutrients** include all other substances in food, such as vitamins and minerals, that regulate the functions of the cells.

---

nutrients   Substances in food that are necessary for good health.

macronutrients   Carbohydrates, fats, and proteins, which are necessary for building and maintaining body tissues and providing energy for daily activities.

micronutrients   Nutrients in food, such as vitamins and minerals, that regulate the functions of the cells.

carbohydrates   One of the macronutrients; they are especially important during many types of physical activity because they are a key energy source for muscular contraction. Dietary sources of carbohydrates are breads, grains, fruits, and vegetables.

glucose   The most noteworthy of the simple sugars because it is the only sugar molecule that can be used by the body in its natural form. All other carbohydrates must first be converted to glucose to be used for fuel.

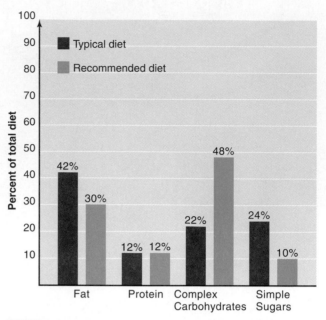

FIGURE 7.1
The recommended nutritionally balanced diet compared with the typical U.S. diet.

MACRONUTRIENTS

A well-balanced diet is composed of approximately 58% carbohydrates, 30% fat, and 12% protein (Figure 7.1).

These macronutrients are called "fuel nutrients" because they are the only substances that can provide the energy necessary for bodily functions. Under normal conditions, carbohydrates and fats are the primary fuels used by the body to produce energy. The primary function of protein is to serve as the body's "building blocks" to repair tissues. However, when carbohydrate is in short supply or the body is under stress, protein can be used as a fuel.

Table 7.1 lists the major food sources and the energy contents of carbohydrates, proteins, and fats. Given the importance of dietary carbohydrates, proteins, and fats to health and fitness, we discuss these macronutrients in more detail.

CARBOHYDRATES   **Carbohydrates** are especially important during many types of physical activity because they are a key energy source for muscular contraction. Dietary sources of carbohydrates are breads, grains, fruits, and vegetables. Carbohydrates can be divided into two major classes and several subclasses. (See Table 7.2 on page 152.)

Simple Carbohydrates. Simple carbohydrates consist of one or two of the simple sugars shown in Table 7.2. **Glucose** is the most noteworthy of the simple sugars because it is the only sugar molecule that can be used by the body in its natural form. To be used for fuel, all other carbohydrates must first be converted to

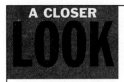

What Is a Calorie?

A **calorie** is the unit of measure used to quantify the energy in foods or the energy expended by the body. Technically, a calorie is the amount of energy necessary to raise the temperature of 1 gram of water 1°C. The amount of energy contained in one serving of a particular food or the amount used during exercise is typically *several hundred thousand calories!* To simplify discussing such large numbers, we measure and report calories contained in foods and energy expended during exercise in thousands of calories, or kilocalories (kcals). For example, one serving of a particular food may contain 100,000 calories, or 100 kcals. Thus, when you read "100 calories" on a food label, this actually refers to 100 kcals. This textbook uses "calorie" and "kcal" interchangeably.

TABLE 7.1
Food Sources and Energy Content of the Macronutrients

Carbohydrate (4 calories/gram)	Protein (4 calories/gram)	Fat (9 calories/gram)
Grains	Meats	Butter
Fruits	Fish	Margarine
Vegetables	Poultry	Oils
Concentrated sweets	Eggs	Shortening
Breads	Milk	Cream
Beans/peas	Beans	
	Rice	

---

glucose. After a meal, glucose is stored by skeletal muscles and the liver as **glycogen,** a molecule composed of a chain of glucose molecules. The glucose remaining in the blood thereafter is often converted to fat and stored in fat cells as a future source of energy.

The body requires glucose to function normally. Indeed, the central nervous system uses glucose almost exclusively for its energy needs. If dietary intake of carbohydrates is inadequate, the body must make glucose from protein. This is undesirable because it results in the breakdown of body protein for use as fuel. Dietary carbohydrate is not only important as a direct fuel source, but also important for its protein-sparing effect.

Other types of simple sugars include fructose, galactose, lactose, maltose, and sucrose. **Fructose,** or fruit sugar, is a naturally occurring sugar found in fruits and in honey. **Galactose** is a sugar found in the breast milk of humans and other mammals. **Lactose** (composed of galactose and glucose) and **maltose** (composed of two glucose molecules linked together) are best known as milk sugar and malt sugar, respectively. **Sucrose** (table sugar) is composed of glucose and fructose. A key point to remember about these simple sugars is that each must be converted to glucose before it can be used by the body.

Complex Carbohydrates. Complex carbohydrates provide both micronutrients and the glucose necessary for producing energy. They are contained in starches

calorie The unit of measure used to quantify food energy or the energy expended by the body. Technically, a calorie is the amount of energy necessary to raise the temperature of 1 gram of water 1°C.

glycogen The storage form of glucose in the liver and skeletal muscles.

fructose Also called *fruit sugar;* a naturally occurring sugar found in fruits and in honey.

galactose A simple sugar found in the breast milk of humans and other mammals.

lactose Also called *milk sugar;* a simple sugar found in milk products; it is composed of galactose and glucose.

maltose Also called *malt sugar;* a simple sugar found in grain products; it is composed of two glucose molecules linked together.

sucrose Also called *table sugar;* a molecule composed of glucose and fructose.

complex carbohydrates Carbohydrates that provide both micronutrients and the glucose necessary for producing energy. They are contained in starches and fiber.

TABLE 7.2
A Classification of Carbohydrates and the Sources of Each

Major Classifications of Carbohydrates	Subclasses of Carbohydrates	Food Sources
Simple carbohydrates (simple sugars)	Fructose	Fruits and honey
	Galactose	Breast milk
	Glucose	All sugars
	Lactose	Milk sugar
	Maltose	Malt sugar
	Sucrose	Table sugar
Complex carbohydrates	Starches	Potatoes, rice bread
	Fiber	Fruits, vegetables, bread

and fiber. **Starches** are long chains of sugars commonly found in foods such as corn, grains, potatoes, peas, and beans. Starch is stored in the body as glycogen and, as previously discussed, is used for that sudden burst of energy we often need during physical activity. **Fiber** is a stringy, nondigestible carbohydrate found in whole grains, vegetables, and fruits in its primary form, cellulose. Because fiber is nondigestible, it is not a fuel source; nor does it provide micronutrients. It is, however, a key ingredient in a healthy diet.

In recent years, nutrition researchers have shown that dietary fiber provides bulk in the intestinal tract. This bulk aids in the formation and elimination of food waste products, thus reducing the time necessary for wastes to move through the digestive system and lowering the risk of colon cancer. Dietary fiber is also thought to be a factor in reducing the risk for coronary heart disease and breast cancer, and in controlling blood sugar in diabetics (3). Some types of fiber bind with cholesterol in the digestive tract and prevent its absorption into the blood, thereby reducing blood cholesterol levels.

Although a minimum of 25 grams of fiber are recommended on a daily basis, excessive amounts of fiber in the diet can cause intestinal discomfort and decreased absorption of calcium and iron into the blood

(3). To increase the fiber in your diet, it is recommended that you:

- Eat a variety of foods.
- Eat at least five servings of fruits and vegetables and three to six servings of whole-grain breads, cereals, and legumes per day.
- Eat less processed food.

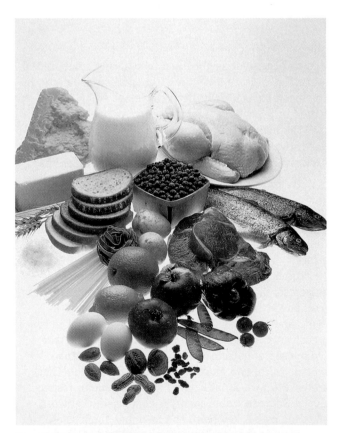

One of the main ingredients of a healthy lifestyle is a well-balanced diet.

starches   Long chains of sugars commonly found in foods such as corn, grains, potatoes, peas, and beans. Starch is stored in the body as glycogen and is used for that sudden burst of energy often needed during physical activity.

fiber   A stringy, nondigestible carbohydrate found in whole grains, vegetables, and fruits in its primary form, cellulose.

- Eat the skins of fruits and vegetables.
- Get your fiber from foods rather than pills or powders.
- Drink plenty of liquids.

FAT   Fat is an efficient storage form for energy, because each gram of fat holds more than twice the energy content of either carbohydrate or protein (Table 7.1). Excess fat in the diet is stored in fat cells (called *adipose tissue*) located under the skin and around internal organs. Fat not only is derived from dietary sources, but also can be formed in the body from excess carbohydrate and protein in the diet. Although fat can be synthesized in the body, fat in the diet should not be totally eliminated. Indeed, dietary fat is the only source of linoleic and linolenic acids, fatty acids that are essential for normal growth and healthy skin.

Fat also gives protection to internal organs and assists in absorbing, transporting, and storing the fat-soluble vitamins A, D, E, and K. Fats are classified as simple, compound, or derived (Table 7.3). Let's discuss each of these subcategories of fat.

Simple Fats. The most common of the simple fats are **triglycerides**. Triglycerides constitute approximately 95% of the fats in the diet and are the storage form of body fat. This is the form of fat that is broken down and used to produce energy to power muscle contractions during exercise.

Fatty acids are the basic structural unit of triglycerides. Though important nutritionally because of their energy content, fatty acids contribute to in cardiovascular disease through their effects on cholesterol. Based on structure, fatty acids are classified as monounsaturated, polyunsaturated, saturated, or trans. Table 7.4 on page 154 lists the dietary sources and effects on cholesterol levels of the various types of fatty acids.

Monounsaturated and polyunsaturated fatty acids are both **unsaturated fatty acids,** which are found in plants (in peas, beans, grains, and vegetable oils) and are liquid at room temperature. Because monounsaturated fatty acids seem to lower bad cholesterol levels, they are thought to be the least harmful fatty acids to the cardiovascular system. Although polyunsaturated fatty acids were favored by nutritional researchers in the early 1980s, recent evidence suggests that polyunsaturated fatty acids may decrease levels of good cholesterol as well as bad cholesterol.

One type of polyunsaturated fatty acid, called **omega-3 fatty acid,** has recently gained widespread attention. This fatty acid, which is found primarily in fresh or frozen mackerel, herring, tuna, and salmon, is reported to lower both blood cholesterol and triglycerides. However, omega-3 fatty acids are not present in canned fish because the canning process destroys the structure of these molecules. Some researchers have argued that one or two servings per week of fish contain-

ing omega-3 fatty acids reduces the risk of heart disease (4). Although this is an exciting possibility, more research is needed to confirm the claim.

Saturated fatty acids, which generally come from animal sources (meat and dairy products), are solid at room temperature. However, some saturated fatty acids, including coconut oil, come from plant sources. It is well accepted that saturated fatty acids increase blood levels of cholesterol. High cholesterol levels, in turn, promote the buildup in the coronary arteries of fatty plaque, which can eventually lead to heart disease (Chapter 9).

Trans fatty acids, which tend to have more complex structures than the other classes of fatty acids, tend to raise total cholesterol in the blood. Trans fatty acids are

---

TABLE 7.3
Major Classes of Fats and Common Examples of Each

Classes of Fat	Example
Simple fats	Triglyceride (one glycerol + three fatty acids)
Compound fats	Lipoprotein
Derived fats	Cholesterol

---

fat   An efficient storage form for energy, because each gram of fat holds over twice the energy content of either carbohydrate or protein. Excess fat in the diet is stored in fat cells (called *adipose tissue*) located under the skin and around internal organs.

triglycerides   The form of fat that is broken down and used to produce energy to power muscle contractions during exercise. Triglycerides constitute approximately 95% of the fats in the diet and are the storage form of body fat.

fatty acids   The basic structural unit of triglycerides that are important nutritionally, not only because of their energy content, but also because they play a role in cardiovascular disease.

unsaturated fatty acid   A type of fatty acid that comes primarily from plant sources and is liquid at room temperature.

omega-3 fatty acid   A type of unsaturated fatty acid that lowers both blood cholesterol and triglycerides and is found primarily in fresh or frozen mackerel, herring, tuna, and salmon.

saturated fatty acid   A type of fatty acid that comes primarily from animal sources (meat and dairy products) and is solid at room temperature.

trans fatty acid   A type of fatty acid that increases cholesterol in the blood and is a major contributor to heart disease.

TABLE 7.4
Classification of Fats According to Fatty Acid Type, and Their Dietary Sources and Effects on Cholesterol Levels

Type of Fatty Acid	Primary Sources	State at Room Temperature	Effect on Cholesterol
Monounsaturated	Canola* and olive oils; foods made from and prepared in them	Liquid	Lowers LDL; no effect on HDL
Polyunsaturated**	Soybean, safflower, corn, and cottonseed oils; foods made from and prepared in them	Liquid	Lowers both LDL and HDL
Saturated	Animal fat from red meat, whole milk, and butter; also, coconut and palm oils	Solid	Raises LDL and total cholesterol
Trans	Partially hydrogenated vegetable oils used in cooking, margarine, shortening, baked and fried foods, and snack foods	Semisolid	Raises LDL and total cholesterol

*Many nutritionists consider canola oil the most healthful vegetable oil because it's low in saturated fat, high in monounsaturated fat, and has a moderate level of omega-3 polyunsaturated fat.

**Contains the omega-3 and omega-6 essential fatty acids that the human body can't make on its own.

Source: Adapted from Fats: The good, the bad, the trans. Health News, *Massachusetts Medical Society*, July 25, 1999, pp. 1–2.

found in baked and fried foods. To date, trans fatty acids are not yet reported on food labels.

Compound Fats. For health considerations, the most important compound fats are the **lipoproteins.** These molecules are combinations of protein, triglycerides, and cholesterol. Although lipoproteins exist in several forms, the two primary types are low-density lipoproteins (LDL cholesterol) and high-density lipoproteins (HDL cholesterol). LDL cholesterol consists of a limited amount of protein and triglycerides but contains large amounts of cholesterol. It is thus associated with promoting the fatty plaque buildup in the arteries of the heart that is the primary cause of heart disease. In contrast, HDLs are primarily composed of protein, have limited amounts of cholesterol, and are associated with a low risk of heart disease. We discuss HDL and LDL cholesterol again in Chapter 9.

Derived Fats. Even though they do not contain fatty acids, **derived fats** are classified as fats because they are not water soluble. The best example of a derived fat is **cholesterol,** which is present in many foods from animal sources, including meats, shellfish, and dairy products (Table 7.5). Although a diet high in cholesterol increases your risk of heart disease, some cholesterol is essential for normal body function. Indeed, cholesterol is a constituent of cells and is used to manufacture certain types of hormones (e.g., male and female sex hormones).

Protein. The primary role of dietary protein is to serve as the structural unit to build and repair body tissues. Proteins are also important for numerous other bodily functions, including the synthesis of enzymes, hormones, and antibodies. These compounds regulate body metabolism and provide protection from disease.

As mentioned earlier, proteins are not usually a major fuel source. Nevertheless, under conditions of low carbohydrate intake (e.g., dieting), proteins can be converted to glucose and used as fuel. During periods of adequate dietary carbohydrate intake, excess proteins consumed in the diet are converted to fats and stored in adipose tissue as an energy reserve.

The basic structural units of proteins are called **amino acids.** Twenty different amino acids exist and can be linked end-to-end in various combinations to create different proteins with unique functions. The

lipoproteins Combinations of protein, triglycerides, and cholesterol in the blood that are important because of their role in promoting heart disease.

derived fats A class of fats that do not contain fatty acids but are classified as fats because they are not soluble in water.

cholesterol A type of derived fat in the body which is necessary for cell and hormone synthesis. Can be acquired through the diet or can be made by the body.

amino acids The basic structural unit of proteins. Twenty different amino acids exist and can be linked end-to-end in various combinations to create different proteins with unique functions.

TABLE 7.5
Cholesterol Content of Selected Foods (listed in ascending order)

Food	Amount of Food	Cholesterol (mg)
Milk, skim	1 cup	4
Mayonnaise	1 T	10
Butter	1 pat	11
Lard	1 T	12
Cottage cheese	1/2 cup	15
Milk, low fat, 2%	1 cup	22
Half and half	1/4 cup	23
Hot dog*	1	29
Ice cream, ~10% fat	1/2 cup	30
Cheese, cheddar	1 oz	30
Milk, whole*	1 cup	34
Oysters, salmon	3 oz	40
Clams, halibut, tuna	3 oz	55
Chicken, turkey	3 oz	70
Beef,* pork,* lobster	3 oz	75
Lamb, crab	3 oz	85
Shrimp	3 oz	125
Heart (beef)	3 oz	164
Egg (yolk)*	1 each	220–275
Liver (beef)	3 oz	410
Kidney	3 oz	587
Brains	3 oz	2637

Leading contributors of cholesterol to the U.S. diet.

Nutritional Links
TO HEALTH AND FITNESS

How Exercise Intensity Affects Fuel Use by the Muscle

The intensity of exercise is the prime determinant of whether fat or carbohydrate is the primary fuel used during exercise. Of course, the intensity of exercise also determines the length of time that you can exercise continuously. Thus, both intensity and duration of exercise will govern the predominant fuel used during an exercise session. The following table illustrates how intensity affects fuel use during endurance-type exercises.

Exercise Intensity	Fuel Used by Muscle
Less than 30% $\dot{V}O_{2max}$	Mainly muscle fat stores
40–60% $\dot{V}O_{2max}$	Fat and carbohydrate equally
75% $\dot{V}O_{2max}$	Mainly carbohydrate
Greater than 80% $\dot{V}O_{2max}$	Nearly 100% carbohydrate

tein intake is one of excess. Protein foods from animal sources are often high in fat (and high in calories), which can lead to an increased risk of heart disease, cancer, and obesity.

MICRONUTRIENTS

The category of nutrients referred to as micronutrients consists of vitamins and minerals. Functionally, micronutrients are as important as macronutrients and are required for sustaining life. Although they do not supply energy, they are essential to the breakdown of the macronutrients.

body can make 11 of these amino acids; because they are not needed in the diet, they are referred to as **nonessential amino acids.** The remaining nine amino acids cannot be manufactured by the body; because they must be obtained in the diet, they are called **essential amino acids.**

Complete proteins contain all of the essential amino acids and are present only in foods of animal origin (meats and dairy products). **Incomplete proteins** are missing one or more of the essential amino acids and are present in numerous vegetable sources. Therefore, vegetarians must be careful to combine a variety of foods in their diet in order to get all of the essential amino acids. (See Figure 7.2 on page 156.)

The dietary need for protein is greatest during the adolescent years, when growth is rapid. During this period, the recommended dietary allowance (RDA) for proteins is 1 gram of protein per kilogram of body weight (3). The recommendation decreases to 0.8 g/kg in women and 0.9 g/kg in men at the end of adolescence (Figure 7.3). Because the average person in industrialized countries consumes more than enough protein in the diet, the nutritional problem associated with pro-

nonessential amino acids Eleven amino acids that the body can make and are therefore not necessary in the diet.
essential amino acids Amino acids that cannot be manufactured by the body and must therefore be consumed in the diet.
complete proteins Contain all the essential amino acids and are found only in foods of animal origin (meats and dairy products).
incomplete proteins Proteins that are missing one or more of the essential amino acids; can be found in numerous vegetable sources.

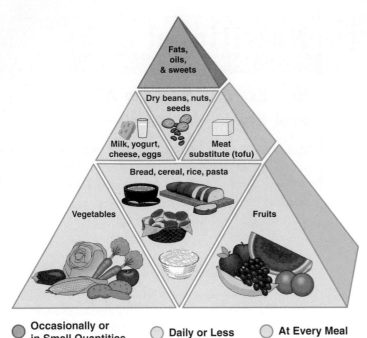

Fats, oils, & sweets

Dry beans, nuts, seeds

Milk, yogurt, cheese, eggs

Meat substitute (tofu)

Bread, cereal, rice, pasta

Vegetables

Fruits

⬤ **Occasionally or in Small Quantities** ◯ **Daily or Less** ◯ **At Every Meal**

FIGURE 7.2
The food guide pyramid for vegetarian meal planning. Eating a healthful vegetarian diet requires that certain combinations of foods are consumed daily so that the diet provides all of the essential amino acids. Planning meals to conform to the proportions shown in the pyramid will result in combinations of foods that enable vegetarians to avoid protein deficiencies.

RDA (g/kg)*		Calculating Your Protein RDA	40 Grams Example (Adult Female)
Adult Males	= 0.9	1. Determine your body weight	1. Weight = 110 lbs
Adult Females	= 0.8	2. Convert pounds to kilograms (pounds divided by 2.2 lb/kg equals kilograms)	2. 110 ÷ 2.2 lbs/Kg = 50 kg
*The RDA is 10 g/day higher during pregnancy, 15 g/day higher during the first six months of lactation, and 12 g/day higher during the remainder of lactation		3. Multiply by 0.8 or 0.9 g/kg (adult RDA) to get an RDA in grams per day	3. 50 Kg × 0.8 g/kg = 40g Results: A 110-lb female would have an RDA of 40g of protein

FIGURE 7.3
Estimated daily protein needs for adults.
(*Source:* From Hales, D. R. *An Invitation to Health.* Copyright © 1994, by The Benjamin/Cummings Publishing Company, Inc. Reprinted by permission of Brooks/Cole Publishing Company, a division of International Thomson Publishing Inc., Pacific Grove, CA 93950.)

VITAMINS **Vitamins** are small molecules that play a key role in many bodily functions, including the regulation of growth and metabolism. They are classified according to whether they are soluble in water or fat. The class of vitamins called *water-soluble vitamins* consists of several B complex vitamins and vitamin C. Because they are soluble in water, these vitamins can be eliminated from the body by the kidneys. The *fat-soluble vitamins* are soluble in fat only and consist of vitamins A, D, E, and K. Because they are stored in body fat, it is possible for these vitamins to accumulate in the body to toxic levels. Table 7.6 on page 158 lists the dietary sources of both water-soluble and fat-soluble vitamins.

vitamins Small molecules that play a key role in many bodily functions, including the regulation of growth and metabolism. They are classified according to whether they are soluble in water or fat.

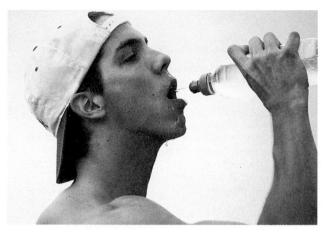

Although often overlooked nutritionally, water should be a key ingredient in any diet.

Most vitamins cannot be manufactured in the body and must therefore be consumed in the diet. The exceptions to this rule are vitamins A, D, and K, which can be produced by the body in small quantities. Vitamins in food can be destroyed in the process of cooking, so eating vegetables raw or lightly steamed is best for retaining their maximum nutritional value. Vitamins exist in almost all foods, and a balanced diet supplies all of the vitamins essential to body function.

Recent research indicates a new function for some vitamins and minerals as protectors against tissue damage (3, 5). This has important implications for individuals engaged in an exercise program. This potential new role for micronutrients is discussed later in this chapter.

MINERALS   **Minerals** are chemical elements such as sodium and calcium that are required by the body for normal function. Like vitamins, minerals are contained in many foods and play important roles in regulating key body functions, such as the conduction of nerve impulses, muscular contraction, enzyme function, and maintenance of water balance. Minerals serve a structural function as well; calcium, phosphorus, and fluoride all are important constituents of bones and teeth.

Table 7.7 on page 160 illustrates the nutritionally important minerals and their functions. Three of the most widely recognized minerals are calcium, iron, and sodium. Calcium is important in its role in bone formation. A deficiency of calcium contributes to the development of the bone disease called osteoporosis. A deficiency of dietary iron may lead to iron-deficiency anemia, which results in chronic fatigue. High sodium intake has been associated with hypertension, a major risk factor for heart disease.

WATER

Approximately 60–70% of the body is water. Because water is involved in all vital processes in the body, it is considered the nutrient of greatest concern to the physically active individual. An individual performing heavy exercise in a hot, humid environment can lose 1 to 3 liters of water per hour through sweating (6). A loss of 5% of body water causes fatigue, weakness, and the inability to concentrate; a loss of 15% can be fatal. Water is important for temperature control of the body, absorption and digestion of foods, formation of blood, and elimination of wastes. Chapter 11 provides guidelines for maintaining proper hydration during exercise training.

Water is contained in almost all foods, especially fruits and vegetables. Combining the water contained in foods and that consumed as beverages, you should consume the equivalent of 8–10 cups of water per day. This does not account for conditions that cause excess fluid loss such as excess sweating, donating blood, diarrhea, or vomiting. Figure 7.4 illustrates the balance between the body's sources of water intake and routes of water output.

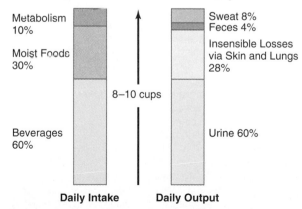

Daily Water Balance in the Body

Metabolism 10%

Moist Foods 30%

Sweat 8%
Feces 4%

Insensible Losses via Skin and Lungs 28%

8–10 cups

Beverages 60%

Urine 60%

Daily Intake   Daily Output

FIGURE 7.4
Daily water intake and output by the body.
(*Source:* Donatelle, R. J., and Davis, L. G., *Access to Health,* 1996. Copyright © 1996 by Allyn & Bacon.)

minerals   Chemical elements (e.g., sodium and calcium) that are required by the body for normal functioning.

TABLE 7.6
Vitamins: Where You Get Them and What They Do

Vitamin	Best Sources	Main Roles	Deficiency Symptoms	Risks of Megadoses
Fat Soluble				
A	Liver; eggs; cheese; butter; fortified margarine and milk; yellow, orange, and dark-green vegetables and fruits (e.g., carrots, broccoli, spinach, cantaloupe)	Assists in the formation and maintenance of healthy skin, hair, and mucous membranes; aids in the ability to see in dim light (night vision); needed for proper bone growth, teeth development, and reproduction.	Night blindness; rough skin and mucous membranes; infection of mucous membranes; drying of the eyes; impaired growth of bones and tooth enamel	Blurred vision, loss of appetite, headaches, skin rashes, nausea, diarrhea, hair loss, menstrual irregularities, extreme fatigue, joint pain, liver damage, insomnia, abnormal bone growth, injury to brain and nervous system
D	Fortified milk; egg yolk; liver; tuna: salmon; cod-liver oil. Made in skin in sunlight.	Aids in the formation and maintenance of bones and teeth; assists in the absorption and use of calcium and phosphorus.	In children, rickets; stunted bone growth, bowed legs, malformed teeth, protruding abdomen; in adults, osteomalacia, softening of the bones leading to shortening and fractures, muscle spasms, and twitching	In infants, calcium deposits in kidneys and excessive calcium in blood; in adults, calcium deposits throughout body, deafness, nausea, loss of appetite, kidney stones, fragile bones, high blood pressure, high blood cholesterol
E	Vegetable oils; margarine; wheat germ; whole-grain cereals and bread; liver; dried beans; green leafy vegetables	Aids in the formation of red blood cells, muscles, and other tissues; protects vitamin A and essential fatty acids from oxidation.	Prolonged impairment of fat absorption; lysis of red blood cells; nerve destruction	None definitely known. Reports of headache, blurred vision, extreme fatigue, muscle weakness; can destroy some vitamin K made in the gut.
K	Green leafy vegetables; cabbage; cauliflower; peas; potatoes; liver; cereals. Except in newborns, made by bacteria in human intestine.	Aids in the synthesis of substances needed for blood clotting; helps maintain normal bone metabolism.	Hemorrhage, especially in newborn infants	Jaundice in babies; anemia in laboratory animals
Water Soluble				
Thiamin (B_1)	Pork (especially ham); liver; oysters; whole-grain and enriched cereals, pasta, and bread; wheat germ; oatmeal; peas; lima beans	Helps release energy from carbohydrates; aids in the synthesis of an important nervous system chemical.	Beriberi: mental confusion, muscular weakness, swelling of the heart, leg cramps	None known. However, because B vitamins are interdependent, excess of one may produce deficiency of others.
Riboflavin (B_2)	Liver; milk; meat; dark-green vegetables; eggs; whole-grain and enriched cereals, pasta, and bread; dried beans and peas	Helps release energy from carbohydrates, proteins, and fats; aids in the maintenance of mucous membranes.	Skin disorders, especially around nose and lips; cracks at corners of mouth; sensitivity of eyes to light	None known. See Thiamin.
Niacin (B_3, nicotinamide, nicotinic acid)	Liver; poultry; meat; fish; eggs; whole-grain and enriched cereals, pasta, and bread; nuts; dried peas and beans	Participates with thiamin and riboflavin in facilitating energy production in cells	Pellagra, skin disorders, diarrhea, mental confusion, irritability, mouth swelling, smooth tongue	Duodenal ulcer, abnormal liver function, elevated blood sugar, excessive uric acid in blood, possibly leading to gout, skin flushing at >100 mg

TABLE 7.6
Vitamins: Where You Get Them and What They Do *(continued)*

Vitamin	Best Sources	Main Roles	Deficiency Symptoms	Risks of Megadoses
Pantothenic acid	Mushrooms; liver; broccoli; eggs	Molecule involved in energy metabolism and fat storage and breakdown	Tingling in hands, fatigue, headache, nausea	None
Biotin	Cheese; egg yolks; cauliflower; peanut butter; liver	Molecule involved in glucose production; fat storage	Dermatitis, tongue soreness, anemia, depression	Unknown
Choline	Lettuce; peanuts; liver, cauliflower	Regeneration of amino acids; nerve function	Liver malfunction	Nausea, diarrhea, vomiting
B_6 (pyridoxine)	Whole-grain (but not enriched) cereals and bread; liver; avocados; spinach; green beans; bananas; fish; poultry meats; nuts; potatoes; green leafy vegetables	Aids in the absorption and metabolism of proteins; helps the body use fats; assists in the formation of red blood cells.	Skin disorders, cracks at corners of mouth, smooth tongue, convulsions, dizziness, nausea, anemia, kidney stones	Dependency on high dose, leading to deficiency symptoms when one returns to normal amounts
B_{12} (cobalamin)	Only in animal foods; liver; kidneys; meat; fish; eggs; milk; oysters; nutritional yeast	Aids in the formation of red blood cells; assists in the building of genetic material; helps the functioning of the nervous system.	Pernicious anemia, anemia, pale skin and mucous membranes, numbness and tingling in fingers and toes that may progress to loss of balance and weakness and pain in arms and legs	None known
Folacin (folic acid)	Liver; kidneys; dark-green leafy vegetables; wheat germ; dried beans and peas. Stored in the body, so daily consumption is not crucial.	Acts with B_{12} in synthesis of genetic material; aids in the formation of hemoglobin in red blood cells.	Megaloblastic anemia; enlarged red blood cells, smooth tongue, diarrhea; during pregnancy, deficiency may cause loss of the fetus or fetal abnormalities. Women on oral contraceptives may need extra folacin.	Body stores it, so it is potentially hazardous. Can mask a B_2 deficiency. Diarrhea; insomnia
C (ascorbic acid)	Citrus fruits; tomatoes; strawberries, melon; green peppers; potatoes; dark-green vegetables	Aids in the formation of collagen; helps maintain capillaries, bones, and teeth; helps protect other vitamins from oxidation; may block formation of cancer-causing nitrosamines.	Scurvy; bleeding gums; degenerating muscles; wounds that don't heal; loose teeth; brown, dry, rough skin. Early symptoms include loss of appetite, irritability, weight loss.	Dependency on high doses, possibly precipitating symptoms of scurvy when withdrawn (especially in infants if megadoses taken during pregnancy); kidney and bladder stones; diarrhea; urinary tract irritation; increased tendency for blood to clot; breakdown of red blood cells in persons with certain common genetic disorders

Source: Reprinted from Jane Brody's Nutrition Book, *with permission of W. W. Norton & Company, Inc. Copyright © 1981 by Jane E. Brody.*

TABLE 7.7
Minerals: Where You Get Them and What They Do

Best Sources	Main Roles	Deficiency Symptoms	Risks of Megadoses
Macrominerals			
Calcium			
Milk and milk products; sardines; canned salmon eaten with bones; dark-green, leafy vegetables; citrus fruits; dried beans and peas	Building bones and teeth and maintaining bone strength; muscle contraction; maintaining cell membranes; blood clotting; absorption of B$_2$; activation of enzymes	In children: distorted bone growth (rickets); in adults: loss of bone (osteoporosis) and increased susceptibility to fractures	Drowsiness; extreme lethargy; impaired absorption of iron, zinc, and manganese; calcium deposits in tissues throughout body, mimicking cancer on X-ray
Phosphorus			
Meat; poultry; fish; eggs, dried beans and peas; milk and milk products; phosphates in processed foods, especially soft drinks	Building bones and teeth; release of energy from carbohydrates, proteins, and fats; formation of genetic material, cell membranes, and many enzymes	Weakness; loss of appetite; malaise; bone pain. Dietary shortages uncommon, but prolonged use of antacids can cause deficiency	Distortion of calcium-to-phosphorus ratio, creating relative deficiency of calcium
Magnesium			
Green, leafy, vegetables (eaten raw); nuts (especially almonds and cashews); soybeans; seeds; whole grains	Building bones; manufacture of proteins; release of energy from muscle glycogen; conduction of nerve impulse to muscles; adjustment to cold	Muscular twitching and tremors; irregular heartbeat; insomnia; muscle weakness; leg and foot cramps; shaky hands	Disturbed nervous system function because the calcium-to-magnesium ratio is unbalanced; catharsis: hazard to persons with poor kidney function
Potassium			
Orange juice; bananas; dried fruits; meats; bran; peanut butter; dried beans and peas; potatoes; coffee; tea; cocoa	Muscle contraction; maintenance of fluid and electrolyte balance in cells; transmission of nerve impulses; release of energy from carbohydrates, proteins, and fats	Abnormal heart rhythm; muscular weakness; lethargy; kidney and lung failure	Excessive potassium in blood, causing muscular paralysis and abnormal heart rhythms
Sulfur			
Beef; wheat germ; dried beans and peas; peanuts; clams	In every cell as part of sulfur-containing amino acids; forms bridges between molecules to create firm proteins of hair, nails, and skin	None known in humans	Unknown
Chlorine			
Table salt and other naturally occurring salts	Regulation of balance of body fluids and acids and bases; activation of enzyme in saliva; part of stomach acid	Disturbed acid-base balance in body fluids (very rare)	Disturbed acid-base balance

☼ IN SUMMARY

- Nutrition is the study of food and its relationship to health and disease.

- A well-balanced diet is composed of approximately 58% complex carbohydrates, 30% fat, and 12% protein; collectively these three components of the diet are called macronutrients.

- The calorie is a unit of measure for quantifying the energy in food or the energy expended by the body.

- Carbohydrates constitute a primary source of fuel for the body. Simple carbohydrates consist of both simple sugars and sugars composed of two simple sugars. Complex carbohydrates include starches (long energy-yielding chains of sugars) and fiber (long nondigestible but essential chains of sugars).

- Fat is an efficient storage form for energy that can either come directly from the diet or be produced from excess carbohydrate and protein in the diet. Fats are either simple fats (e.g., triglycerides),

---

TABLE 7.7
Minerals: Where You Get Them and What They Do (continued)

Best Sources	Main Roles	Deficiency Symptoms	Risks of Megadoses
Trace Minerals			
Iron			
Liver; kidneys; red meats; egg yolk; green, leafy vegetables; dried fruits; dried beans and peas; potatoes; blackstrap molasses; enriched and whole-grain cereals	Formation of hemoglobin in blood and myoglobin in muscles, which supply oxygen to cells; part of several enzymes and proteins	Anemia, with fatigue, weakness, pallor, and shortness of breath	Toxic buildup in liver, pancreas, and heart
Copper			
Oysters; nuts; cocoa powder; beef and pork liver; kidneys; dried beans; corn-oil margarine	Formation of red blood cells; part of several respiratory enzymes	In animals: anemia; faulty development of bone and nervous tissue; loss of elasticity in tendons and major arteries; abnormal lung development; abnormal structure and pigmentation of hair	Violent vomiting and diarrhea. Cooking acid foods in unlined copper pots can lead to toxic accumulation of copper.
Zinc			
Meat; liver; eggs; poultry; seafood; milk; whole grains	Constituent of about 100 enzymes	Delayed wound healing; diminished taste sensation; loss of appetite; in children: failure to grow and mature sexually; prenatally: abnormal brain development	Nausea, vomiting; anemia; bleeding in stomach; premature birth and stillbirth; abdominal pain; fever. Can aggravate marginal copper deficiency. May produce atherosclerosis.
Iodine			
Seafood; seaweed; iodized salt; sea salt	Part of thyroid hormones; essential for normal reproduction	Goiter (enlarged thyroid with low hormone production); newborns: cretinism, retarded growth, protruding abdomen, swollen features	Not known to be a problem, but could cause iodine poisoning or sensitivity reaction.
Fluorine			
Fish; tea; most meats; fluoridated water; foods grown with or cooked in fluoridated water	Formation of strong, decay-resistant teeth; maintenance of bone strength	Excessive dental decay; possibly osteoporosis	Mottling of teeth and bones; in larger doses, a deadly poison
Manganese			
Nuts; whole grains; vegetables and fruits; tea; instant coffee; cocoa powder	Functioning of central nervous system; normal bone structure; reproduction; part of important enzymes	None known in human beings; in animals: poor reproduction; retarded growth; birth defects; abnormal bone development	Masklike facial expression; blurred speech; involuntary laughing; spastic gait; hand tremors

Source: Adapted from Jane Brody's Nutrition Book, *with the permission of W. W. Norton & Company, Inc.* Copyright © 1981 by Jane E. Brody.

---

compound fats (e.g., lipoproteins), or derived fats (e.g., cholesterol).

- Protein consumed in the diet serves as the structural unit for building and repairing cells in the body. Proteins are composed of amino acids, which are either made by the body (nonessential amino acids) or must be consumed in the diet (essential amino acids).

- Vitamins serve many important functions in the body. The water-soluble vitamins include several B

complex vitamins and vitamin C. The fat-soluble vitamins are vitamins A, D, E, and K.

- Minerals are chemical elements in foods that, like vitamins, play important roles in many body functions.

- Water is the nutrient of greatest concern to physically active individuals because approximately 60% of body weight is water. It is recommended that people consume 8–10 cups of fluids each day.

✺ Guidelines for a Healthy Diet

Several national health agencies have suggested guidelines for healthy diets. Although they don't agree on all points, in essence, they do agree on the following, as suggested by the U.S. Department of Agriculture's "Dietary Guidelines for Americans, 2000":

Aim for fitness . . .

- Aim for a healthy weight.
- Be physically active each day.

Build a healthy base . . .

- Let the Pyramid guide your food choices.
- Choose a variety of grains daily, especially whole grains.
- Choose a variety of fruits and vegetables daily.
- Keep food safe to eat.

Choose sensibly . . .

- Choose a diet that is low in saturated fat and cholesterol and moderate in total fat.
- Choose beverages and foods to moderate your intake of sugars.
- Choose and prepare foods with less salt.
- If you choose to drink alcoholic beverages, do so in moderation.

The following sections provide general rules for selection of the macro- and micronutrients to meet the goals of a healthy diet. In addition, we discuss how to critically analyze your diet using a dietary record.

NUTRIENTS

The general rule for meeting the body's need for macronutrients is that an individual should consume approximately 58% of needed calories from carbohydrates (48% complex carbohydrates and 10% simple sugars), 30% or less in fats (approximately 10% saturated and 20% unsaturated fats), and 12% in proteins (3). Again, the daily protein requirement for adults is approximately 0.8 grams of protein per kilogram (2.2 lbs) of body weight.

To meet the need for micronutrients, the National Academy of Science (7) has established guidelines concerning the quantities of each micronutrient required to meet the minimum needs of most individuals. These Recommended Dietary Allowances (RDAs) are contained in Table 7.8 on page 164.

Once you know the recommended daily requirements for nutrients, the key question is, "How do I choose foods to meet these goals?" Previous dietary guidelines suggested choosing foods from four basic food groups: fruits and vegetables; poultry, fish, meat, and eggs; beans, grains, and nuts; and dairy products. Although these guidelines are still generally acceptable, they do not represent the most desirable proportions of different foods. Government health agencies responsible for setting nutritional guidelines (7) have altered their recommendations about how we should choose foods from these groups. Figure 7.5 illustrates these latest

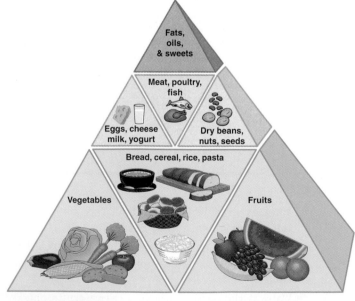

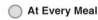

FIGURE 7.5

The "eating-right pyramid." The basic diet should consist primarily of those foods on the lower two tiers of the pyramid, with decreasing amounts of foods from the top.

(*Source:* Donatelle, R. J., and L. G. Davis, *Access to Health,* 2002. Copyright © 2002. Reprinted by permission of Allyn & Bacon.)

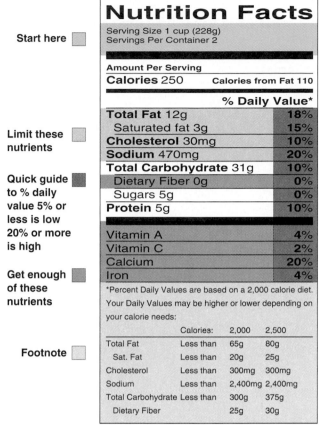

FIGURE 7.6
How to read a "Nutrition Facts" label, in this case a label from a box of macaroni and cheese. Labels in the food labeling system are required to list both the total amount and the % Daily Value of each nutrient shown on this sample label. Note that daily values are based on a 2000-calorie diet.
(*Source*: U.S. Department of Agriculture. *Dietary Guidelines for Americans, 2000*. Washington, DC: U.S. Government Printing Office, 2000.)

recommendations for a healthy diet using the "eating-right pyramid."

The use of the eating-right pyramid in forming a diet accomplishes two important goals. First, the relative proportions of foods known to promote disease are minimized. Second, "nutrient-dense" foods—that is, foods high in micronutrients per calorie—are maximized. Thus, by following the pyramid approach, you are assured of getting the proper balance of macro- and micronutrients.

Until recently, nutrition labeling provided little help in choosing the right foods. Labels were required on only 60% of packaged foods, making it difficult to follow the RDA guidelines. Further, the terms used on labels were often undefined, poorly organized, and misleading. In 1994, consumer groups and major health organizations prompted the U.S. Food and Drug Adminis-

tration to adopt a new set of requirements for food labeling. As illustrated in Figure 7.6, the labeling system now enables consumers to choose foods based on current, accurate, and easy-to-understand information.

CALORIES

The number of calories in the diet is a key consideration for developing good eating habits. As mentioned, the problem with most U.S. diets is not the lack of nutrients, but excess caloric content. Therefore, monitor your total caloric intake to prevent overconsumption of food energy.

When monitoring your dietary calories, remember these two important points. First, most people consume too many calories from simple sugars. The primary simple sugar in most diets is sucrose (i.e., table sugar). The principal nutritional problem related to simple sugars is that they contain many calories but few micronutrients. A second concern when determining caloric intake is the amount of fat in the diet. Fat is high in calories, often rich in cholesterol, and contains over twice as many calories as a gram of carbohydrate or protein (1 gram of fat = 9 calories; 1 gram of carbohydrate = 4 calories; and 1 gram of protein = 4 calories). Limiting fat in the diet both reduces the risk of heart disease and helps avoid excess caloric intake. We discuss how to determine the optimal caloric intake for a healthy body weight in much greater detail in Chapter 8.

DIETARY ANALYSIS

From the preceding discussions, it is clear that eating a balanced diet is the key to good nutrition. Now the critical question is, "How do I know if I'm eating a well-balanced diet?" The answer is to perform a dietary analysis by keeping a 3-day record of everything you eat. It is a good idea to include both weekdays and weekends in your record (two weekdays and one weekend day are generally recommended). At the end of each day, look up the nutrient content of each food (Appendices B and C) and record this information in the tables provided in Laboratory 7.1. The process of analyzing your diet in this way is often time-consuming and can be simplified by using computerized dietary analysis software.

When you have recorded the nutritive values for each day of your 3-day record, compare your average nutrient intake with the recommended dietary allowances for your age and gender (Laboratory 7.1). These results will provide you with a good index of your dietary strengths and limitations. If you find your diet to be deficient in any macro- or micronutrient (compared with RDA values), you should modify your diet to include foods that will provide adequate amounts of that nutrient. In contrast, if you find your diet to be

TABLE 7.8
Recommended Dietary Allowances of Selected Micronutrients (with upper limits in parentheses)
Revised 2001

Life Stage and Gender	Vit A μg^e μg^e	Thiamin (B$_1$) mg	Riboflavin (B$_2$) mg	Niacin (B$_3$) mg	Pantothenic Acid mg	Biotin μg	Vit B$_{12}$ μg	Folate μg	Vit B$_6$ mg	Vit C$^\#$ mg	Vit D μg^e	Vit E^c μg^e
Infants												
0–6 mos	400 (600)	0.2*	0.3*	2*	1.7*	5*	0.1*	65*	0.4*	40	5* (25)	4
7–12 mos	500 (600)	0.3*	0.4*	4*	1.8*	6*	0.3*	80*	0.5*	50	5* (25)	5
Children												
1–3 yr	300 (600)	0.5	0.5	6 (10)	2*	8*	0.5 (30)	150 (300)	0.9 (400)	15 (50)	5*	6 (200)
4–8 yr	400 (900)	0.6	0.6	8 (15)	3*	12*	0.6 (40)	200 (400)	1.2	25 (650)	5* (50)	7 (300)
Males												
9–13 yr	600 (1700)	0.9	0.9	12 (20)	4*	20*	1.0 (60)	300 (600)	1.8	45 (1200)	5* (50)	11 (600)
14–18 yr	900 (2800)	1.2	1.3	16 (30)	5*	25*	1.3 (80)	400 (800)	2.4	75 (1800)	5* (50)	15 (800)
19–30 yr	900 (3000)	1.2	1.3	16 (35)	5*	30*	1.3 (100)	400 (1000)	2.4	90 (2000)	5* (50)	15 (1000)
31–50 yr	900 (3000)	1.2	1.3	16 (35)	5*	30*	1.3 (100)	400 (1000)	2.4	90 (2000)	5* (50)	15 (1000)
51–70 yr	900 (3000)	1.2	1.3 (35)	16	5*	30*	1.7 (100)	400 (1000)	2.4*	90 (2000)	10* (50)	15 (1000)
>70 yr	900 (3000)	1.2	1.3 (35)	16	5*	30*	1.7 (100)	400 (1000)	2.4*	90 (2000)	15* (50)	15 (1000)
Females												
9–13 yr	600 (1700)	0.9	0.9	12 (20)	4*	20*	1.0 (60)	300 (600)	1.8	45 (1200)	5* (50)	11 (600)
14–18 yr	700	1	1	14 (30)	5*	25*	1.2 (80)	400^a (800)	2.4	65 (1800)	5* (50)	15 (800)
19–30 yr	700	1.1	1.1	14 (30)	5*	30*	1.3 (100)	400^a (1000)	2.4	75 (2000)	5* (50)	15 (1000)
31–50 yr	700	1.1	1.1	14 (30)	5*	30*	1.3 (100)	400^a (1000)	2.4	75 (2000)	5* (50)	15 (1000)
51–70 yr	700 (3000)	1.1	1.1	14 (30)	5*	30*	1.5 (100)	400^a (1000)	2.4^b	75 (2000)	10* (50)	15 (1000)
>70 yr	700 (3000)	1.1	1.1	14 (30)	5*	30*	1.5 (100)	400^a (1000)	2.4^b	75 (2000)	15* (50)	15 (1000)
Pregnant												
<19 yr	750	1.4	1.4	18 (30)	6*	30*	1.9 (80)	600 (800)	2.6	80	5* (50)	15 (800)
≥19 yr	770	1.4	1.4	18 (35)	6*	30*	1.9 (100)	600 (1000)	2.6	85	5* (50)	15 (1000)
Lactating												
<19 yr	1200	1.4	1.6	17 (30)	7*	35*	2.0 (80)	500 (800)	2.8	115	5* (50)	19 (800)
≥19 yr	1300	1.4	1.6	17 (35)	7*	35*	2.0 (100)	500 (1000)	2.8	120	5* (50)	19 (1000)

* Asterisk indicates Adequate Intake (AI) values because the RDA is unknown. RDA meets ~98% of needs and AI is at or above that value. See "A Closer Look" on page 166 for further explanation.

\# Smokers should consume an additional 35 mg/day.

^{a} Women capable of becoming pregnant should consume 400 ug of folate from supplements or fortified foods in addition to intake from a varied diet.

^{b} Food-bound B$_{12}$ may have inadequate absorption. Therefore, those over age 50 should consume foods fortified with B$_{12}$ or a supplement.

^{c} Alpha-tocopherol (other forms of vitamin E do not have the same effects); Vitamin E as alpha-tocopherol (1 mg = 1.5 IU).

^{d} The upper limit (UL) for magnesium represents intake from supplement only and does not include food or water.

^{e} Vitamin A: 1 μg = 1 retinol equivalent (RE) = 3.3 international units (IU).

(Source: Reprinted with permission from Recommended Dietary Allowances, 11th edtion. Copyright © 2001 by National Academy of Sciences. Courtesy of the National Academy Press, Washington, D.C.)

Minerals

Vit K μg	Choline mg (g)	Calcium mg (g)	Iodine μg	Iron mg	Magnesium mg	Phosphorus mg (g)	Selenium μg	Zinc mg	Chromium mg	Fluoride mg
2.0*	125*	210*	110*	0.27* (40)	30*	100*	15 (450)	2.0*	0.2*	0.01* (0.7)
2.5*	150*	270*	130*	11 (40)	75*	275*	20 (60)	3	5.5*	0.5* (0.9)
30* (1g)	200*	500* (2.5g)	90 (200)	7 (40)	80 (65)	460 (3g)	20 (90)	3	11*	0.7* (1.3)
55*	250* (1g)	800* (2.5g)	90 (300)	10 (40)	130 (110)	500 (3g)	30 (150)	5	15*	1.0* (2.2)
60*	375* (2g)	1300* (2.5)	120 (600)	8 (40)	240 (350	1250 (4g)	40 (280)	8	25*	2* (10)
75*	550* (3g)	1300* (2.5)	150 (900)	11 (45)	410 (350)	1250 (4g)	55 (400)	11	35*	3* (10)
120*	550* (3.5g)	1000* (2.5)	150 (1100)	8 (45)	400 (350)	700 (4g)	55 (400)	11	35*	4* (10)
120*	550* (3.5g)	1000* (2.5)	150 (1100)	8 (45)	420 (350)	700 (4g)	55 (400)	11	35*	4* (10)
120*	550* (3.5g)	1200* (2.5)	150 (1100)	8(45)	420 (350)	700 (4g)	55 (400)	11	30*	4* (10)
120*	550* (3.5g)	1200* (2.5)	150 (1100)	8 (45)	420 (350)	700 (4g)	55 (400)	11	30*	4* (10)
60*	375* (2g)	1300* (2.5g)	120 (600)	8 (40)	240 (350)	1250 (4g)	40 (280)	8	21*	2* (10)
75*	400* (3g)	1300* (2.5g)	150 (900)	15 (45)	360 (350)	1250 (4g)	55 (400)	9	24*	3* (10)
90*	425* (3.5g)	1000* (2.5g)	150 (1000)	18 (45)	310 (350)	700 (4g)	55(400)	8	25*	3* (10)
90*	425* (3.5g)	1000* (2.5g)	150 (1100)	18 (45)	320 (350)	700 (4g)	55 (400)	8	25*	3* (10)
90*	425* (3.5g)	1200* (2.5g)	150 (1100)	8 (45)	320 (350)	700 (4g)	55 (400)	8	20*	3* (10)
90*	425* (3.5g)	1200* (2.5g)	150 (1100)	8 (45)	320 (350)	700 (4g)	55 (400)	8	20*	3* (10)
75*	450* (3g)	1300* (2.5g)	220 (900)	27 (45)	400 (350)	1250 (3.5g)	60 (400)	13	29*	3* (10)
90*	450* (3.5g)	1000* (2.5g)	220 (1100)	27 (45)	360 (350)	700 (3.5g)	60 (400)	11	30*	3* (10)
75*	550* (3g)	1300* (2.5g)	290 (900)	10 (45)	360 (350)	1250 (3.5g)	70 (400)	14	44*	3* (10)
90*	550* (3.5g)	1000* (2.5g)	290 (1100)	9 (45)	320 (350)	700 (4g)	70 (400)	12	45*	3* (10)

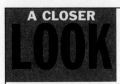

New Recommended Dietary Allowances of Nutrients

Recommended Dietary Allowances (also known as RDAs) are the daily amounts of the different food nutrients the National Academy of Sciences deems adequate for healthy individuals. Great effort has been made over the last few years to define these amounts more precisely, and an updated list of nutrients has now been published (7).

Over the past decade our increased knowledge about nutritional needs and the boom in the use of supplements have prompted the Academy to revise the way in which the values are reported. People now ask, "What are the minimal amounts of nutrients I need?" and "What are the maximal amounts that are safe?"

Even today, RDAs for some nutrients are not known. Thus, the Academy has changed the way in which recommendations are reported. In 1997 they issued several indices to guide people in monitoring their diets. They refer to these indices as Dietary Reference Intakes (DRIs). The new DRIs are divided into four categories, each of which addresses a different nutritional issue. (See the figure below.) The new DRIs are:

- **Recommended Dietary Allowance (RDA):** Unlike their predecessors, these RDAs are the amount of nutrient that will meet the needs of almost every healthy person in a specific age and gender group. Also, these RDAs are meant to reduce disease risk, not just prevent deficiency.

- **Adequate Intake (AI):** This value is used when the RDA is not known because the scientific data aren't strong enough to produce a specific recommendation, yet there is enough evidence to give a general guideline. Thus, it is an "educated guess" at what the RDA would be if it were known.

- **Estimated Average Requirement (EAR):** This is a value that is estimated to provide one-half of the RDA for that nutrient. It is primarily used to establish the RDA. In addition, it is used for evaluating and planning the diets of large groups of people (such as the army), not individuals.

- **Tolerable Upper Intake Level (UL):** This is the maximal amount that a person can take without

risking "adverse health effects." Anything above this amount might result in toxicity. In most cases this number refers to the *total* intake of the nutrient—from food, fortified foods, and nutritional supplements.

The new guidelines have changed the categorization of nutrients to more closely group them according to the functional properties of each. The following list shows the groups, the year of the latest update, and the nutrients in each.

- **Micronutrients (2001):** Vitamin A, vitamin K, arsenic, boron, chromium, copper, iodine, iron, manganese, molybdenum, nickel, silicon, vanadium, and zinc

- **The B Vitamins and Choline (2000):** Thiamin (B_1), riboflavin (B_2), niacin (B_3), vitamin B_6, folate, vitamin B_{12}, pantothenic acid, biotin, and choline

- **Antioxidants (2000):** Vitamin C, vitamin E, selenium, and carotenoids

- **Calcium and Related Nutrients (1999);** Calcium, phosphorus, magnesium, vitamin D, and fluoride

Source: National Academy of Sciences. *Dietary Reference Intakes: Applications in Dietary Assessment.* Washington, DC: National Academy Press, 2001.

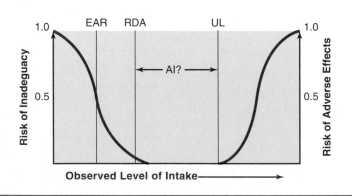

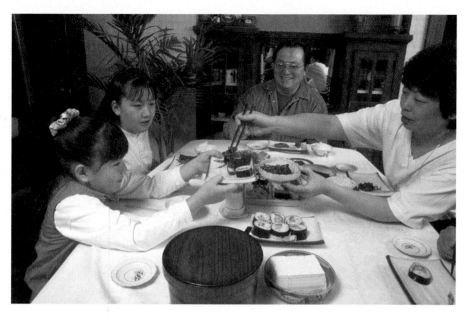

Family and cultural influences often dictate the foods we choose.

excessive in any macro- or micronutrient, modify it to reduce the values to those suggested elsewhere in this chapter.

A careful and honest dietary analysis is a critical step in modifying a poor diet and planning a well-balanced one. It is also an eye-opening experience, because most of us are not aware of the nutrient contents of common foods. After performing a 3-day dietary analysis, many people are surprised by their high fat intake. The average U.S. diet contains approximately 42% fat (% of total calories), which is well above the recommended 30% (Figure 7.1). As mentioned earlier, a high fat intake results in an increased risk of disease and obesity.

Thus, the most likely deficiency you will encounter in dietary analysis is too few micronutrients in your diet. The most likely problem of excess you may encounter is overconsumption of fat, simple sugars, and calories. Remember, by following the eating-right pyramid and counting calories, you can protect your diet against these common pitfalls.

FOODS TO AVOID

Now that we have outlined the macro- and micronutrients that should be included in your diet, remember that several foods should be minimized in order to maintain a healthy diet. Even if you do not have the health problems that will be discussed next, determine whether close relatives have these problems. If they do, you may be a prime candidate for developing the problem later in life if you do not change your eating habits now.

First and foremost on the list of foods to avoid are those with a high fat content. Both saturated and unsaturated fats are linked to heart disease, obesity, and certain cancers. In addition, it is often overlooked that

---

TABLE 7.9
Guidelines for Cutting Fat from the Diet

- Read food labels. Keep in mind that 30% or less of total calories should come from fat, and that no more than 10% should be saturated fat.

- Many foods are now fat free or low in fat and should be chosen over high-fat foods.

- For baking and sautéing, choose vegetable oils, such as olive oil, that do not raise cholesterol levels.

- Choose margarines with the *lowest* levels of trans fatty acids.

- Choose only lean meats, fish, and poultry. Always remove the skin before eating, and bake or broil meats whenever possible. Meats that are the most well-done have fewer calories and are less likely to cause food poisoning. Drain off all oils from meats after cooking.

- Eliminate most cold cuts from your diet (e.g., bacon, sausage, hot dogs). Beware of meat products that claim to be "95% fat-free," because they may still have a high fat content.

- Select nonfat dairy products whenever possible. Part skim milk cheeses such as mozzarella, farmer's, lappi, and ricotta are the best choices.

- Substitute other products for butter, margarine, oils, sour cream, mayonnaise, and salad dressings when cooking. Chicken broths, wine, vinegar, and low-calorie dressings make good flavorings and/or cooking ingredients.

- Think of food intake as an average over a day or couple of days. A high-fat breakfast can be offset by a low-fat lunch or dinner.

---

dietary fat contributes more to body fat than does protein or carbohydrate (3). Table 7.9 provides guidelines to help you cut fat intake from your diet.

TABLE 7.10
The Cholesterol/Saturated Fat Index: Which Foods Promote Cardiovascular Disease?

The cholesterol/saturated fat index (CSI) compares the saturated fat in foods with the amount of cholesterol. The CSI value listed for each food indicates the relative contribution of that food to promoting cardiovascular disease. The lower the saturated fat and cholesterol, the lower the CSI. However, because saturated fat poses a greater risk than cholesterol in the diet, it is given a heavier weight in calculating CSI. For example, fruits and vegetables have a CSI of zero (the best). A food that is high in cholesterol but low in saturated fat would have an intermediate CSI value. Shrimp, for example, with 182 mg of cholesterol but virtually no saturated fat, has a CSI of 6. In contrast, lean hamburger, with approximately 95 mg of cholesterol and 6.3 grams of fat, has a CSI of 10 and carries a greater risk for promoting cardiovascular disease. For a healthy diet, the total daily CSI should range from 22 to 50, depending on the caloric content of your diet (22 for a 1200-calorie diet; 50 for a 2800-calorie diet).

	Cholesterol (mg)	Saturated Fat (g)	CSI
Fish, shellfish, cooked (3.5 oz)			
Sole	50	3	4
Salmon	74	1.5	5
Shrimp, crab, lobster	182	0.2	6
Poultry, no skin (3.5 oz.)	84.7	1	6
Beef, pork, lamb (3.5 oz.)			
15% fat (ground round)	94.6	6.3	10
30% fat (ground beef)	88.6	11.4	18
Cheeses (3.5 oz)			
1–2% fat (low-fat, cottage cheese)	7.9	1.2	1
5–10% fat (cottage cheese)	15.1	2.8	6
32–38% fat (cheddar, cream cheese)	104.7	20.9	26
Eggs			
Whites (3)	0	0	0
Whole (1)	246	2.41	15
Fats (1/4 cup, 4 tablespoons, or 55 g)			
Most vegetable oils	0	7	8
Soft vegetable margarines	0	7.8	10
Stick margarines	0	8.5	15
Butter	124	28.7	37
Frozen desserts (1 serving)			
Frozen low-fat yogurt	*	*	2
Ice milk	13.6	2.4	6
Ice cream (10% fat)	60.6	9	13
Specialty ice cream (22% fat)	*	*	34

*Varies according to brand.

Source: Adapted with permission of Simon & Schuster Inc. from The New American Diet by Sonja L. Connor, M.S., R.D. and William E. Connor, M.D. Copyright © 1986 by Sonja L. Connor, M.S., R.D., and William E. Connor, M.D.

Although cholesterol is a substance that the body needs to function properly, too much contributes to heart disease. Lowering blood cholesterol by dietary modifications can lower your risk of heart disease. Improvement in one's coronary heart disease risk is closely related to a decrease in dietary cholesterol, and a 1% reduction in cholesterol results in a 2% reduction in risk (Chapter 9). The new food labeling system will help identify foods high in cholesterol; however, the cholesterol content of some unlabeled foods may surprise you. Many foods that are high in cholesterol are also high in fat. Table 7.10 will help you determine your cholesterol/saturated fat index in order to rate the cardiovascular risks of certain foods.

Although salt (sodium chloride) is a necessary micronutrient, the body's daily requirement is small (less than 1/4 of a teaspoon). For very active people who perspire a great deal, this need may increase to over 1.5 teaspoons/day. To put this into perspective, the average diet in the United States ranges from 3 to 10 teaspoons/day! Most people are totally unaware of the amount of salt in some foods. Figure 7.7 illustrates the "hidden" salt in an average pizza.

An excess of salt should be avoided because it is a complicating factor in people with high blood pressure. In countries where salt is not added to foods, either during cooking or at the table, high blood pressure is virtually unknown. Thus, even if you don't already have high blood pressure, you should limit salt in your diet to only the minimal daily requirements.

It has been estimated that half of the dietary carbohydrate intake of the average U.S. citizen is in the form of simple sugars as sucrose (table sugar) and corn syrup (commercial sweetener)(3). This represents more than 80 pounds of table sugar and 45 pounds of corn syrup per person each year! Sucrose and corn syrup are used to make cakes, candies, and ice cream, as well as to sweeten beverages, cereals, and other foods. Although overconsumption of these simple sugars has been linked to health problems—from hyperactivity in children to diabetes—there is little evidence to support these claims. However, several effects from overconsumption of these simple sugars should be avoided. First, the amount of sugar in sweets adds a tremendous amount of calories to the diet. This leads to obesity, which contributes to many health problems (e.g., diabetes). In addition, calories from sweets are considered "empty" calories because they provide little of the micronutrients the body needs to metabolize the macronutrients. Thus, complex carbohydrates are preferred because they are "loaded" with micronutrients. Second, sugar in sweets also leads to tooth decay. Although brushing your teeth after eating sweets can prevent this problem, it will not solve the other problems of overconsumption of sugar. One way of avoiding sucrose in the diet is to use fructose as a sweetener. Fructose is twice as sweet as sucrose, so you get equal sweetness for fewer calories.

Like table sugar, alcohol provides empty calories. In addition, chronic alcohol consumption tends to deplete the body's stores of some vitamins, which could lead to severe deficiencies. Thus, if for no other reason, alcohol consumption should be limited because it adds empty calories to your diet.

YOUR NEW DIET

Now that we have presented the guidelines for a healthy diet, let's put these principles into practice and illustrate how to construct a new diet. As we discuss the steps for choosing the right foods, refer to Table 7.11 on page 170, which presents a sample healthful 1-day diet for a college-age woman weighing 110 pounds. Assuming light daily activities, her projected daily caloric need is approximately 1690 calories. For your use of this diet plan, adjust the quantities accordingly.

Because the diet should consist of mainly complex carbohydrates, let's start each meal with a selection of food from the lower two levels of the eating-right pyra-

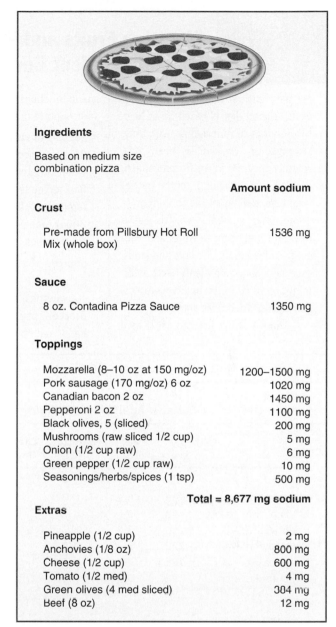

Ingredients

Based on medium size combination pizza

	Amount sodium
Crust	
Pre-made from Pillsbury Hot Roll Mix (whole box)	1536 mg
Sauce	
8 oz. Contadina Pizza Sauce	1350 mg
Toppings	
Mozzarella (8–10 oz at 150 mg/oz)	1200–1500 mg
Pork sausage (170 mg/oz) 6 oz	1020 mg
Canadian bacon 2 oz	1450 mg
Pepperoni 2 oz	1100 mg
Black olives, 5 (sliced)	200 mg
Mushrooms (raw sliced 1/2 cup)	5 mg
Onion (1/2 cup raw)	6 mg
Green pepper (1/2 cup raw)	10 mg
Seasonings/herbs/spices (1 tsp)	500 mg
Total = 8,677 mg sodium	
Extras	
Pineapple (1/2 cup)	2 mg
Anchovies (1/8 oz)	800 mg
Cheese (1/2 cup)	600 mg
Tomato (1/2 med)	4 mg
Green olives (4 med sliced)	304 mg
Beef (8 oz)	12 mg

FIGURE 7.7
The "hidden" salt in a typical medium pizza.
(*Source:* Donatelle, R. J., and L. G. Davis, *Access to Health*, 2002. Copyright © 2002 by Allyn & Bacon.)

mid. This will provide mainly carbohydrates, which should be greater than 58% of the total caloric intake, or 980 calories. These calories may be spread out over the day in any proportion you choose. We will use foods from the upper two levels of the pyramid to "fill in" where certain nutrients are needed.

Breakfast. Our subject first chooses a banana, a cup of milk, yogurt, and a cup of apple juice, which provide plenty of complex carbohydrates from fruits and dairy products. The bran flakes add lots of vitamin A and iron. The grapefruit adds plenty of vitamin C.

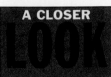

A CLOSER LOOK

Choosing Fruits and Vegetables for High Nutrient Content

As the "eating-right pyramid" suggests, a good diet is based on at least two servings of fruit and at least three servings of vegetables each day, whether they are fresh, frozen canned, or dried. Often, the brighter the fruit or vegetable, the higher the content of vitamins and minerals. So, to eat a healthful diet, choose fruits and vegetables of a variety of colors and kinds, especially dark-green leafy vegetables, bright orange fruits and vegetables, and cooked dried peas and beans.

The following list can serve as a guide for choosing the best sources of four important nutrients:

• **Sources of vitamin A (carotenoids)**
Bright orange vegetables (carrots, sweet potatoes, pumpkins)
Dark-green leafy vegetables (spinach, collards, turnip greens)
Bright orange fruits (mangoes, cantaloupes, apricots)

• **Sources of vitamin C**
Citrus fruits and juices, kiwis, strawberries, and cantaloupes
Broccoli, peppers, tomatoes, cabbage, and potatoes

Leafy greens (romaine lettuce, turnip greens, spinach)

• **Sources of folate**
Cooked dried beans and peas
Oranges, orange juice
Dark-green leafy vegetables (spinach, mustard greens)

• **Sources of potassium**
Potatoes, sweet potatoes, spinach, winter (orange) squash
Bananas, plantains, many dried fruits, orange juice

Source: National Academy of Sciences. *Dietary Reference Intakes: Applications in Dietary Assessment.* Washington, DC: National Academy Press, 2001.

TABLE 7.11
Sample Diet for a College-Age Female Weighing 110 Pounds, Assuming Light Daily Activities

	kcal	Fat (g)	Sat. Fat (g)	Chol. (mg)	Sod. (mg)	CHO (g)	Pro (g)	Vit A (RE)	Vit C (mg)	Ca (mg)	Iron (mg)
Breakfast											
1/2 grapefruit	38	0.1	0.02	0	0	9.7	0.8	2	41.3	14	0.1
2/3 cup bran flakes	90	0	0	0	220	18	3	380	1.2	20	18
1 cup whole milk	150	8.2	5.1	33	120	11.4	8	65	2.3	291	0.1
1 cup lowfat yogurt	225	2.6	1.7	10	121	42	9	20	1.4	314	0.1
1 banana	105	0.6	0.2	0	1	26.7	1.2	35	10.3	7	0.4
1 cup apple juice	92	0.5	0.02	0	1	24	0.3	24	7.8	16	1.4
Lunch											
Turkey sandwich with mustard	171	3.7	0.7	9	784	25	9.4	0	0	78	2.2
1 slice pizza	327	10.3	4.6	51	643	44	17	48	14	150	2
1 cup carrots (raw)	48	0.2	0.04	0	38	11.2	1.1	1400	10.2	30	0.54
1 cup low-fat milk	102	2.6	1.6	10	123	11.7	8	38	2.4	300	0.1
Dinner											
Baked fish with mushrooms (3 oz)	112	1.9	0.3	46	83	1.6	21	2	5.5	120	1.4
Baked potato	116	0.14	0.04	0	7	27	2.3	0	10	10	0.4
2 tsp margarine	100	11.4	2.1	0	150	0	0	32	0.02	3.75	0
3 slices tomato	12	0.15	0.02	0	5	2.4	0.5	62	11	3.9	0.3
1 diet cola	1	0	0	0	63	0.2	0	0	0	0	0.1
TOTALS	1689	42	16	159	2359	255	81.6	2108	117	1358	27
RDA	1690	<30%	<10%	<300	<3000	>58%	40	700	75	1000	18
% of RDA	100	76	90	53	79	105	204	300	156	135	150

Abbreviations: Sat. Fat, saturated fat; Chol., cholesterol; Sod., sodium; CHO, carbohydrate; Pro., protein; RE, retinol equivalents; Ca, calcium.

Nutritional Links

Choosing Your Fast Food More Wisely

As our lifestyles become faster, fast food has become a way of life. According to the May 1996 issue of *American Demographics,* the average American adult eats at a fast-food restaurant six times each month. The typical fast-food meal is high in fat and calories, factors that are major contributors to heart disease and obesity, so it is important to know how to choose foods during your next stop at the drive-through window. Keep the following guidelines in mind the next time you decide to grab a quick meal out:

- **Order small.** Don't "supersize" your meal. Consider these numbers: Depending on the restaurant, a double cheeseburger may contain 600–700 calories, 30–40 grams fat, 120–140 mg cholesterol, and 1000–1200 mg sodium.

- **Ask for sauce on the side.** Typically, tartar sauce contains about 20 grams of fat and about 220 mg sodium per tablespoon. Ketchup or pickle relish make a healthier sauce.

- **Order grilled meat instead of fried.** Breaded chicken typically contains double the amount of fat than if that same piece is broiled.

- **Share fries with a friend.** A medium serving of French fries may contain more fat than a cheeseburger! Consume a cheeseburger and fries, and you've eaten more fat in one meal than you need in almost an entire day.

- **Order salads without the dressing.** Most fast-food restaurants are adding more and more salad options. A side salad is an excellent way to include vegetables in your drive-through meal. Opting for a salad entree will provide a meal with less fat and sodium if you choose a nonfat salad dressing. However, you must choose wisely: At one fast-food restaurant, one serving of reduced calorie light Italian dressing contains 170 calories and 18 grams of fat!

On your next "drive-through," ask for the nutrition information sheet that most restaurants offer. Then you'll be able to choose fast food that is appealing to you *and* meets your dietary goals.

Lunch. Our subject can't resist a slice of pizza for lunch and gets approximately one-fourth of her daily salt, fat, and cholesterol. This is not as bad as it may seem if consumed in small quantities. She also gets protein, complex carbohydrates, and some micronutrients. The lunch also includes a turkey sandwich, which adds considerably to the salt load but also adds other needed nutrients. The carrots add considerably to the vitamin A and C totals. In addition, low-fat milk gives more of the much needed calcium.

Dinner. Any nutritional needs that are not met during the day should be met at dinner. The fish provides a low-fat source of concentrated protein as well as calcium, which is so important for our subject. This dinner provides an excellent example of how foods such as margarine and diet cola provide so little nutrient value. The margarine provides mainly fat and calories, and the cola provides only sodium.

SPECIAL DIETARY CONSIDERATIONS

Several conditions require special dietary considerations, especially as they pertain to people who lead an active lifestyle. Following is a list of nutrients that may need to be supplemented, depending on your individual needs. Use these concepts to help complete Laboratory 7.2 on page 189.

VITAMINS As mentioned previously, healthy people who eat a balanced diet generally do not need vitamin supplements. Some individuals, however, may not be getting proper nutrition because of poor diet or disease. Therefore, the following people may find a multivitamin supplement helpful:

- strict vegetarians
- people with chronic illnesses that depress appetite or the absorption of nutrients
- people on medications that affect appetite or digestion
- athletes engaged in a rigorous training program
- pregnant women or women who are breast-feeding infants
- individuals on prolonged low-calorie diets
- the elderly

IRON Iron is an essential component of red blood cells, which carry oxygen to all our tissues for energy production. A deficiency of iron can result in decreased oxygen transport to tissues and thus an energy crisis. Getting enough iron is a major problem for women who are menstruating, pregnant, or nursing. Indeed, only one-half of all women of child-bearing age get the necessary 15 mg of iron per day (3). Five percent suffer from iron-deficiency anemia! Although these individuals should not take iron supplements unless their physician prescribes them, they can modify their diets to assure getting the RDA of iron. To meet this requirement, the following dietary modifications should be undertaken:

- Eat legumes, fresh fruits, whole-grain cereals, and broccoli, all of which are high in iron.
- Also eat foods high in vitamin C, which helps iron absorption.
- Eat lean red meats high in iron at least two or three times per week.
- Eat iron-rich organ meats, such as liver, once or twice per month.
- Don't drink tea with your meals; it interferes with iron absorption.

CALCIUM Calcium, the most abundant mineral in the body, is essential for building bones and teeth, as well as for normal nerve and muscle function. Adequate calcium is especially important for pregnant or nursing women. There is some evidence that calcium may help in the prevention of colon cancer (3).

The most recent RDAs call for a significant increase in calcium intake for both sexes beginning at age 9. Whereas the previous RDA for calcium for adults was 800 mg, now 1300 mg of calcium are recommended each day for individuals between 9 and 18 years of age. Adequate calcium intake during those years may be a crucial factor in preventing osteoporosis in later years, which strikes one of every four women over the age of 60 (8). The following recommendations can help you get the calcium you need:

- Add dairy products to your diet, but remember, choose those low in fat.
- Choose other calcium-rich alternatives, such as canned fish (packed in water), turnip and mustard greens, and broccoli.
- Eat foods rich in vitamin C to boost absorption of calcium.
- Use an acidic dressing, made with citrus juices or vinegar, to enhance calcium absorption from salad greens.
- Add a supplement if you can't get enough calcium in the foods you like. However, beware of supplements made with dolomite or bone meal, as they may be contaminated with lead.

☀ IN SUMMARY

- The basic goals of developing good nutritional habits are to maintain ideal body weight; eat a variety of foods following the "eating-right pyramid"

model; avoid consuming too much fat, saturated fat, and cholesterol; eat foods with adequate starch and fiber; avoid consuming too much simple sugar; avoid consuming too much sodium; and if you drink alcohol, do so in moderation.

- The general rule for meeting the body's need for macronutrients is that an individual should consume approximately 58% of needed calories in carbohydrates (about 48% complex carbohydrates and 10% simple sugars), 30% or less in fats (approximately 10% saturated and 20% unsaturated fats), and 12% in proteins.
- The calorie is a unit of measure of the energy value of food or the energy required for physical activity.

☀ Nutritional Aspects of Physical Fitness

The number of myths about physical fitness and nutrition increases every year. Radio, T.V., newspaper, and magazine advertisements create a never-ending source of fallacies. Successful athletes are often viewed as experts by the public, and their endorsements of various nutritional products are attempts to convince the public that a particular food or beverage is responsible for their success. Even though most of the claims made in commercial endorsements are not supported by research, the claims are so highly publicized that they often become accepted as fact. The truth is, there are no miracle foods to improve physical fitness or exercise performance. In the paragraphs that follow we discuss the specific needs of individuals engaging in a regular exercise program.

CARBOHYDRATES

The increased energy expenditure during exercise creates a greater demand for fuel. Recall that the primary fuels used to provide energy for exercise are carbohydrates and fat. Because even very lean people have a large amount of energy stored as fat, lack of fat for fuel is not a problem during exercise. In contrast, the carbohydrate stores in the liver and muscles can reach critically low levels during intense or prolonged exercise (6) (Figure 7.8).

Because carbohydrates play a critical role in providing energy during exercise, some exercise scientists have suggested that people participating in daily exercise programs should increase the complex carbohydrates in their diet from 58–70% of the total calories consumed (fat intake is then reduced to 18% of total caloric intake) (6). If exercise is intense, carbohydrates can be depleted from the liver and muscles, and the result is fatigue. The intensity of the exercise dictates whether carbohydrates or fat is the predominant source of energy production (6, 9).

Manufacturers of sweets have perpetrated the notion that candy can give you a quick burst of energy when needed. Does a candy bar consumed prior to exercise provide a quick burst of energy? The answer is "no." In fact, there are at least two potential problems with this type of carbohydrate consumption. First, simple sugar in the form of sweets contains only minimal amounts of the micronutrients necessary for energy production. Second, consumption of candy results in a rapid rise in blood glucose, which promotes hormonal changes that reduce blood glucose levels below normal and can create a feeling of fatigue. In this case, the effect is opposite of the one intended. Increasing the percentage of complex carbohydrates in the diet and maintaining sufficient caloric intake can ensure that an adequate supply of energy from carbohydrates is stored in the muscles and the liver to meet the needs of a rigorous exercise training program.

PROTEIN

Another common myth among individuals involved in strength training programs is that additional amounts of protein are necessary to promote muscular growth. In fact, many bodybuilders consume large quantities of protein to supplement their normal dietary protein. Research has shown that the protein requirements of most bodybuilders is met by a normal, well-balanced diet (10, 11). Therefore, the increased caloric needs of an individual engaged in a strength training program should come from additional amounts of food from the

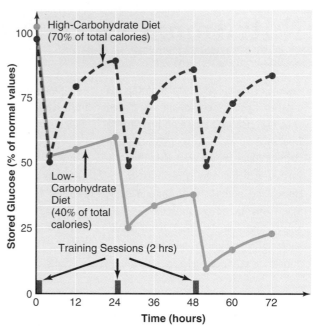

FIGURE 7.8
The importance of a high-carbohydrate diet during exercise training. With a low-carbohydrate diet (solid line), glucose stored in muscles as glycogen is depleted by daily training sessions. If a high-carbohydrate diet is consumed (dashed line), muscle glycogen levels are maintained at near normal levels.
(*Source:* Neiman, David C. *Fitness and Sports Medicine: An Introduction.* Palo Alto, CA: Bull Publishing, 1995. Used with permission.)

bottom three levels of the eating-right pyramid and not simply from additional protein. In this way, not only are the extra macronutrients supplied, but also the micronutrients necessary for energy production.

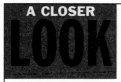

How to Control Cravings for Sweets

The following guidelines can help in your quest to control your sweet tooth.

- Know how to spot sugar. When you see terms such as *sucrose, glucose, maltose, dextrose, fructose,* or *corn syrup* on food labels, beware. These are all forms of sugar.
- If sugar or its "pseudos" are in the first three ingredients on a label, avoid the product. It has a high sugar content by weight.

- Cut back on all sugars, including honey, brown sugar, and white sugar.
- Eat graham crackers, yogurt, fresh fruits, popcorn, and other healthy substitutes for high-sugar sweets when you have the munchies.
- Buy cereals that do not have sugars listed among their top ingredients. Shredded Wheat®, Cheerios®, and oatmeal are among the best choices.

- When baking, try cutting the sugar in recipes by one-fourth or more; you can also substitute fruit juices for sweetness or use spices such as cinnamon, anise, ginger, and nutmeg for flavorings.
- If you can't resist sweets, at least eat foods that give you some nutritional value. For example, put bananas on your oatmeal rather than brown sugar, or make oatmeal cookies rather than sugar cookies.

Source: Boyle, M., and G. Zyla. *Personal Nutrition.* St. Paul, MN: West Publishers, 1991.

Nutritional Links

Do Antioxidants Prevent Muscle Injury or Fatigue?

Recent research suggests that the increased muscle metabolism associated with exercise may cause an increase in free radical production (12). Several studies have shown that this increase in free radicals may contribute to fatigue, and perhaps even muscle damage. The obvious question is, Do active individuals need to increase their consumption of antioxidants?

Several preliminary studies have indicated a positive role for antioxidants, primarily vitamin E, in neutralizing exercise-produced free radicals. In fact, recent reports have demonstrated a reduction in muscle fatigue following administration of antioxidants (13). Several researchers have suggested that an additional 400 I.U. of vitamin E be consumed daily to protect against free radical damage. However, you should consult your pharmacist or nutritionist before consuming more than the RDA of fat-soluble vitamins. Remember: Fat-soluble vitamins are stored in the body, and their accumulation may lead to toxicity.

VITAMINS

Some vitamin manufacturers have argued that megadoses of vitamins can improve exercise performance. This belief is based on the notion that exercise increases the need for energy and, because vitamins are necessary for the breakdown of foods for energy, an extra load of vitamins should be helpful. There is no evidence to support this claim (14). The energy supplied for muscle contraction is not enhanced by vitamin supplements. In fact, megadoses of vitamins may interfere with the delicate balance of other micronutrients and can be toxic as well (3).

ANTIOXIDANTS

Although large doses of vitamins may be counterproductive, recent research has discovered a new function for some vitamins and other micronutrients (3). These vitamins and micronutrients provide protection to cells by working as antioxidants. **Antioxidants** are chemicals that prevent a damaging form of oxygen (called *oxygen free radicals*) from causing damage to the cells. Although free radicals are constantly produced by the body, excess production of these has been implicated in cancer, lung disease, heart disease, and even the aging process (15). If cellular antioxidants can combine with the free radicals as they are produced, the free radicals become neutralized before they cause damage. Therefore, increasing the level of antioxidants may be beneficial to health. Several micronutrients, including vitamins A, E, and C, beta-carotene, zinc, and selenium, have been identified as potent antioxidants.

☼ IN SUMMARY

- The intensity of exercise dictates the relative proportions of fat and carbohydrate that are consumed as fuel during exercise.
- The extra energy needed for strength training should not come solely from increased protein intake.
- Excess vitamin intake does not improve exercise performance.
- Antioxidants are chemicals that prevent oxygen free radicals from combining with cells and damaging them. To date, vitamins A, E, and C, beta-carotene, zinc, and selenium have been identified as potent antioxidants.

☼ Do Supplements Provide an Edge for Health and Performance?

What are supplements? Should I take them? Are they safe? Millions of people concerned about health, disease prevention, and exercise performance are asking these questions. Over the past decade the use of nutritional and pharmaceutical supplements has become common in the United States. The search for a speedy path to health, wellness, and fitness led Americans to double what they spent on dietary supplements during

---

antioxidants Chemicals that prevent a damaging form of oxygen (called *oxygen free radicals*) from causing destruction to cells. Although free radicals are constantly produced by the body, excess production of these compounds has been implicated in cancer, lung disease, heart disease, and even the aging process.

1991–1996 to over $6 billion (Figure 7.9). In the following sections we examine what supplements are, how they are regulated, and which ones might have the potential to be beneficial.

WHAT IS A DIETARY SUPPLEMENT?

Due to the widespread marketing of dietary supplements over the past two decades, Congress has intervened by defining the term *dietary supplement*. According to the Dietary Supplement Health and Education Act (DSHEA) of 1994, a dietary supplement:

- is a product (other than tobacco) that is intended to supplement the diet and bears or contains one or more of the following dietary ingredients: a vitamin, a mineral, an herb, or other botanical; an amino acid; a dietary substance for use by humans to supplement the diet by increasing the total daily intake; or a concentrate, metabolite, constituent, extract, or combinations of these ingredients.

- is intended for ingestion in pill, capsule, tablet, or liquid form.

- is not represented for use as a conventional food or as the sole item of a meal or diet.

- is labeled as a "dietary supplement."

- includes products such as an approved new drug, certified antibiotic, or licensed biologic that was marketed as a dietary supplement or food before approval, certification, or license (unless the Secretary of Health and Human Services waives this provision).

GOVERNMENT REGULATIONS CONCERNING SUPPLEMENTS

The U.S. Food and Drug Administration (FDA) administers the DSHEA and is responsible for regulating dietary supplements. Regulation of dietary supplements is different from that of foods and prescription and over-the-counter drugs. The DSHEA dictates that manufacturers, not the government, are responsible for the safety of supplements. Moreover, supplement manufacturers are not required to get FDA approval before they market their products.

The DSHEA allows supplement manufacturers to claim effects on the "structure or function" of the body, but disallows claims concerning the treatment, prevention, cure, or diagnosis of disease. The FDA instituted the "structure/function rule" in 2000 to distinguish disease claims, which require that evidence of safety and benefit be demonstrated to the FDA before marketing, from structure/function claims, which have no such requirement. The rule prohibits both express disease claims (such as "prevents heart disease") and implied disease claims (such as "prevents bone fragility

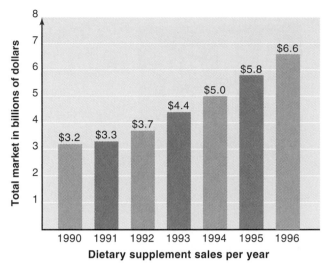

FIGURE 7.9
The steady growth in the use of dietary supplements in the United States. The growing popularity of supplements helped this billion-dollar industry double its sales between 1991 and 1996.
(*Source:* FDA Consumer. *An FDA Guide to Dietary Supplements.* Washington, DC: U.S. Government Printing Office, 1999.)

in post-menopausal women") without prior FDA review. However, the rule permits health-maintenance claims (such as "maintains healthy bones"), other claims not related to disease (such as "for muscle enhancement"), and claims for the relief of common minor symptoms associated with life stages (such as "for common symptoms of PMS").

Since its initial release, the rule has been modified both to expand the number of acceptable structure/function claims and to narrow the definition of "disease" to disallow structure/function claims pertaining to aging, pregnancy, menopause, and adolescence. Under the DSHEA, supplement manufacturers are required to keep on file substantiation of any structure/function claims they make. Keep in mind, however, the FDA neither examines nor substantiates the "legitimacy" of this documentation. Manufacturers must also include on their labels a disclaimer stating that their dietary supplements are not drugs and received no FDA approval before marketing. Additionally, manufacturers must notify the FDA of a product claim within 30 days of marketing it. All this means that dietary supplements are not well regulated. The consumer is responsible for determining whether a given supplement is needed or safe.

THE ROLE OF SUPPLEMENTATION IN A HEALTHFUL DIET

The FDA estimates that more than 25,000 products are available as dietary supplements. It is important to note that there is no scientific evidence to validate most of

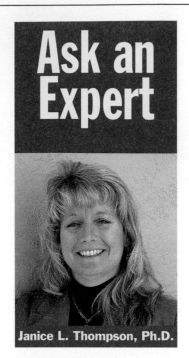

Ask an Expert

Janice L. Thompson, Ph.D.

Nutrition, Exercise, and Metabolism

Dr. Thompson is an internationally renowned researcher in the Department of Internal Medicine at the University of New Mexico. She is best known for her work describing the interactions of nutrition and physical activity on chronic diseases. She has published many scientific papers, books, and book chapters related to diet, nutrition, and exercise. In the accompanying interview, Dr. Thompson addresses several hot topic questions related to diet and exercise.

Q: There are hundreds of supplements on the market for replenishment of protein and carbohydrates after exercise. Is there any benefit to this type of supplement over the normal diet?

A: Active people need to eat a relatively high carbohydrate diet, or at least 60% of total energy as carbohydrate. Very little protein is used for energy during exercise; however, protein supports the growth and repair of body tissues and helps recovery from exercise. Unless you are exercising more than 60 to 90 minutes each day at a high training intensity, you probably do not need to consume supplements. If you do eat a "normal" diet, you should consume enough carbohydrate and protein to support exercise and recovery from exercise. Women and men who are dieting, highly active people who do not eat a balanced diet, and athletes who train many hours each day are at risk for getting too little carbohydrate and protein and may benefit from supplements.

Q: Weight-training is my primary means of activity. I am concerned that I may not be getting enough protein in my diet. Should I supplement my diet with a protein powder?

A: One of the most prevalent myths in the strength training world is that people who lift weights have very high protein needs. In reality, studies of strength athletes show that they need 1.6 to 1.7 grams of protein each day for every kilogram of body weight, about two times the current protein recommendation for the average adult. Endurance athletes also need more protein than the average person, requiring about 1.2 to 1.4 grams of protein each day for every kilogram of body weight. Most people in the United States eat at least two times the recommendation for protein in their normal diet with no effort, so supplementing your diet with protein powder is not necessary.

Q: I have seen a great deal written about phytochemicals. What are they? Should I be concerned about getting enough in my diet?

A: Phytochemicals are substances found in plants that may protect us against diseases such as heart disease and cancer and are naturally found in fruits, vegetables, grains, legumes, seeds, soy, and green tea. The study of phytochemicals is still new, and we do not yet know the complete story on how these substances can prevent disease. Although we have started to study hundreds of these substances, there could be thousands remaining in food yet to be discovered. Your best approach is to eat more fruits and vegetables, at least two fruits and three vegetables each day.

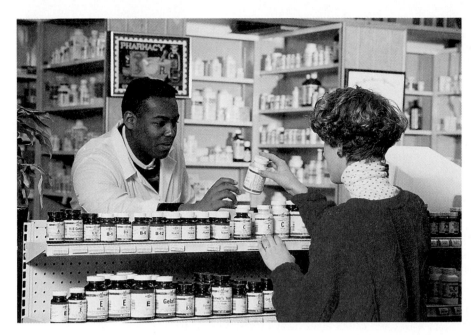

Many special considerations such as age, gender, size, and activity must be assessed in determining vitamin requirements. Consult your pharmacist or a registered dietician when considering any dietary supplementation.

the claims that supplements improve health or exercise performance. Table 7.12 lists and evaluates a few of the more popular supplements currently marketed for improving health and enhancing exercise performance.

Our knowledge of the relationship between diet and disease points out the importance of micronutrients and macronutrients, as well as the need to ensure adequate nutrient consumption while avoiding dietary excesses. However, not much is known about newly discovered, unclassified, and naturally occurring micronutrient components of food and the subsequent effects on health and disease. For example, several studies have identified numerous plant compounds, called phytochemicals, that when ingested by humans in small amounts may protect against a variety of diseases. (See Nutritional Links to Health and Fitness, p. 180.) We still don't know whether phytochemicals, in the large amounts typically present in supplements, are safe or effective. Given our current incomplete knowledge, eating a wide variety of foods and avoiding excesses or imbalances that can potentially result from relying too much on dietary supplements are the best ways to obtain adequate amount of beneficial food constituents. As previously explained, following the Dietary Guidelines for Americans (7) and the recommendations of the eating-right pyramid can help you consume a variety of foods, which reduces the risks of both inadequate and excessive dietary intake.

☼ IN SUMMARY
- The use of dietary supplements has grown tremendously over the last decade, with Americans spending over $6 million a year on the products.

- The FDA defines a dietary supplement as a product that contains a vitamin, mineral, herb, or other botanical, an amino acid, a dietary substance for use by humans to supplement the diet by increasing the total daily intake, or a concentrate, metabolite, constituent, extract, or combinations of these ingredients. The FDA mandated that the supplement should be in pill, capsule, tablet, or liquid form and labeled as a supplement.

- Regulations also mandate that the only claims that can be made about the supplement must relate to effects on "structure or function" of the body.

- Manufacturers can make no claims about the effects of a supplement on disease.

- Because dietary supplements are poorly regulated, consumers should be cautious when choosing and using such supplements. When doubts about a product arise, a nutritionist should be consulted.

- Supplements should never be relied on as major sources of dietary nutrients.

☼ Current Topics in Food Safety

Many aspects of nutrition, such as food safety, have significant effects on health. In recent years there have been increased reports of illness and death due to improperly stored and prepared foods. Let's examine some of the latest suggestions for improving food safety.

FOODBORNE INFECTIONS

According to the Institute of Food Technologists, approximately 80 million cases of foodborne bacterial disease occur each year. These illnesses produce nausea,

TABLE 7.12
Comparison of Dietary Supplements

Supplement	Origin	Benefits Claimed	Evidence of Effectiveness
Androstenedione	Made by the body as part of testosterone production	Enhances the production of testosterone and causes an increase in muscle mass	Evidence suggests that it does not increase testosterone, and it may increase female hormones in men.
Antioxidants	Produced by cells to protect against free radical production. Some vitamins, minerals, and other chemicals in foods also have antioxidant properties.	Buffer free radical damage, which could help prevent fatigue and/or muscle damage during exercise. Also, could help protect against some diseases.	No evidence to suggest enhancement of exercise performance. Some evidence to suggest a benefit in preventing damage to tissues. Growing evidence to suggest benefits in fighting many conditions such as cancer, heart and lung disease, and aging.
Caffeine	Compound found in coffee, cola, candy, stimulants, weight-loss products.	Used to increase muscle fiber activation to increase strength, or to increase fat metabolism and endurance.	Increases endurance in events lasting greater than 20 min. No consistent effects on strength.
Carbohydrates	Component of most food. Usually found as a dietary supplement in the form of beverages or bars.	Increase in stored glucose in muscle and liver and increase in endurance.	Improves endurance in events longer than 90–120 minutes. Also helps restore glucose after exercise.
L-Carnitine	Made by the body and ingested in meat products.	Increases transport of fat in cells, reduces lactate accumulation.	Carnitine is in adequate supply in the cells, and additional amounts provide no benefit before, during, or after exercise.
Chromium picolinate	Chromium is a trace element found in several foods; picolinate is added to supplements to aid absorption in the gut.	Helps insulin action and is thought to aid glucose metabolism, blood fats, and have anabolic effects.	No good evidence for any benefits. *Side effects: Stomach upset, anemia, genetic damage, kidney damage.*
Coenzyme Q-10	Made by the body as a component of the biochemical pathway that makes ATP.	Enhances ATP production.	No evidence suggests a benefit during or after exercise.
Creatine	Made by the body and also obtained by eating meat products.	Decreases fatigue in short, intense exercise. Increases muscle size and strength.	Increases endurance in short, intense exercise. Causes water gain in muscle but not increases in strength.
Echinacea	Herbal supplement.	Reduces duration of colds, boosts immune system, heals wounds.	Some evidence suggests it may be beneficial for these conditions. *Side effects: Uncommon, but possible GI upset, chills, nausea.*
Ginkgo Biloba	Extracts of dried leaves of *Ginkgo* plant.	Used for antioxidant properties and to improve blood flow and memory.	Does have antioxidant properties that may be beneficial in improving blood flow, improving neural function, and reducing production of stress hormones. *Side effects: nausea, headache, dizziness, skin rash, hemorrage if used with blood thinners.*
B-Hydroxy Methyl Butyate (HMB)	By-product of amino acid breakdown. Also ingested in some food.	Inhibition of protein breakdown.	Scant evidence suggests some increase in muscle mass.
Ribose	Naturally occurring sugar that is now mass produced.	Used to delay fatigue during high-volume type training.	Much evidence to suggest benefits in heart muscle but very little evidence for effects on skeletal muscle.
St. John's Wort	Plant extract.	Used to treat depression and external wounds, burns, and muscle aches.	Some evidence suggests that it is beneficial for treating these conditions.

Detecting Supplement Fraud

Most of the dietary supplements on the market today are useless. Advertisements for fraudulent products are everywhere—in newspaper and magazine ads, on TV "infomercials," on the Internet, and accompanying products sold in stores and through mail-order catalogues. And consumers, in their desire to cure an ailment, improve their well-being, or improve athletic performance, respond by spending billions of dollars each year on fraudulent health products. The products they buy often do nothing more than cheat them out of their money or steer them away from products that have been proven useful. Some supplement products may do more harm than good.

How can you avoid being scammed by the maker of a worthless supplement? Marketers have sophisticated ways of making their products attractive to potential buyers, but you can protect yourself by learning about marketing ploys. Beware of the following techniques, claims, or catch-phrases:

- **The product "does it all."** Be suspicious of any supplement that claims to have multiple benefits. No one product is likely to be capable of so great a range of effectiveness.
- **The product is supported by personal testimonials.** Testimonials are quite often simply stories that have been passed from person to person, and sometimes they are completely made up. Because testimonials are difficult to prove, they may be a "tip" to the possibility of fraud.
- **The product provides a "quick fix."** Be skeptical of products that claim to produce immediate results. Among the tip-offs are ambiguous language like "provides relief in days" or "you'll feel energized immediately." Unscrupulous marketers use such phrases to protect themselves against any subsequent legal action.
- **The product is "natural."** The term *natural,* which is clearly an attention-grabber, suggests that the product is safer than conventional treatments. However, *any* product—whether synthetic or natural—that is potent enough to produce a significant physiological effect is potent enough to cause side effects.
- **The product is "a new, time-tested treatment."** A product is usually one or the other, but be suspicious of any product that claims to be both a breakthrough and a decades-old treatment. If a product that claims to be an "innovation," an "exclusive product," or a "new discovery" were really so revolutionary, it would be widely reported in the media and pre-scribed by health professionals, not featured in obscure ads.
- **Your "satisfaction is guaranteed."** Money-back guarantees are often empty promises. To evade cheated customers, scam artists move often, rarely staying in one place for long. And the makers of this claim know most people won't go to all the trouble involved in trying to get a refund of only $9.95 or so.
- **The product's ads contain meaningless medical jargon.** The use of scientific-sounding terms as "aerobic enzyme booster" may seem impressive and may even contain an element of truth, but these terms likely cover up a lack of scientific data concerning the product.

Always ask yourself, Does this claim seem too good to be true? If it does, then the product is probably a fraud. If you're still not sure, talk to your doctor or other health professional. The Better Business Bureau or your state attorney general's office can tell you whether other consumers have lodged complaints about a product or its marketers. If a product is promoted as being helpful for a specific condition, check with the appropriate professional group—for example, consult the American Heart Association about products that claim some effectiveness concerning heart disease.

vomiting, and diarrhea from 12 hours to 5 days after infection (8). The severity of the illness depends on the microorganism ingested and the victim's overall health. Indeed, foodborne infections can be fatal in people with compromised immune systems or those in ill health.

One of the most common types of food poisoning is caused by the bacterium *Salmonella.* It is usually found in undercooked chicken, eggs, and processed meats. A relatively uncommon but sometimes fatal form of food poisoning is *botulism,* which usually results from

Nutritional Links

Do Phytochemicals Protect Against Disease?

Besides nutrients, plant foods—legumes, vegetables, fruits, and whole grains—contain a whole other "crop" of chemicals called *phytochemicals* (*phyto* means "plant"). These substances, which plants produce naturally to protect themselves against viruses, bacteria, and fungi, may help protect us from diseases as well.

Phytochemicals include hundreds of naturally occurring substances, including carotenoids, flavenoids, including indoles, isoflavones, capsaicin, and protease inhibitors. And just as occurs with vitamins and minerals, different plant foods contain different kinds and amounts of phytochemicals.

Even though the exact ways phytochemicals promote health are not yet clear, certain phytochemicals appear to protect against some cancers, heart disease, and other chronic health conditions. Research into their roles is ongoing, so stay tuned! Until more is known, the nutrition bottom line still applies: Eat a wide variety of fruits, vegetables, legumes, and whole grains, and count on food, not diet supplements, to get the nutrients your body needs. That way, you'll reap the potential benefits of the many phytochemicals found in all kinds of plant foods.

Source: Duyff, R. L. *The American Dietetic Association's Complete Food and Nutrition Guide,* Minnetonka, MN: Chronimed Publishing, 1996.

improper home-canning procedures. Use the following guidelines for preventing food poisoning:

- Clean food thoroughly. Wash all produce and raw meats, and make sure cans show no sign of leaks or bulges.
- Drink only pasteurized milk.
- Don't eat raw eggs.
- Cook chicken thoroughly.
- Cook pork to an internal temperature of 170°F to kill parasites called trichina.
- Cook all shellfish thoroughly; steaming them open may not be sufficient.
- Be wary of raw fish; it may contain parasitic roundworms. Keep fish frozen and cook until well done.
- Wash utensils, plates, cutting boards, knives, blenders, and other cooking equipment with soap and very hot water after preparing raw poultry.

FOOD ADDITIVES

Food additives are substances added to food to lengthen its storage time, change its taste or color, or otherwise make it more appealing. Although they can provide these benefits, they may also pose a risk. One example is nitrites, which are found in foods such as bacon, sausages, and lunch meats. Nitrites inhibit spoilage and prevent botulism, but they also form cancer-causing agents (nitrosamines) in the body.

organic   Refers to foods that are grown without pesticides.

ORGANICALLY GROWN FOODS

Each year, over one million pounds of commercial pesticides are used in the United States. Although these chemicals can save crops from disease and pests, they may also endanger human health. In recent years, many people have begun to purchase organically grown foods. **Organic** in this context refers to foods that are grown without the use of pesticides. Organically grown foods are more expensive than foods commonly supplied by supermarkets.

In the near future, look for new genetics techniques in biology to spawn a new world of pest- and insecticide-free foods. These new techniques combine the genetic material from various plants, in an effort to produce strains of high-yield crops that are resistant to diseases and pests, high in nutritional quality, and free of chemicals. Whether these new plants will live up to expectations remains to be seen.

IRRADIATED FOODS

Irradiation is the use of radiation (high-energy waves or particles, including radioactivity and X-rays) to kill microorganisms that grow on or in food. When radioactivity is used, the food does not become radioactive; instead the irradiation serves to prolong the shelf life of the food (16). Indeed, irradiated food can be stored for years in sealed containers at room temperature without spoiling. In addition, irradiation can delay the sprouting of vegetables such as potatoes and onions and delay the ripening of fruits such as bananas, mangoes, tomatoes, pears, and avocados. This can result in significant cost savings.

Are these irradiated foods safe to eat? Currently, the best answer is a qualified "yes." All research indicates

Nutritional Links
How to Handle Take-out Food Safely

Whether from restaurants, supermarkets, or quick-service establishments, take-out foods have become a part of our way of life. But in order to avoid foodborne illnesses, these foods must be handled with care. The next time your order take-out, keep the following recommendations in mind.

For Hot Foods:
- Hot foods must be kept above 140°F. First, make sure the food is hot when you pick it up or it's delivered. You can cover food with foil (to keep it moist) and keep it warm—140°F or above—in the oven (check the food's temperature with a meat thermometer). Using a

crockpot is another option for some foods. It's best to eat food within 2 hours of preparation.

- If the food won't be eaten for more than 2 hours, refrigerate in shallow, covered containers. Before serving, reheat it in an oven to 165°F or until it's hot and steaming. If you prefer, reheat food in a microwave oven—cover and rotate—and then let it stand for 2 minutes to ensure thorough, even heating.

For Cold Foods:
- Cold foods must be kept at 40°F or below.
- If cold, take-out foods are not eaten right away, refrigerate them

as soon as possible. Transport and store cold foods in chilled, insulated coolers.

- Discard any foods kept at room temperature for more than 2 hours. If conditions are warmer than 90°F, toss the food after only 1 hour.
- Keep deli platters that stay out—as is the practice in buffet dining—on bowls of ice.

Source: Duyff, R. L. *The American Dietetic Association's Complete Food and Nutrition Guide.* Minnetonka, MN: Chronimed Publishing, 1996.

that the foods are safe and nutritional content is maintained, but only limited data exist (16). In addition, most studies have used very low radiation levels to irradiate foods. This raises the question, "What is a safe level of radiation for the treatment of foods?"

ANIMALS TREATED WITH ANTIBIOTICS AND HORMONES

In recent years, consumers have grown suspicious of eating meat from animals that have been treated with antibiotics to prevent infections. Concern has developed because of the possibility that eating such meat could lead to the development of antibiotic-resistant bacteria in humans. At present, a definitive answer to this issue is not available.

Another recent concern has been the use of hormones to increase production of meat and milk. Most notably, a form of growth hormone, bovine somatotropin, has been used to increase milk production in

dairy cows. Some people fear that the presence of hormones in food may result in health problems that have not yet been determined. Many supermarkets are restricting the sale of milk produced with the aid of hormone supplements.

☀ IN SUMMARY
- Proper food storage and preparation are the keys to preventing food poisoning. Select foods that appear clean and fresh; keep foods cold or frozen to prevent bacteria from growing; clean fresh fruits, vegetables, and meats (especially chicken) thoroughly; cook all meats thoroughly; order meats well done when dining out.
- Consumption of organically grown foods may be beneficial if you are concerned about pesticides used to grow grains, fruits, and vegetables.
- Future use of food irradiation and genetic manipulation of plants and animals will likely increase yield and enhance safety of food.

Summary

1. Nutrition is the study of food and its relationship to health and disease. The current primary problem in nutrition in industrialized countries is overeating.

2. A well-balanced diet is composed of approximately 58% complex carbohydrates, 30% fat, and 12% protein. These macronutrients are also called the fuel nutrients, because they are the only substances that can be used as fuel to provide the energy (calories) necessary for bodily functions.

3. Carbohydrate is a primary fuel used by the body to provide energy. The calorie is a unit of measure of the energy value of food or the energy required for physical activity.

4. Simple carbohydrates consist of a single sugar (glucose, fructose, sucrose) or two sugars linked together (galactose, lactose, and maltose).

5. The complex carbohydrates consist of starches and fiber. Starches are composed of chains of simple sugars. Fiber is a nondigestible but essential form of complex carbohydrates contained in whole grains, vegetables, and fruits.

6. Fat is an efficient storage form for energy, because each gram contains over twice the energy content of 1 gram of either carbohydrate or protein. Fat can be derived from dietary sources or formed from excess carbohydrate and protein consumed in the diet. Fat is stored in the body in adipose tissues located under the skin and around internal organs. Fats are classified as either simple, compound, or derived. The triglycerides are the most notable of the simple fats. Fatty acids, the basic structural unit of triglycerides, are classified as either saturated or unsaturated, depending on their chemical structures. For nutritional considerations, the most important of the compound fats are the lipoproteins. Cholesterol is the best example of the class of fats called derived fats.

7. The primary role of protein consumed in the diet is to serve as the structural unit for building and repairing cells in all tissues of the body. Protein consists of amino acids made by the body (11 nonessential amino acids) and those available only through dietary sources (nine essential amino acids).

8. Vitamins serve many important functions in the body, including regulation of growth and metabolism. The class of water-soluble vitamins consists of several B-complex vitamins and vitamin C. The fat-soluble vitamins are A, D, E, and K.

9. Minerals are chemical elements contained in many foods. Like vitamins, minerals serve many important roles in regulating body functions.

10. Approximately 60–70% of the body is water. Water is involved in all vital processes in the body and is the nutrient of greatest concern to the physically active individual. In addition to the water contained in foods, it is recommended that an additional 8–10 cups of water be consumed daily.

11. The basic goals of developing good nutritional habits are to maintain ideal body weight; eat a variety of foods, following the "eating-right pyramid" model; avoid consuming too much fat, saturated fat, and cholesterol; eat foods with adequate starch and fiber; avoid consuming too much simple sugar; avoid consuming too much sodium; and if you drink alcohol, do so in moderation.

12. The general rule for meeting the body's need for macronutrients is that an individual should consume approximately 58% of needed calories in carbohydrates (48% complex carbohydrates and 10% simple sugars), 30% or less in fats (approximately 10% saturated and 20% unsaturated fats), and 12% in proteins.

13. In order to have a healthy diet, fats (especially saturated or animal fats), cholesterol, salt, sugar/corn syrup, and alcohol should be minimized.

14. The intensity of exercise dictates the relative proportions of fat and carbohydrate that are consumed as fuel during exercise. In general, the lower the intensity of exercise, the more fat is used as a fuel. Conversely, the greater the intensity of exercise, the more carbohydrate is used as a fuel.

15. Antioxidants are nutrients that prevent oxygen free radicals from combining with cells and damaging them. The micronutrients that have been identified as potent antioxidants are vitamins E and C, beta-carotene, zinc, and selenium.

16. Food storage and preparation is key to the prevention of food poisoning. Select foods that appear clean and fresh; keep foods cold or frozen to prevent bacteria from growing; thoroughly clean fresh fruits, vegetables, and meats (especially chicken); cook all meats thoroughly, and order well-done meats when dining out.

Study Questions

1. What is the role of carbohydrates in the diet?
2. List the major food sources of dietary carbohydrates.
3. List the various subcategories of carbohydrates.
4. Compare the three classes of fats.
5. Define *triglyceride* and discuss its use in the body.

6. Distinguish between saturated and unsaturated fatty acids.

7. What are omega-3 fatty acids?

8. Discuss the role of protein in the diet.

9. Distinguish between essential and nonessential amino acids.

10. What are the classes of vitamins, and what is the role of vitamins in body function?

11. Outline the role of minerals in body function.

12. Discuss the importance of water in the diet.

13. What approximate proportions of carbohydrate, fat, and protein in the diet are recommended daily?

14. Discuss the "eating-right pyramid" and its role in the selection of foods for the diet.

15. How many calories are contained in 1 gram of carbohydrate, fat, and protein, respectively?

16. Discuss the special need for carbohydrate in an individual who is engaging in an exercise training program.

17. Discuss the special need for protein for an individual who is engaging in an exercise training program.

18. Define the following:
    antioxidants
    calorie

19. What is the potential role of antioxidants in the diet?

20. Discuss the impact of the following on heart disease:
    high-density lipoproteins (HDL cholesterol)
    low-density lipoproteins (LDL cholesterol)

21. Define "dietary supplement" and give an example.

22. Discuss the "structure/function" rule pertaining to dietary supplements.

23. How does the FDA "police" the marketing of dietary supplements?

24. Compare and contrast dietary supplementation with a good, well-rounded diet.

Suggested Reading

Nutrition Reviews. Dietary supplements: Recent chronology and legislation. *Nutrition Reviews* 53:31–36, 1995.

Wood, O. B., and C. M. Bruhn. Position of American Dietetic Association: Food irradiation. *Journal of the American Dietetic Association* 100(2):246–253, 2000.

Position of the American Dietetic Association, Dietitians of Canada, and the American College of Sports Medicine: Nutrition and athletic performance. *Journal of the American Dietetic Association* 100(12):1543–1556, 2000.

Wardlaw, G. M. *Perspectives in Nutrition*. Dubuque, IA: McGraw-Hill, 1999.

For links to the Web sites below visit Web Links at www.aw.com/fitness and choose Powers/Dodd Web Links from the drop-down menu.

MEDLINEplus

Contains a wealth of up-to-date, quality nutrition information from the world's largest medical library, the National Library of Medicine at the National Institutes of Health. MEDLINEplus is for anyone with a nutrition or medical question.

Food and Drug Administration

In the summer of 2001, the FDA began publishing a quarterly newsletter titled "Dietary Supplement and Food Labeling Electronic Newsletter." The newsletter's goal is to provide interested parties access to key information and updates about regulatory actions related to food labeling, nutrition, and dietary supplements, as well as educational materials and important announcements. To subscribe to the letter, visit the link.

Nutrition Café

Contains several intriguing nutritional games, including one in which you build a meal from the menu and then get nutritional information about your selections.

FoodSafety

Gateway to government food safety information. Includes news and safety alerts, consumer advice, national food safety programs, and food-borne pathogens.

Ask the Dietician

Presents sound nutritional advice on many diet-related questions. Includes an excellent "Health Body Calculator" for formulating diet and exercise programs.

USDA Center for Nutrition Policy and Promotion

Provides governmental guidelines for diets and use of the Food Guide Pyramid.

USDA Food Safety Publications

Contains articles about all aspects of safety in food preparation, storage, and handling.

Fast Food Finder

Enables you to search for desired fast food (by restaurant or food) and find nutritional information.

Fat-Free Recipe Center

Contains a large collection of fat-free recipes.

Veggies Unite! On-line guide to vegetarianism

Includes recipes, books, articles, and discussions.

American Dietetic Association

Presents nutritional resources, FAQs, links, and more.

Crunch Your Numbers

When it comes to health, everything really does add up. So here are 34 fun, easy-to-use calculators. Learn your ideal weight, determine your protein needs, assess your heart rate, determine how many calories your favorite sport will burn and more.

References

1. Guyer, B., M. A. Freedom, D. M. Strobino, and E. J. Sordik. Annual summary of vital statistics: Trends in the health of Americans during the 20th century. *Pediatrics* 106(6): 1307, 2000.

2. U.S. Department of Health and Human Services. *The Surgeon General's report on nutrition and health.* DHHS (PHS) Publication No. 88-50211. Washington, DC: U.S. Government Printing Office, 1994.

3. Wardlaw, G. M. *Perspectives in Nutrition.* IA: McGraw-Hill, 1999.

4. Von Schacky, C., P. Angerer, K. Wolfgang, T. Kothny, and H. Mudra. The effect of dietary omega-3 fatty acids on coronary atherosclerosis. *Annals of Internal Medicine* 130(7):554, 1999.

5. Kromhout, D. Diet and cardiovascular diseases. *Journal of Nutrition, Health and Aging* 5(3):144–149, 2001.

6. Powers, S., and E. Howley. *Exercise Physiology: Theory and Application to Fitness and Performance,* 4th ed. Dubuque, IA: McGraw-Hill, 2001.

7. National Academy of Sciences. *Dietary Reference Intakes: Applications in Dietary Assessment.* Washington, DC: National Academy Press, 2001.

8. Donatelle, R. J. *Access to Health,* 7th ed. Pearson Education, Inc., publishing as Benjamin Cummings. San Francisco, 2002.

9. Jones, N. L., and K. J. Killian. Exercise limitation in health and disease. *New England Journal of Medicine* 343(9):632–641, 2000.

10. Tipton, K. D., and R. R. Wolfe. Exercise, protein metabolism, and muscle growth. *International Journal of Sport Nutrition and Exercise Metabolism* 11(1):109–132, 2001.

11. Lemon, P. W. Beyond the zone: Protein needs of active individuals. *Journal of the American College of Nutrition* 19(5 Suppl):513S–521S, 2000.

12. Jenkins, R. R. Free radical chemistry: Relationship to exercise. *Sports Medicine* 5:156–170, 1988.

13. Kanter, M. Free radicals and exercise: Effects of nutritional antioxidant supplementation. *Exercise and Sports Sciences Reviews* 23:375–398, 1995.

14. Williams, M. H. Vitamin supplementation and athletic performance. *International Journal for Vitamin and Nutrition Research* 30(Suppl):163–191, 1989.

15. Young, I. S., and J. V. Woodside. Antioxidants in health and disease. *Journal of Clinical Pathology* 54(3):176–186, 2001.

16. Lee, P. Irradiation to prevent foodborne illness. *Journal of the American Medical Association* 272(4):261, 1994.

17. Powers, S. K., and S. L. Lennon. Analysis of cellular responses to free radicals: Focus on exercise and skeletal muscle. *Proceedings of the Nutrition Society* 58(4):1025–1033, 1999.

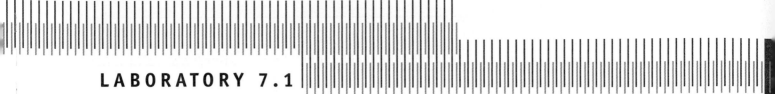

Diet Analysis

NAME _____ DATE _____

The purpose of this exercise is to analyze eating habits during a 3-day period.

DIRECTIONS

For a 3-day period (two weekdays and one weekend day), eat the foods that typically constitute your normal diet. At the end of each day, record on the following chart the foods eaten for that day and the amounts of the listed nutrients contained in each. Most packaged foods now have the amounts of the nutrients listed on the package. See the appendix for the listings of the nutrients contained in various foods. Total the values for each nutrient at the bottom of the chart. Transfer the total to the next chart. At the end of the 3-day period, total the daily values and divide by 3 to get the average dietary intake for each of the nutrients analyzed. Compare your average intake for each of the nutrients with those recommended at the bottom of the page for your sex and age group. Remember that this analysis is only as representative of your normal diet as the foods you eat over the 3-day period.

WRITE-UP

In the space provided, list the strengths and weaknesses in your diet and discuss the steps that can be taken to improve it.

continued on next page

Daily Nutrient Intake

NAME: _____ DATE: _____

Foods	Amount	kcals (total)	kcals from fat	Protein (gm)	CHO (gm)	Fiber (gm)	Fat (gm)	Fat % (kcal)	Sat. Fat (gm)	Chol. (mg)	Sodium (mg)	Vit. A (I.U.)	Vit. C (mg)	Calcium (mg)	Iron (mg)	Vit. B₁ (mg)	Vit. B₂ (mg)	Niacin (mg)
Totals																		

Look in your Behavioral Change Log Book for an additional three-day nutrient intake log.

186

Three-Day Nutrient Summary

NAME: _____   DATE: _____

Day	kcals Total	kcals from Fat	Protein (gm)	CHO (gm)	Fiber (gm)	Fat (gm)	Fat % (kcal)	Sat. Fat (gm)	Chol. (mg)	Sodium (mg)	Vit. A (I.U.)	Vit. C (mg)	Calcium (mg)	Iron (mg)	Vit. B_1 (mg)	Vit. B_2 (mg)	Niacin (mg)
One																	
Two																	
Three																	
Totals																	
Average																	

Recommended Dietary Allowances*

- Kcal total (total daily energy expenditure) is body weight multiplied by kcals per pound per day:

$$\text{Body weight in lbs} \times \underline{\text{kcals per lb per day}} = \textbf{kcal total (total daily energy expenditure)}$$
$$\text{(from Table 8.1)}$$

- Kcals from fat should be less than 30% of total calories per day:

$$30\% \, (0.3) \times \underline{\text{kcals per day}} = \textbf{recommended MAXIMUM kcals from fat}$$

- Protein intake is 0.8 gms per kg of body weight (0.36 gms per lb). (Pregnant women should add 15 gms, and lactating women should add 20 gms):

$$0.36 \text{ gms} \times \underline{\text{body weight in lbs}} = \textbf{recommended protein intake}$$

- Carbohydrate intake should be more than 58% of total calories per day:

$$58\% \, (0.58) \times \underline{\text{kcals per day}} = \textbf{recommended carbohydrate intake}$$

Fat <30% of diet; Fiber ~30% of diet; Saturated fat <10% of diet: Cholesterol <300 mg.; Sodium <3000 mg

* See Table 7.8 on pages 164 and 165 for information on vitamin and mineral RDA values.

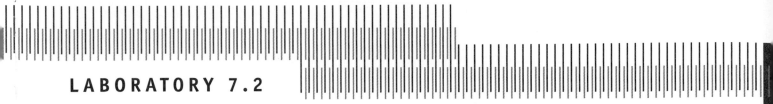

Construct a New Diet

NAME _____ DATE _____

The purpose of this exercise is to construct a new diet using the principles outlined in Chapter 7.

DIRECTIONS

After completing Laboratory 7.1, you should have a general idea of how your diet may need modification. Follow the example given in Table 7.11 and the discussion in the text to choose foods to construct a new diet that meets the recommended dietary goals presented in this chapter. Fill in the blanks on the following chart with the requested information obtained from Appendices B and C or package labels. Use the totals for each column and the RDA for each nutrient in Laboratory 7.1 or Table 7.7 to determine your percent of RDA for each nutrient.

	Kcal (g)	Fat (g)	Sat. Fat (g)	Chol (mg)	Sod. (mg)	CHO (g)	Pro (g)	Vit A (I.U.)	Vit C (mg)	Ca (mg)	Iron (mg)
Breakfast											
Lunch											
Dinner											
Totals											
RDA	*	<30%	<10%	<300	3000	>58%	**	1000	60	1200	12
% of RDA											

* See Chapter 8 for determination of kcal requirements.

**Protein intake should be 0.8 g/kg of body weight (0.36 g/lb). Pregnant women should add 15 g, and lactating women should add 20 g.

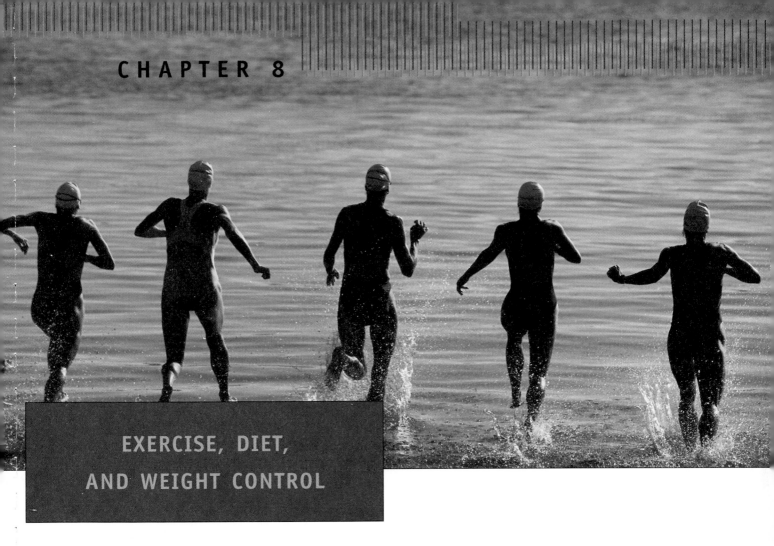

CHAPTER 8

EXERCISE, DIET, AND WEIGHT CONTROL

After studying this chapter, you should be able to:

1. Define obesity and discuss potential causes of obesity.

2. Explain the relationship between obesity and the risk of disease.

3. Explain the concept of optimal body weight.

4. Discuss the energy balance theory of weight control.

5. Explain the roles of resting metabolic rate and exercise metabolic rate in determining daily energy expenditure.

6. Outline a simple method to estimate your daily caloric expenditure.

7. List and define the four basic components of a weight loss program.

8. Discuss several weight loss myths.

9. Describe the eating disorders anorexia nervosa and bulimia.

10. Discuss strategies to gain body weight.

Millions of people in the United States believe they are too fat. This is evidenced by the fact that 30–40% of adult women and 20–25% of adult men are currently trying to lose weight (1). Interest in weight loss has opened the door to numerous commercial weight loss programs and a billion-dollar industry. Many commercial weight loss programs advertise that they are highly successful in promoting individual weight loss. Unfortunately, research demonstrates that if no other treatment is given, only 5% of individuals maintain the weight loss for 5 years after completion of the program (2).

A key element in any weight loss program is education. This chapter, therefore, provides a general overview of body fat control. Specifically, we will discuss the principles of determining an ideal body weight for health and fitness; ways to achieve loss of body fat, using a combination of diet, exercise, and behavior modification; and the principles involved in maintaining a desirable body weight throughout life. We begin with an overview of body weight gain and an introduction to obesity.

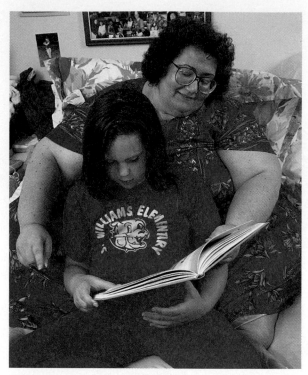

Obesity tends to run in families.

Obesity

Obesity is a term applied to individuals with a high percentage of body fat, generally over 25% for men and over 30% for women (3–7). Obesity is a major health problem in the United States, and numerous diseases have been linked to being too fat (A Closer Look, p. 194). Current estimates for the United States suggest that over 65 million people meet the criteria for obesity (1, 8).

What causes obesity? There is no single answer. Obesity is related to both genetic traits and characteristics of a person's lifestyle (9, 10). Studies have demonstrated that children of obese parents have a greater potential to become obese than children of nonobese parents (10). Further, adopted children with low genetic potential for obesity have a greater chance of becoming obese if their adoptive parents are obese (10).

The link between genetics and obesity is poorly understood. Researchers continue to search for specific genes that could influence body fatness (Fitness and Wellness for All, p. 194). In contrast, the tie between lifestyle and obesity is well defined. Nutritional studies have demonstrated that families consuming high-fat meals have a greater risk of obesity than families who

eat low-fat diets (4, 5, 9). Similarly, children raised in households where physical activity is not encouraged have a greater potential for obesity than children reared in homes where physical activity is encouraged (4, 11).

Many individuals who do not have a genetic link to obesity may gradually add fat over the years and become obese at some point in their lives. This slow increase in body fat is often called **creeping obesity** because it gradually "creeps up" on us (12). This type of weight gain is usually attributed to poor diet (including increased food intake) and a gradual decline in physical activity (12). Figure 8.1 illustrates the process of creeping obesity over a 5-year period. In this example, the individual is gaining one-half pound of fat per month (6 pounds per year), resulting in a total weight gain of 30 pounds over 5 years.

Regional Fat Storage

Recall from Chapter 2 that much of our body fat is stored beneath the skin (Figure 8.2). The fact that different people can have very different regional patterns of fat storage is well known. What factor determines where body fat is stored? The answer is genetics. We inherit specific fat storage traits that determine the regional distribution of fat. This occurs due to the fact

---

obesity   A term applied to individuals with a high percentage of body fat, generally over 25% for men and over 30% for women.
creeping obesity   A slow increase in body fat over a period of several years.

Body Weight (pounds)

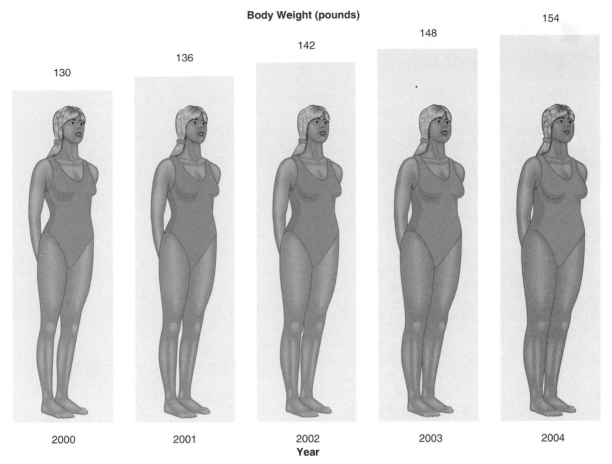

FIGURE 8.1
The concept of creeping obesity.

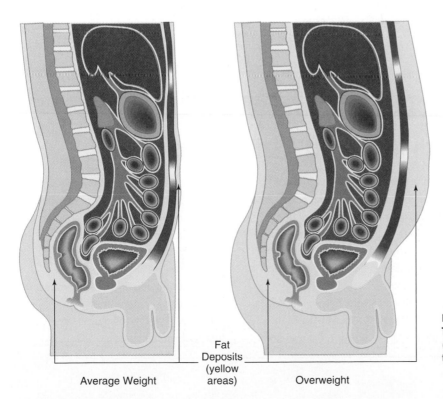

FIGURE 8.2
The sites of fat storage. Much of our body fat (shown in yellow) is stored directly beneath the skin.

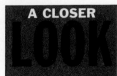

A CLOSER LOOK

Obesity and the Risk of Disease

Obesity increases the risk of developing at least 26 diseases (8, 12, 13), among the most serious of which are heart disease, colon cancer, hypertension (high blood pressure), kidney disease, arthritis, and diabetes (12). For example, obesity increases the risk of heart attack by 60–80% (14). Further, a high correlation exists between the onset of type II diabetes and body fatness; over 80% of type II diabetics are obese (1). In light of this strong link between obesity and disease, the National Institutes of Health has estimated that obesity directly accounts for 15–20% of the deaths in the United States (13).

Even though the biological link between obesity and a specific disease is not always clear, new research has linked obesity to diabetes via a hormone called *resistin* (15). This hormone, which is produced by fat cells and released into the blood, in- hibits glucose uptake into cells. Thus it is not surprising that obese individuals, who have a large number of fat cells, also have high blood levels of resistin. The resulting inhibition of glucose uptake into cells produces high blood sugar (hyperglycemia) and type II diabetes.

Obesity may also contribute to emotional disorders in individuals (particularly adolescents and young adults) whose negative feelings about their body image and being overweight lowers their self-esteem and thus reduces their quality of life.

---

that fat cells are unequally distributed throughout the body. For example, many men have a high number of fat cells in the upper body, which results in a predominance of fat storage within the abdominal area (i.e., waist area). In contrast, most women contain a high number of fat cells in the lower body, resulting in fat storage in the waist, hips, and thighs. As we have seen, people who carry body fat primarily in the abdominal or waist area are at greater risk for development of heart disease than are those who store body fat in the hips or lower part of the body. Therefore, obtaining a desirable body weight with proper fat distribution is a primary health goal (1,16).

Optimal Body Weight

Almost everyone has an idea about how much they should weigh for optimal physical appearance. However, a key question is, *"What is my optimal body weight for health and fitness?"* Although researchers disagree on the answer to this question, some guidelines are available. In general, optimal body fat for health and fitness in men ranges from 10–20%, whereas the optimal range of body fat for women is 15%–25% (11, 17–21) (Figure 8.3). These ranges allow for individual differences in physical activity and appearance and are associated with limited risk of the diseases linked to body fatness.

FITNESS AND WELLNESS FOR ALL

The Search for Obesity-related Genes

Even though obese individuals are found in every segment of the U.S. population, certain subsets of Americans experience the greatest prevalence of obesity. For example, compared to the U.S. population as a whole, the risk of becoming obese is greatest among Mexican-American women, African-American women, some Native Amer- icans (for example, Pima Indians), and children from low-income families. The high prevalence of obesity in these populations places individuals in those groups at the greatest risk of developing obesity-related diseases.

Research efforts to understand the roles of genetics in the high prevalence of obesity in these popu- lations are expanding. One large investigation, called the Heritage Family Study, is searching for the genes responsible for both obesity and weight loss (22). Results from this and other genetics studies are expected to provide important information for developing programs that can prevent and treat obesity in high-risk populations.

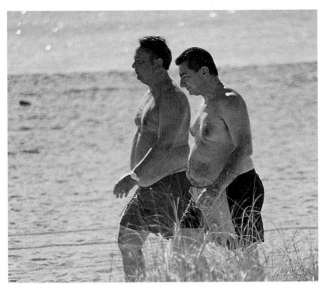

Men tend to store body fat in the upper body.

Men

Too Fat	Optimal Body Weight	Too Lean	

% Fat 30 25 20 15 10 5 0

Women

Too Fat	Optimal Body Weight	Too Lean	

% Fat 35 30 25 20 15 10 5

FIGURE 8.3
The concept of ideal body weight based on a desirable percent of body fat.

OPTIMAL BODY WEIGHT BASED ON PERCENT FAT

A variety of methods and equipment is available for estimating body fat composition, including the skinfold caliper technique discussed in Chapter 2. (For a brief review of what's available on the market, see Fitness-Wellness Consumer, p. 197). Once we know how to compute percent body fat and the optimal range of body fat, how can we determine the desired range of body weight? Consider the following example of a male college student who has 25% body fat and weighs 185 pounds. What is the optimal range of body weight for health and fitness in this individual? The calculations can be done in two simple steps:

Step 1. Compute *fat-free weight*—that is, the amount of total body weight contained in bones, organs, and muscles:

Total body weight − fat weight = fat-free weight
       100%   −   25%   =   75%

This means that 75% of total body weight is fat-free weight. Therefore, the fat-free weight for this student is

75% × 185 pounds = 138.8 pounds

Step 2. Calculate the optimal weight (which for men is 10–20% of total body weight): The formula to compute optimum body weight is

Optimum weight = fat-free weight ÷ (1 − optimal % fat)

Note that % fat should be expressed as a decimal. Thus, for 10% body fat,

Optimum weight = 138.8 ÷ (1 − 0.10) = 154.2 pounds

For 20% body fat,

Optimum weight = 138.8 ÷ (1 − 0.20) = 173.5 pounds

Hence, the optimal body weight for this individual is between 154.2 and 173.5 pounds. Laboratory 8.1 on page 215 provides the opportunity to compute your optimal body weight, using both percent body fat and body mass index (introduced in Chapter 2).

☀ IN SUMMARY

- Obesity refers to individuals with a high percentage of body fat, generally over 25% for men and over 30% for women.
- Much of an individual's body fat is stored directly beneath the skin. The different regional patterns of fat storage in different individuals result from genetic differences.
- The ranges of optimal body fat for health and fitness are 10–20% for men and 15–25% for women.

☀ Physiology of Weight Control

Before we discuss how to begin a weight loss program, let's outline some key physiological concepts associated with weight loss. Although the details of how body fat stores are regulated are beyond the scope of this text, Figure 8.4 presents a simplified overview of the processes involved. Simply stated, body fat stores are regulated by two factors: (1) the rate at which fat is synthesized and stored, and (2) the rate at which energy is expended and fat is metabolized (broken down). In general, fat stores increase when energy intake exceeds energy expenditure, and decrease when energy expenditure exceeds energy intake. Note in Figure 8.4a

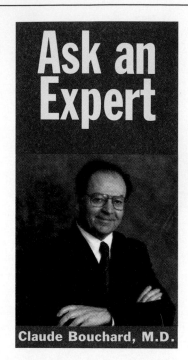

Claude Bouchard, M.D.

Obesity and Weight Loss

Dr. Bouchard is professor and Director of the Pennington Biomedical Research Institute at Louisiana State University School of Medicine. Dr. Bouchard is an internationally known expert regarding the cause and treatment of obesity. Indeed, Dr. Bouchard has published many scientific papers, books, and book chapters related to physical activity, diet, genetics. and weight loss. In the following interview, Dr. Bouchard addresses several hot topic questions related to obesity and weight loss.

Q: Having a low resting metabolic rate is generally accepted as a major contributing factor to obesity. Based on current research, what percent of obese individuals actually suffer from an abnormally low resting metabolic rate?

A: There is no universal agreement on the notion that a low resting metabolic rate is a cause of obesity. The hypothesis is supported by a study on Pima Indians but is not supported in several other reports. It is unlikely that a low resting metabolic rate is a important cause of the predisposition to become obese over time. Most likely, low resting metabolic rate plays only a minor role in the cause of obesity.

Q: How important is daily exercise in the prevention and treatment of obesity?

A: A low level of daily energy expenditure from physical activity is one of the factors contributing to the current epidemic of overweight and obesity cases. Over the last century we have continued to consume about the same number of calories in the presence of a decreasing level of energy expenditure as a result of major changes in transportation, work environment, household and other chores, as well as in discretionary time. As a result of decreasing energy expenditure, a growing number of people are gaining body fat (weight) until their weight reaches a new level that matches energy balance. The only way to prevent this weight gain is to reduce calorie intake or to become physically active. A reasonable volume of weekly physical activity, say about 200 min per week, is an excellent way to prevent unwarranted weight gain.

Q: You are currently the principal investigator of a very important research study aimed at determining the role of genetics in obesity. What are some of the most important findings of this work?

A: The main finding is that obesity is seldom caused by one simple deficiency in one specific gene. A genetic predisposition to obesity is generally brought about by multiple deficiencies of multiple genes. In other words, the genetic predisposition to gain weight for prolonged periods of time is not the prime determinant of obesity. In most cases, the predisposition can be opposed by reducing calorie intake and increasing calorie expenditure.

FITNESS-WELLNESS
CONSUMER

Commercial Devices for Measuring Body Composition

Public interest in measuring body fat has prompted several companies to develop and sell a variety of devices, which range in price from under $20 to over $30,000. As discussed in Chapter 2, one of the least expensive and most accurate techniques involves measuring fat beneath the skin using skinfold calipers.

Several companies sell high-quality metal calipers that maintain a standard amount of tension when the calipers are closed up around the skinfold (cost: generally above $300). Such standardized tension is critical to the accurate measurement of skinfold thickness. In contrast, some companies market plastic calipers (cost: $20–$50), some of which generate too much or too little tension when in use. Therefore, before you purchase a lower-cost plastic caliper, do some homework and choose calipers that have been scientifically proven to provide accurate skinfold measurements.

Several companies are also marketing bathroom scales that contain electronic instruments designed to estimate body fat rapidly and noninvasively (cost: $70–$2500). Most of these devices use the principle of bioelectric impedance analysis (BIA) and measure the conductance of electricity in your body. Put simply, because fat-free (lean) tissues (such as skeletal muscle) contain large amounts of electrolytes (such as sodium and potassium) and water, lean tissue is a good conductor of electricity. In contrast, fat contains limited water and therefore is a poor conductor of electricity. Accordingly, an individual with a high percentage of body fat conducts electricity more poorly than someone with a lower percentage of body fat. These instruments are calibrated to estimate the amount of lean tissue in the body based on the electrical conductance they measure.

But are BIA devices accurate? Unfortunately, a direct answer to this question is not available, but it's clear that some of them are more accurate than others. Before you purchase any BIA device for home use, consult some of the excellent published reviews on BIA, including Going and Davis (2001) (cited in Suggested Readings at the end of this chapter).

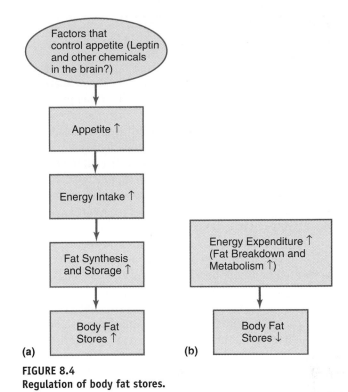

FIGURE 8.4
Regulation of body fat stores.

that an increase in energy intake in response to increased appetite leads to increases in fat synthesis and storage. In contrast, fat stores are reduced when fat is broken down for use as a source of energy for the body (Figure 8.4b).

We discuss energy expenditure and fat metabolism later in this chapter; here the focus is on the rate of energy intake. Because the key factor determining the rate of energy intake is appetite, it is not surprising that the factors that regulate hunger are the subjects of intense research. In 1994, scientists discovered in fat cells a new gene, called the obese (Ob) gene, that produces the hormone leptin, which appears to depress appetite by acting on areas of the brain that control hunger (23). Research revealed that obese mice had very low blood levels of leptin, and when obese mice injected with leptin became lean, researchers became hopeful that leptin might become a cure for obesity in humans. However, those hopes were dashed when it was later discovered that many obese people produce abnormally high levels of leptin, and that leptin is but one of several interacting chemicals involved in appetite (23). Perhaps ongoing research will soon provide a clearer picture of what controls appetite.

During the past two decades, two scientifically sound approaches to weight loss have emerged: the energy balance concept of weight control, and the fat deficit concept of weight control. Let's examine these two approaches next.

ENERGY BALANCE CONCEPT OF WEIGHT CONTROL

The energy balance theory of weight control is simple and can be illustrated by the energy balance equation (Figure 8.5). To maintain a constant body weight, your food energy intake (expressed in calories) must equal your energy expenditure, a condition called **isocaloric balance** (Figure 8.5a). If you consume more calories than you expend, you gain body fat. Consuming more calories than you expend results in a **positive caloric balance** (Figure 8.5b). Finally, if you expend more calories than you consume, you lose body fat and have a **negative caloric balance** (Figure 8.5c).

From the energy balance equation presented in Figure 8.5, you might conclude that weight gain can be prevented by either decreasing your energy (food) intake or increasing your energy (exercise) expenditure. In practice, good weight loss programs include both a reduction in caloric intake and an increase in caloric expenditure achieved through exercise (7, 21, 24, 25).

ENERGY EXPENDITURE   Estimating your daily energy expenditure is a key factor in planning a weight loss program and adjusting the energy balance equation. The daily expenditure of energy involves both the resting metabolic rate and exercise metabolic rate. Let's examine each of these individually.

Resting metabolic rate (RMR) is the amount of energy expended during all sedentary activities. That is, RMR includes the energy required to maintain necessary bodily functions (called the *basal metabolic rate*) plus the additional energy required to perform such activities as sitting, reading, typing, and digestion of food. The RMR is an important component of the energy balance equation because it represents approximately 90% of the total daily energy expenditure in sedentary individuals (26).

Exercise metabolic rate (EMR) represents the energy expenditure during any form of exercise (walking, climbing steps, weight lifting, and so on). In sedentary individuals, EMR constitutes only 10% of the total daily

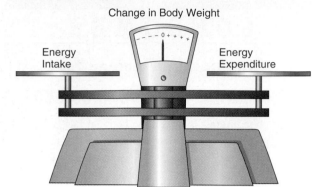

(a) Isocaloric Balance

Change in Body Weight

Energy Intake   Energy Expenditure

Energy Intake = Energy Expenditure

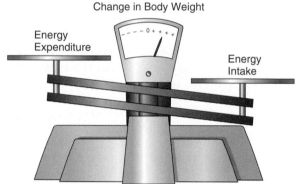

(b) Positive Balance

Change in Body Weight

Energy Expenditure   Energy Intake

Energy Intake > Energy Expenditure

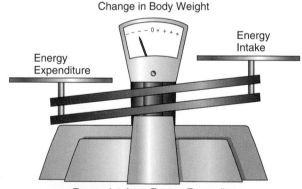

(c) Negative Caloric Balance

Change in Body Weight

Energy Expenditure   Energy Intake

Energy Intake < Energy Expenditure

FIGURE 8.5
The concept of energy balance. (a) Isocaloric balance; (b) a positive caloric balance; and (c) a negative caloric balance.

energy expenditure. By comparison, EMR can account for 20–40% of the total daily energy expenditure in active individuals (26). For example, during heavy exercise, EMR may be 10–20 times greater than RMR (21). Therefore, increased daily exercise results in an

---

isocaloric balance   Condition when food energy intake equals energy expenditure.

positive caloric balance   Condition when more calories are consumed than are expended.

negative caloric balance   Condition when more calories are expended than are consumed.

resting metabolic rate (RMR)   The amount of energy expended during all sedentary activities.

exercise metabolic rate (EMR)   The energy expenditure during any form of exercise.

TABLE 8.1
Estimation of Daily Caloric Expenditure Based on Body Weight and Physical Activity

To compute your estimated daily caloric expenditure, multiply your body weight in pounds by the calories per pound that corresponds to your activity level.

Activity Level	Description	Calories per Pound of Body Weigth Expended during a 24-hour Period
1	Very sedentary (restricted movement, such as a patient confined to a house)	13
2	Sedentary (most U.S. citizens; light work or office job)	14
3	Moderate activity (many college students; some daily activity and weekend recreation)	15
4	Very physically active (vigorous activity at least 3–4 times/week)	16
5	Competitive athlete (daily activity in high-energy sport)	17–18

increase in the EMR and is a key factor in weight control programs.

ESTIMATING DAILY ENERGY EXPENDITURE Dieting is widespread in the United States as people try to reduce body fat by decreasing energy intake. The obvious goal of dieting is to consume less energy than is expended and therefore create a negative energy balance and resulting weight loss. The first step in this process is to estimate your daily caloric expenditure. One of the simplest ways to do so is presented in Table 8.1, which provides estimates of daily caloric energy expenditure based on body weight and physical activity. For example, let's compute the estimated daily caloric expenditure for a college-age woman whose body weight is 120 pounds and who is involved in only moderate physical activity on weekends. Using Table 8.1, we locate her activity level on the left (i.e., level 3) and her estimated calories expended per pound of body weight (15 calories per pound per day) in the right-hand column. To calculate her total daily energy expenditure, we multiply her body weight by her caloric expenditure:

Daily caloric expenditure = 120 pounds × 15 calories/pound/day = 1800 calories/day

Do this same calculation for your own daily caloric expenditure. If you need to lose weight, you are now prepared to create a negative energy balance by reducing your energy intake. Note that after losing 5 pounds of body weight, you should recalculate your estimated caloric expenditure; this is necessary because the weight loss results in a lower daily energy expenditure (Laboratory 8.2, p. 217).

FAT DEFICIT CONCEPT OF WEIGHT CONTROL

The general concept that weight loss occurs due to a negative caloric balance is straightforward and easy to understand. Nonetheless, recent evidence suggests that creating a fat deficit is another essential factor in weight loss that is often overlooked (27). For instance, it is now accepted that dietary fat is more easily stored as body fat than are either carbohydrate or protein (27). This occurs because dietary fat is not used as a body fuel as rapidly as is carbohydrate or protein. For example, if a positive caloric balance is created by eating large amounts of carbohydrate or proteins, many of the excess calories are used to repair body tissues, replace body carbohydrate stores, or provide body energy. In contrast, if excess calories are consumed as fat, they are more likely to be stored as body fat (27).

The importance of a low-fat diet in weight control can best be illustrated by the fact that body fat gain is a result of a continual imbalance of fat intake and fat metabolism (fat burned in the body). In other words, if you ingest more fat than you burn during the day, you gain weight (Figure 8.6a). It follows that if you consume and burn equal amounts of fat, your weight remains constant (Figure 8.6b). Finally, if you burn more fat than you consume (a fat deficit), you lose body fat and weight (Figure 8.6c). Thus, losing body fat is not as simple as creating an energy deficit; your diet must provide a caloric deficit that also results in a fat deficit. We will discuss how to design a diet plan that is low in fat and calories and high in carbohydrates shortly.

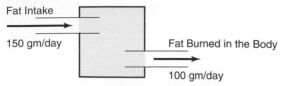

(a) Positive Fat Balance

Fat Intake

150 gm/day

Fat Burned in the Body

100 gm/day

Fat Intake > Fat Metabolism (weight gained)

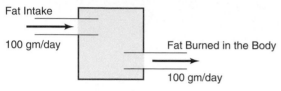

(b) Iso Fat Balance

Fat Intake

100 gm/day

Fat Burned in the Body

100 gm/day

Fat Intake = Fat Metabolism (no weight gained)

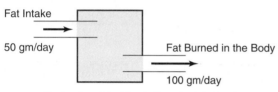

(c) Negative Fat Balance

Fat Intake

50 gm/day

Fat Burned in the Body

100 gm/day

Fat Intake < Fat Metabolism (weight loss)

FIGURE 8.6
Importance of a low-fat diet in creating a fat deficit and promoting weight loss.

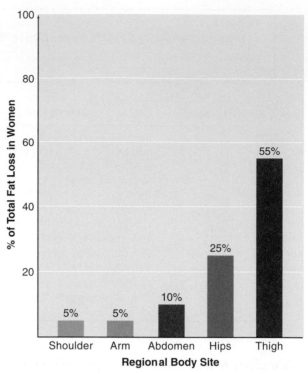

FIGURE 8.7
Fat loss from different areas of the body in women. In both sexes, fat is lost from those areas that store the most fat.
(Source: Data from King, M., and F. Katch. Changes in body density, fatfolds, and girths at 2.3 kg increments of weight loss. *Human Biology* 58:709, 1986.)

WHAT IS A SAFE RATE OF WEIGHT LOSS?

Before we discuss how to design a weight loss program, we should address two general points about weight loss. First, the maximum recommended rate for weight loss is 1 to 2 pounds per week. Diets resulting in a weight loss of more than 2 pounds per week are associated with a significant loss of lean body mass (i.e., muscle and body organs). In general, a weight loss goal of 1 pound per week is a safe and reasonable goal. The negative energy balance required to lose 1 pound per week is approximately 3500 calories. Therefore, a negative energy balance of 500 calories per day would theoretically result in a loss of 1 pound of fat per week (3500 calories/week ÷ 7 days/week = 500 calories/day).

A second general point about weight loss is that the rate of loss during the first several days of dieting will be greater than later in the dieting period. This is true because at the onset of a diet, in addition to fat loss there is an initial reduction in body carbohydrate and water stores, which also results in some weight loss (21). Further, some lean tissue, such as muscle, may also be lost during the beginning of any diet; the caloric content of lean tissue is less than fat. Therefore, more than 1 pound will be lost during the first 3500-calorie deficit. However, as the diet continues, weight loss will

occur at a slower rate. This fact should not discourage you, because subsequent weight loss will be primarily from body fat stores. Sticking with your weight plan for several weeks will result in a significant fat loss, and you will like the associated changes.

WHERE ON THE BODY DOES FAT REDUCTION OCCUR?

A key weight loss question is, "Where on the body do changes occur when fat is lost?" The answer is that most weight loss occurs in body areas that contain the greatest fat storage. Figure 8.7 illustrates this point in a study of obese women who completed a 14-week weight loss program that resulted in each participant losing approximately 20 pounds of fat (28). At the beginning of the study, regional fat storage was assessed using skinfold measurements, and it was determined that the largest percentage of fat was stored in the thighs, hips, and abdomen. At the completion of the study, regional fat storage was reassessed to determine where the fat loss occurred. Approximately 90% of the fat loss occurred in the body regions with the highest fat storage (Figure 8.7). This is good news because most people want to lose fat from those areas.

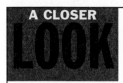

Short-Term and Long-Term Weight Loss Goals

Short-term weight loss goals are designed to provide weight loss targets that can be achieved within a 2- to 4-week period. For example, an initial short-term weight loss goal might be to lose 2 pounds during the first 2 weeks of your weight loss program. Achievement of each short-term goal provides the motivation to establish another short-term goal and continue the weight loss program. (See the box figure.)

Long-term weight loss goals generally focus on reaching the desired percent of body fat. For instance, a long-term goal for a male college student might be to reach 15% body fat within the first year of his weight loss program. After reaching this long-term goal, his objective then becomes the maintenance of this desired body composition.

The relationship between short-term and long-term weight loss goals.

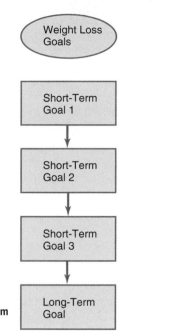

☀ IN SUMMARY

- To maintain a constant body weight, your food energy (caloric) intake must equal your caloric expenditure; this is called an isocaloric balance.
- Consuming more calories than you expend results in a positive caloric balance and weight gain.
- Consuming fewer calories than you expend results in a negative caloric balance and weight loss.
- Daily energy expenditure can be estimated by considering both your resting metabolic rate and your exercise caloric expenditure.
- While it is true that weight loss generally occurs due to a caloric deficit, new evidence also indicates that creating a fat deficit is another essential factor in the loss of body fat. A fat deficit is created when the amount of fat burned in the body exceeds the dietary intake of fat.

☀ Establishing a Successful Weight Loss Program

With proper knowledge and motivation, almost anyone can design a weight loss program. The four basic components of a comprehensive weight control program are establishment of weight loss goals; a reduced caloric diet stressing balanced nutrition, high carbohydrate intake, and low fat intake; an exercise program designed to increase caloric expenditure and maintain or increase mus-

cle mass; and a behavior modification program aimed at changing eating habits that contribute to weight gain.

WEIGHT LOSS GOALS

The establishment of weight loss goals is a key component of any weight loss program. The first step is to decide where your percent body fat should be within the optimal range (10–20% for men, 15–25% for women). Many people who are beginning a comprehensive weight loss program choose a long-term weight loss goal that will place them in the middle of the optimal weight range (15% body fat for men, 20% body fat for women). After choosing your long-term goal, it is also useful to establish short-term weight loss goals—usually expressed in the number of pounds lost per week (A Closer Look and Laboratory 8.3, on p. 219).

ROLE OF DIET IN WEIGHT LOSS

Bookstore shelves are filled with diet books, and television and radio advertisements promote "miracle" diets. While some of these diets may promote weight loss, many do not provide balanced nutrition. When assessing new diets, a general rule of thumb is to avoid diets that promise fast and easy weight loss (Nutritional Links to Health and Fitness, p. 202). If you have concerns about the safety or effectiveness of a published diet, you can either contact your local branch of the American Dietetic Association for information or approach a dietitian at a hospital or college. By learning

Nutritional Links

Frequently Asked Questions About Weight Loss Diets

Question: Does the "grapefruit diet" promote rapid weight loss?

Answer: Among the numerous myths circulated about the value of consuming large quantities of grapefruit to promote weight loss is one suggesting that the ingestion of highly acidic grapefruit dissolves fat and results in rapid loss of body weight. Although eating citrus fruit as a part of a healthful diet is a good idea, there is nothing magic about grapefruit that promotes fat loss. In fact, no food can magically assist in weight loss.

Question: What is the "Mayo Clinic Diet", and was it developed at the Mayo Clinic?

Answer: A number of Mayo Clinic Diets have surfaced over the years. One recent version is a 2-week plan that claims to help users lose 20 pounds by eating large amounts of grapefruit. According to Mayo Clinic researchers, however, the Mayo Clinic has never developed a diet plan, and none of the so-called "Mayo diets" are approved by this prestigious medical facility.

Question: What is the "Sugar Busters Diet," and how does it relate to the "glycemic index" of food?

Answer: The Sugar Busters Diet comes from a popular book authored by H. L. Steward and others. This diet is like many others in that it advocates a low carbohydrate intake to promote weight loss. The authors argue that the problem with eating diets that are high in carbohydrates is that they promote increased levels of the hormone insulin, which is counterproductive to weight loss because insulin promotes both fat storage and a reduction in the use of fat as a body fuel. The "glycemic index" is a measure of the amount of insulin released when a given food is consumed. Foods that produce the greatest release of insulin are assigned a high glycemic index, so the Sugar Busters Diet is designed to help users avoid foods with high glycemic indexes.

Question: Which diets are low-carbohydrate diets, and are they safe and effective ways to lose fat?

Answer: Among the many low-carbohydrate diets that have been popularized over the years are the Zone Diet, the Atkins New Diet Revolution, Calories Don't Count, the Sugar Busters Diet, and the Scarsdale Diet. Although new ones appear all the time, they are all essentially the same.

All low-carbohydrate diets promote similar physiological responses, and each of the diets mentioned in the previous paragraph enjoyed a surge of popularity because of the initial weight loss that occurs with low-carbohydrate diets. They make sales pitches like "You never feel hungry" and "You'll lose weight fast!" Both claims are true, but misleading. For example, even though low-carbohydrate diets can cause loss of appetite in some people, it does not occur in everyone. Further, the rapid loss in body weight most people experience immediately after beginning these diets is not due to a loss of fat, but instead to a loss of water. Unfortunately, the water is rapidly regained as soon as a normal diet is resumed (29).

The answer to the question of whether low-carbohydrate diets are safe is "No!" Among the many health hazards associated with low-carbohydrate diets are high blood cholesterol, hypoglycemia, mineral imbalances, and other metabolic disorders. Because some low-carbohydrate diets can be very dangerous, they are never recommended by knowledgeable practitioners.

---

the basic nutrition principles contained in this chapter and in Chapter 7, you should be able to critically evaluate most diet plans.

Table 8.2 presents a brief summary of some of the major types of diets used in weight loss programs (21). Of these, only the last plan is a nutritionally balanced, low-calorie diet; it is the only one recommended. Any safe and nutritionally sound diet should adhere to the following guidelines (4–7, 12, 19, 30):

- The diet should be low in calories but provide all the essential nutrients the body requires.
- The diet should be low in fat (less than 30% of total calories) and high in complex carbohydrates (approximately 60% of total calories). Remember, a

diet low in fat is essential to creating a fat deficit. Establishing a diet that creates a negative caloric balance with less than 30% of the total calories coming from fat will ensure that each day you metabolize more fat than you take in.

- The diet should contain a variety of foods to appeal to your tastes and to prevent hunger between meals.
- The diet should be compatible with your lifestyle, and the foods should be easily obtainable.
- The diet should be a lifelong diet; that is, it should be one that you can follow for the remainder of your life. This type of diet greatly increases your chances of maintaining an ideal weight in the future.

TABLE 8.2
Examples of Weight Loss Diets

Type of Diet	Description/Comments	Recommended?
Low-carbohydrate diet	Has high fat or protein content, but is nutritionally unbalanced; not safe for long-term use	No (See Nutritional Links to Health and Fitness.)
Low-calorie liquid diet	Although nutritionally balanced, is monotonous and unsatisfying	No
Very-low-calorie liquid diet	Protein/carbohydrate mixture that provides only 300–600 calories/day; is nutritionally unbalanced and not safe for long-term use	No
Balanced low-calorie diet	Is nutritionally balanced; high in carbohydrates (approximately 60% of total caloric intake) and low in fat (less than 30% of total calories); provides a caloric deficit of 500–1000 calories/day	Yes

- The diet should provide foods that adhere to the principles of eating for health.

In addition to these diet guidelines, here are some helpful reminders (some of which were covered in Chapter 7) for planning a successful balanced diet:

- Avoid high-calorie, low-nutrient foods such as those high in sugar (e.g., candy bars, cookies). Instead, select low-calorie, nutrient-dense foods such as fruits, vegetables, and whole-grain breads.

- Reduce the amount of fat in your diet. High-fat foods are high in calories. For example, eat less butter and choose meats that are low in fat, such as lean cuts of beef, chicken, and fish. Avoid fried foods; broil, bake, or microwave your food. If you must use oil in your cooking, use monosaturated oils such as olive oil or peanut oil.

- Although dairy products are excellent sources of protein, they may be high in calories unless the fat has been removed. Use nonfat or low-fat milk, low-fat cottage cheese, and similar products.

- Select fresh fruits and vegetables whenever possible, and avoid fruits that are canned in heavy syrup.

- Limit salt intake. Use herbs and other seasonings as substitutes for salt.

- Drink fewer alcoholic beverages. Alcoholic beverages are low in nutrients and high in calories.

- Eat three meals per day, and do not snack in between.

Remember that a negative energy balance of 500 calories/day will result in a weight loss of approximately 1 pound per week. The key to maintaining a caloric deficit of 500 calories/day is careful planning of meals and accurate calorie counting.

EXERCISE AND WEIGHT LOSS

Exercise plays a key role in weight loss for several reasons (25, 31). First, increased physical activity elevates your daily caloric expenditure and therefore assists you

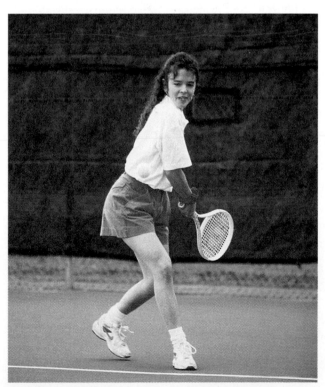

Exercise is a key component of any weight loss program.

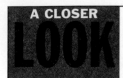

What Intensity of Aerobic Exercise Is Best for Burning Fat?

Many people assume that the intensity of aerobic exercise (running, cycling, and so on) must be maintained at a low level if fat is to be burned as fuel, and it is true that fat is a primary fuel source during low-intensity exercise. But as the figure in this box shows, the total amount of fat burned during exercise varies with the intensity of exercise, and for a given exercise duration, more total fat is metabolized during moderate-intensity exercise. Therefore, moderate-intensity exercise (that is, approximately 50% $\dot{V}O_{2max}$) is typically the optimal intensity of exercise for burning the most fat during an endurance exercise workout. For more details on this topic, see reference 32 in the Suggested Reading list at the end of this chapter.

(*Source:* Coyle, E. Fat metabolism during exercise. *Sports Science Exchange* (Gatorade Sports Science Institute) 8:6, 1995.)

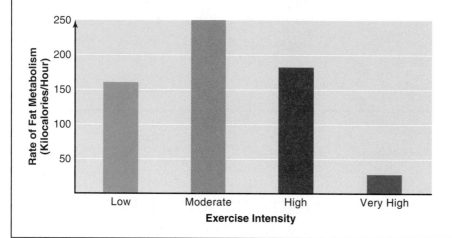

The rates of fat metabolism at low-intensity (20% $\dot{V}O_{2max}$), moderate-intensity (50% $\dot{V}O_{2max}$), high-intensity (80% $\dot{V}O_{2max}$), and very-high-intensity (100% $\dot{V}O_{2max}$) exercise. While this figure is not intended to reveal any "ideal" exercise intensity for all individuals, it indicates that moderate-intensity exercise is often optimal for maximizing the amount of fat metabolized during exercise.

in creating a negative energy balance. Second, regular cardiorespiratory exercise training improves the ability of skeletal muscles to burn fat as energy. Third, regular resistance exercise (such as weight training) can reduce the loss of muscle that occurs during dieting. This is important because your primary goal in dieting is not to lose muscle mass but to promote fat loss. Finally, increasing your muscle mass by weight training results in an increased resting metabolic rate, which further aids in weight loss (33).

What type of exercise should be performed to assist in weight loss? A sound recommendation is that both cardiorespiratory training (i.e., running, cycling, swimming, and so on) and strength training be performed while dieting. (See A Closer Look, above, for some details about the relationship between exercise and fat metabolism.) The combination of these two types of training will maintain cardiorespiratory fitness and reduce the loss of muscle.

How much exercise must be performed during a weight loss program? In general, exercise sessions designed to promote weight loss should expend in excess of 250 calories. Further, it is recommended that the negative caloric balance should be shared equally by exercise and diet. For instance, if an individual wishes to achieve a 500-calorie/day deficit, this should be done by increasing energy expenditure (exercise) by 250 calories/day and by decreasing caloric intake by 250 calories.

Although intensity of exercise is an important factor in improving cardiorespiratory fitness, it is the total amounts of energy expended and fat burned that are important in weight loss. Some authors have argued that low-intensity prolonged exercise is better than short-term high-intensity exercise (e.g., sprinting 50 yards) in burning fat calories and promoting weight loss (34, 35). However, recent evidence clearly demonstrates that both high- and low-intensity exercise can promote fat loss (21). Nonetheless, for the sedentary or obese individual, low-intensity exercise is the proper choice because it can be performed for longer time periods and results in an increase in the ability of skeletal muscle to metabolize fat as an energy source (21, 36). A brief discussion of the energy cost of various activities follows.

Table 8.3 contains estimates of the caloric costs of several types of physical activities. To compute your caloric expenditure (per minute) during an activity, simply multiply your body weight in kilograms (2.2 pounds = 1 kilogram) by the values in the Cal/min./kg column in Table 8.3 and by the exercise time. For example, suppose a 70-kilogram (kg) individual plays 20 minutes

TABLE 8.3
Energy Costs for Selected Sporting Activities

	Cal/min./kg	Cal/min.*	METs**
Archery (American Round)	0.0412	2.8	2.3
Bowling (with three other bowlers)	0.0471	3.2	2.7
Golf (playing in a foursome)	0.0559	3.8	3.2
Walking (17-min. mile on a grass surface)	0.0794	5.4	4.5
Cycling (6.4-min. mile)	0.0985	6.7	5.6
Canoeing (15-min. mile)	0.1029	7.0	5.8
Swimming (50-yd./min.)	0.1333	9.1	7.6
Running (10-min. mile)	0.1471	10.0	8.0
Cycling (5-min. mile)	0.1559	10.6	8.5
Handball (singles)	0.1603	10.9	9.1
Skipping rope (80 turns/min.)	0.1655	11.3	9.5
Running (8-min. mile)	0.1856	12.6	10.0
Running (6-min. mile)	0.2350	16.0	12.8

These values are for a 150-lb (68-kg) person.

**1 MET equals your resting metabolic rate.*

Source: From Getchell, B., 1992. Physical Fitness: A Way of Life. Copyright © 1992. Reprinted with permission from Benjamin Cummings.

of handball. How many calories did he or she expend during the time of play? The total estimated caloric expenditure is computed as follows:

$$\text{Caloric expenditure} = 70 \text{ kg} \times 0.1603 \text{ calories/kg/min} \times 20 \text{ min} = 224 \text{ calories}$$

EXERCISE AND APPETITE

A common question is, Does exercise increase appetite? Although the high-intensity training programs used by many athletes may increase appetite, it is generally believed that when a moderate exercise program is introduced to sedentary or obese individuals, appetite does not increase (37). In fact, moderate exercise training may diminish appetite (37).

BEHAVIOR MODIFICATION

Research demonstrates that behavior modification plays a key role in both achieving short-term weight loss and maintaining weight loss over the years (4–7). **Behavior modification** is a technique used in psychological therapy to promote desirable changes in behavior. The rationale behind it is that many behaviors are learned. For example, attending movies at the theater elicits, in many people, a response of eating popcorn and candy. Because these types of responses are learned, they can also be eliminated (unlearned). In regard to weight control, behavior modification is used primarily to reduce or (ideally) eliminate social or environmental stimuli that promote overeating.

The first step in a diet-related behavior modification program is to identify those social or environmental factors that promote overeating. This can be done by keeping a written record of daily activities for 1 or 2 weeks to identify factors associated with consumption of high-calorie meals. In recording your daily eating habits, consider the following social or environmental factors (12):

- *Activities.* What activities are associated with eating? You may find a correlation between specific types of activities, such as watching TV and eating snacks.

- *Emotional behavior before or during eating.* What emotions are associated with eating? For instance, do you overeat when you are depressed or under stress? (*Overeating* is defined as the consumption of high-calorie meals that leads to a positive calorie balance).

- *Location of meals.* Where do you eat? Are specific rooms associated with snacks?

- *Time of day and level of hunger.* Do you eat at specific times of the day? When you eat, are you always hungry?

behavior modification   A technique used in psychological therapy to promote desirable changes in behavior.

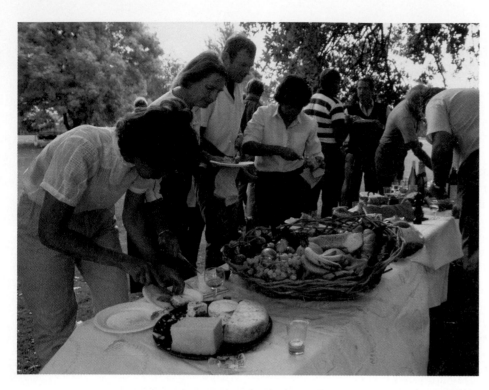

Avoid parties or social gatherings that encourage overeating.

- *People involved*. With whom do you eat? Are specific people associated with periods of overeating?

After identifying the factors that influence your eating behavior, start a program aimed at correcting those behaviors that contribute to weight gain. The following weight control techniques have been used successfully for many years. Although it is not essential to use each of them, adhering to many will make weight control easier (12).

- *Make a personal commitment to losing weight*. This is the first step toward behavior modification and weight loss. The establishment of realistic short-term and long-term weight loss goals assists in maintaining a lifelong commitment to weight control.

- *Develop healthy low-calorie eating patterns*. Avoid eating when you are not hungry. Learn to eat slowly and only while sitting at the table. Finally, keep food quantities to the minimum amount within your caloric guidelines.

- * *Avoid social settings where overeating is encouraged*. If you go to parties where high-calorie foods are served, don't go to these functions hungry. Eat a low-calorie meal before going.

- *Avoid snacking*. If snacks must be eaten, eat low-calorie foods such as carrots or celery.

- *Engage in daily exercise*. Regular exercise that uses large-muscle groups can play an important role in increasing your daily caloric expenditure and can therefore assist in weight control.

- *Reward yourself for successful weight loss with non-food rewards*. Rewards or positive feedback are an important part of behavior modification. For example, after reaching part of your weight loss goal, reward yourself by doing something you like to do (going to the beach, going hiking, or buying a new CD.)

- *Think positively*. Avoid negative thinking about how difficult weight loss can be. Positive thinking promotes confidence and maintains the enthusiasm necessary for a lifetime of successful weight control.

☀ IN SUMMARY

- Designing and executing a successful weight loss program requires knowledge and motivation.
- Establishing weight loss goals is a key component of any weight loss program.
- A safe and nutritionally sound diet should adhere to the guidelines of good nutrition.
- Both exercise and behavior modification play a key role in weight loss.

☀ Lifetime Weight Control

The good news about weight loss is that anybody with the proper motivation can lose body fat. The bad news is that there is no simple way of losing body fat and keeping the fat off forever. Weight control over the course of a lifetime is only accomplished by the proper combination of diet, exercise, and behavior modification. The key factors in long-term weight control are a positive attitude toward weight control, regular exercise, and a personal commitment to maintaining a desired body composition.

Like many other facets of personal or professional life, weight control has its ups and downs. Be prepared for occasional setbacks. For instance, gaining weight during holiday periods is common and experienced by everyone at some time. When this type of weight gain occurs, avoid self-criticism, quickly reestablish your personal commitment to a short-term weight loss goal, and develop a new diet and exercise plan to lose the undesired fat. Remember, any amount of weight gain can be lost by applying the principles discussed in this chapter.

Finally, the importance of family and friends in lifetime weight control cannot be overemphasized. Their encouragement and support can both assist you in maintaining good eating habits and provide the needed support to sustain a lifetime commitment to exercise. It is much easier to lose weight if your close associates are trying to help you achieve your goals rather than tempting you to eat improperly. Therefore, surround yourself with friends that support you in your weight control goals. See Kroll (2001) in the Suggested Reading list for more tips on lifetime weight control.

☀ Weight Loss Myths

Numerous weight loss myths cause confusion among people who are attempting to lose weight. Several common myths are discussed next.

DIET PILLS REALLY WORK

A number of over-the-counter diet pills are available on the market, and most of them contain caffeine and other mild stimulants (Fitness-Wellness Consumer, above right). Unfortunately, none of these products has been scientifically shown to assist in achieving safe and permanent weight loss. One study of individuals using commercially available diet pills reported that fewer than 3% of users lost weight and retained this weight loss longer than 12 months (2).

SPOT REDUCTION CAN OCCUR

The notion that exercise applied to a specific region of the body will result in fat loss in that region is called **spot reduction.** Will performing sit-ups, for example, result in a reduction in abdominal fat? Unfortunately, the answer is "no." To date, there is no scientific evidence to show that exercise promotes fat loss in local regions of the body (38). As we have seen, the evidence suggests that when a caloric deficit exists, fat loss will occur from the largest sites of fat stores and not from specific areas (28).

FITNESS-WELLNESS
CONSUMER
Are Diet Pills Safe and Effective?

Many of the hundreds of weight loss products available for purchase are nonprescription diet pills that claim to promote weight loss by raising the body's metabolic rate and by reducing appetite. Apparently many people believe these unsubstantiated advertising claims, because billions of diet pills are consumed in the United States each year. Still, as with many weight loss products, safety is a concern. While small doses of two major components of most diet pills—the stimulants caffeine and ephedrine— are not harmful to most people, these substances can cause significant health problems for some individuals. For this reason, and because diet pills are not an effective way to lose weight, you should always consult a physician before considering the purchase of *any* weight loss product. And remember, there is no quick fix for losing weight.

EATING BEFORE BEDTIME MAKES YOU FATTER

Some people believe that eating immediately prior to going to bed at night results in a greater fat gain than if the same meal were consumed during the day. These rumors are probably unfounded. Although eating a late-night meal or snack might not be a good dietary habit, this practice does not result in a greater weight gain than if the same meal had been consumed at another time during the day. Remember, it is the total daily caloric intake that determines fat gain, not the timing of the meal (4, 5).

CELLULITE IS A SPECIAL TYPE OF FAT

It is commonly believed that two kinds of body fat exist: cellulite and regular fat (19). The term **cellulite** refers to the "lumpy" hard fat that often gives skin a dimpled

---

spot reduction The false notion that exercise applied to a specific region of the body will result in fat loss in that region.
cellulite The "lumpy" hard fat that often gives skin a dimpled look. Cellulite is just plain fat and not a special category of fat.

look. In reality, cellulite is just plain fat, not a special type of fat. The "dimpled" appearance comes from fat accumulating into small clusters beneath the skin.

Some health spas have advertised that vigorous massages provided by machines can remove cellulite and improve the appearance of your skin. Nonetheless, no scientific evidence exists that massage techniques are effective in promoting body fat loss or altering skin appearance.

FAT-DISSOLVING CREAMS ARE EFFECTIVE

Over the years, numerous companies have marketed "weight loss creams" that are claimed to cause spot reduction of fat when applied to the skin. This is an attractive idea, as evidenced by the fact that companies have made millions of dollars from selling these products. Despite the boastful claims made by manufacturers, only limited scientific evidence suggests that these creams are effective in promoting fat loss.

SAUNAS, STEAMBATHS, AND RUBBER SUITS CAN AID IN LONG-TERM WEIGHT LOSS

Another myth related to the loss of body fat is the notion that sitting in saunas or steambaths and/or running in a rubber suit melts body fat. Although saunas and steambaths do temporarily increase your metabolic rate, they do not melt away fat, nor do they significantly contribute to weight loss (7). For similar reasons, exercising in a rubber suit does not promote greater fat loss than would be achieved by performing the same exercise in comfortable clothes.

These three methods do result in body water loss due to sweating, however. The accompanying body weight loss has been believed by some to be a loss of fat, but this is not the case. The weight temporarily lost in this way is regained as soon as body water is restored to normal levels.

Using saunas or steambaths and exercising while wearing a rubber suit may increase body temperature well above normal. This puts additional stress on the heart and circulatory system and could increase the risk of cardiac problems for older individuals or anyone with heart problems.

---

anorexia nervosa   A common eating disorder that is unrelated to any specific physical disease. The end result of extreme anorexia nervosa is a state of starvation in which the individual becomes emaciated due to a refusal to eat.

☀ Eating Disorders

The low social acceptance of individuals with a high percentage of body fat and an emphasis on having the "perfect" body have increased the incidence of eating disorders. Two of the more common ones that affect young adults are anorexia nervosa and bulimia. Because of the relatively high occurrence of both disorders in female college students, we will discuss both the symptoms and health consequences of each.

ANOREXIA NERVOSA

Anorexia nervosa is a common eating disorder that is unrelated to any specific physical disease. The end result of extreme anorexia nervosa is a state of starvation in which the individual becomes emaciated due to a refusal to eat. The psychological cause of anorexia nervosa is unclear, but it seems to be linked to an unfounded fear of fatness that may be related to familial or societal pressures to be thin (12).

The incidence of this eating disorder has grown in recent years. Individuals with the highest probability of developing anorexia nervosa are upper-middle-class

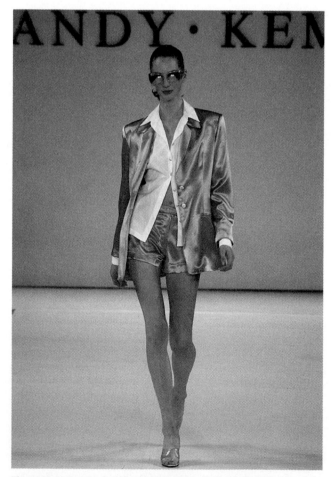

There are enormous societal pressures to be lean.

young women who are extremely self-critical. It is estimated that the incidence of anorexia nervosa is as high as one of every 200 adolescent girls (39, 40).

Anorexics may use a variety of techniques to remain thin, including starvation, exercise, and laxatives. The effects of anorexia include excessive weight loss, cessation of menstruation, and, in extreme cases, death. Because anorexia is a serious mental and physical disorder, medical treatment by a team of professionals (physician, psychologist, nutritionist) is needed to correct the problem. Treatment may require years of psychological counseling and nutritional guidance. The first step in seeking treatment for anorexia is recognizing a problem exists. The following are common symptoms of anorexia:

- An intense fear of gaining weight or becoming obese
- Feeling fat even at normal or below-normal body fatness because of a highly distorted body image
- In women, the absence of three or more menstrual cycles
- The possible development of odd behaviors concerning food; for example, the preparation of elaborate meals for others but of only a few low-calorie foods for their own consumption

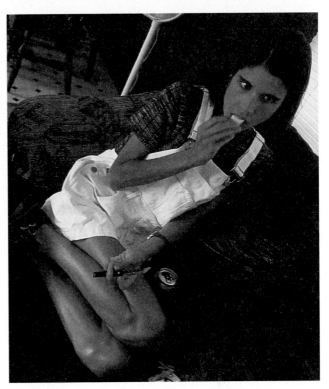

People with anorexia often have distorted body images.

BULIMIA

About 50% of all anorexics eventually come to suffer **bulimia,** which is overeating (called *binge eating*) followed by vomiting (called *purging*). In essence, bulimics repeatedly ingest large quantities of food and then force themselves to vomit in order to prevent weight gain. Bulimia may result in damage to the teeth and the esophagus due to frequent vomiting of stomach acids. Like anorexia nervosa, bulimia is most common in young women, has a psychological origin, and requires professional treatment when diagnosed. Several authors have indicated that the prevalence of bulimia may be as low as 1% or as high as 20% among U.S. girls and women aged 13 to 23 years (39, 40).

Most bulimics look "normal" and are of normal weight. However, even when their bodies are slender, their stomachs may protrude due to being stretched by frequent eating binges. Other common symptoms of bulimia include the following (41):

- Recurrent binge eating
- A lack of control over eating behavior
- Regular self-induced vomiting and use of diuretics or laxatives
- Strict fasting or use of vigorous exercise to prevent weight gain
- Averaging two or more binge-eating episodes a week during a 2- to 3-month period
- Overconcern with body shape and weight

Although maintaining an optimal body composition is a primary health goal, eating disorders are not appropriate means of weight loss. If you or any of your friends exhibit one or more of the symptoms cited here, please seek professional advice and treatment.

IN SUMMARY

- Numerous weight loss myths add to confusion about weight loss.
- Even though many nonprescription diet pills are available, research indicates that the diet pill approach to weight loss is not successful for most people.
- Research indicates that exercise applied to a specific region of the body will not result in a "spot reduction" of body fat.
- The prevalence of two common eating disorders, anorexia nervosa and bulimia, is relatively high among female college students in the United States.

bulimia An eating disorder that involves overeating (called *binge eating*) followed by vomiting (called *purging*).

☀ Exercise and Diet Programs to Gain Weight

The major focus of this chapter has been how to lose body fat. However, a small number of people, who consider themselves to be too thin, want to gain body weight. Both men and women can suffer from self-image problems if they feel they are too skinny. Although current social attitudes stress leanness in women, many women agree that some degree of body curvature is desirable. Also, many men want a muscular body because of the improved self-image that comes with increased muscularity (12).

Body weight gain can be achieved in two ways. First, you can create a positive caloric balance and a positive fat balance and gain additional body fat. Second, you can increase your body weight by increasing your muscle mass through a weight-training program. Let's discuss each of these types of body weight gain.

GAINING BODY FAT

Before deciding to gain body fat, you should determine if your current body composition is within the desired range (Chapter 2). If your percent body fat is below the recommended range (fewer than 8% of people fall into this category), it may be desirable for you to add body fat to reach the optimal percent body fat. Nonetheless, before looking at a dietary means for gaining fat, you should examine the cause of your being too lean (12).

Several lifestyle problems could contribute to a low percentage of body fatness (12). For example, are you getting enough sleep? If not, you may be burning large amounts of energy and creating a negative caloric balance. Do you drink large amounts of coffee? Coffee can influence body weight in two ways. First, more than three to five cups of coffee can reduce your appetite. Second, consumption of coffee or other caffeine-containing beverages increases your resting metabolism for several hours. Further, do you skip meals? Failing to eat regularly may result in a negative caloric balance and fat loss. Finally, do you have an eating disorder?

If lifestyle is not the problem, consult with your physician to rule out the possibility that the cause of your low body fat is hormonal imbalances or other diseases that influence body weight. After discussing with your physician your desire to gain fat and obtaining medical clearance to do so, consider the following recommendations:

1. Establish a weight gain goal that will place you at the low end of the recommended percent body fat range.

2. Create a positive caloric balance. This is accomplished by increasing your total caloric intake to exceed your daily expenditure. A positive caloric balance of 500 calories per day will generally result in a weight gain of 1 pound of fat per week, a reasonable goal.

3. To create a positive caloric balance, compute your daily caloric expenditure, and increase your caloric intake to exceed expenditure. When creating a positive caloric diet, use the basic principles of nutrition discussed in Chapter 7. That is, increase your total caloric intake by using the "eating-right pyramid," so that you adhere to the recommended guidelines for fat, carbohydrate, and protein intake.

4. Consult a physician and a nutritionist. Although anyone can gain weight while eating a positive caloric diet, the safest means of gaining body fat is with the assistance of these professionals.

GAINING MUSCLE MASS

If your percent of body fat is within the recommended range and you wish to increase your body mass, your goal should be to gain muscle mass, not fat. Unfortunately, there are no over-the-counter products or short-cuts for gaining muscle (Nutritional Links to Health and Fitness). The key to gaining muscle mass is a program of rigorous weight training combined with the increase in caloric intake needed to meet the increased energy expenditure and energy required to synthesize muscle. Exercise programs designed to improve muscular strength and size are discussed in Chapter 5 and are not addressed here. The focus here is on the dietary adjustments needed to optimize gains in muscle mass. Again, in order to gain muscle mass, you need to create a small positive caloric balance to provide the energy required to synthesize new muscle protein. Nonetheless, before we provide dietary guidelines, let's discuss how much energy is expended during weight training, and how much energy is required to promote muscle growth.

How much energy is expended during weight training? Energy expenditure during routine weight training is surprisingly small. For instance, a 70-kg man performing a 30-minute weight workout probably burns fewer than 70 calories (12). The reason for this low caloric expenditure is that during 30 minutes in the weight room, the average person spends only 8 to 10 minutes actually lifting weights; much time is spent in recovery periods between sets.

How much energy is required to synthesize 1 pound of muscle mass? Current estimates are approximately 2500 calories, of which about 400 calories (100 grams) must be protein (12). To compute the additional calories required to produce an increase in muscle mass, you must first estimate your rate of muscular growth. This is difficult because the rate of muscular growth during weight training varies among people. While relatively large muscle mass gains are possible in some

Nutritional Links

Do Protein Supplements Have a Role in Promoting Muscle Growth?

Many of the numerous nutritional products that are advertised as "wonder drugs" for promoting muscle growth are high-protein (and often high-calorie) drinks. But are they effective? There is no scientific evidence to support the notion that any of these products result in increases in muscular size or strength. The only proven and safe method of building muscle mass is regular weight training coupled with a nutritionally sound diet. (See reference 21 for a review of this topic.)

But do you even need such high intakes of protein to promote muscle growth? Although consumption of small quantities of high-protein drinks may not be harmful, if you are eating a typical U.S. diet you don't need to increase your protein intake to achieve muscle growth (12, 21). Here's why: To achieve normal growth and development, the RDA for protein is 0.8 gram per kilogram (kg) of body weight, which means that a 70-kg man needs 56 grams of protein per day (70 kg × 0.8 gram/kg/day = 56 grams/day). But because the average daily U.S. diet contains about 100 grams of protein, which is well above the RDA, no protein supplementation is needed to promote muscle growth.

muscle gain is 0.25 pound per week and that 2500 calories are required to synthesize one pound of muscle, a positive caloric balance of less than 100 calories per day is needed to promote muscle growth (0.25 pound/week × 2500 calories/ pound = 625 calories/week; therefore, 625 calories/week ÷ 7 days/ week = 90 calories/day).

What are the dietary guidelines for gaining muscle mass? The major adjustments in diet are an increased caloric intake and assurance that you are obtaining adequate amounts of dietary protein. If you follow the dietary guidelines discussed in Chapter 7 while producing a positive caloric balance, your diet will contain enough protein to support an increase in muscle mass. When planning your diet, consider the following points:

- To increase your caloric intake, use the "eating-right pyramid" presented in Chapter 7. This will ensure that your diet meets the criteria for healthful living and provides adequate protein for building muscle.

- Avoid intake of high-fat foods, and limit your positive caloric balance to approximately 90 calories per day. Increasing your positive caloric balance above this level will not promote a faster rate of muscular growth but will result in increased body fat.

- If you discontinue your weight-training program, lower your caloric intake to match your daily energy expenditure.

☀ IN SUMMARY

- Gaining body fat can be achieved by creating a positive caloric balance. Before deciding to gain body fat, you should consider whether your current body composition is within your desired range.

- Gaining muscle mass cannot be attained by over-the-counter products alone; it must be achieved by combining exercise with proper nutrition.

individuals, studies have shown that most men and women rarely gain more than 0.25 pound of muscle per week during a 20-week weight training program (3 days/ week, 30 minutes/day). If we assume that the average

Summary

1. Millions of people in the United States carry too much body fat for optimal health.

2. Obesity is defined as a high percentage of body fat—that is, over 25% for men and over 30% for women.

3. Obesity is linked to many diseases, including heart disease, diabetes, and hypertension.

4. The optimal percent body fat for health and fitness is believed to be 10–20% for men and 15–25% for women.

5. The energy balance theory of weight control states that to maintain your body weight, your energy intake must equal your energy expenditure.

6. Evidence suggests that creating a fat deficit is an essential factor in weight loss. This is because dietary fat is more easily stored as body fat than are either carbohydrate or protein. The importance of a low-fat diet in weight control is illustrated by the fact that body fat gain results when fat intake continually exceeds fat metabolism.

7. Total daily energy expenditure is the sum of resting metabolic rate and exercise metabolic rate.

8. The four basic components of a comprehensive weight control program are weight loss goals; a reduced-calorie diet stressing balanced nutrition; an exercise program designed to increase caloric expenditure and maintain muscle mass; and a

behavior modification program designed to modify those behaviors that contribute to weight gain.

9. Weight loss goals should include both short-term and long-term goals.

10. Numerous weight loss myths exist. This chapter has discredited weight loss myths concerning diet pills, spot reduction, grapefruit diets, cellulite reduction, and the use of saunas, steam baths, and rubber exercise suits.

11. Two relatively common eating disorders, anorexia nervosa and bulimia, are serious medical conditions that require professional treatment.

12. Weight training and a positive caloric balance are required to produce increases in muscle mass.

Study Questions

1. What is obesity? What diseases are linked to obesity?

2. Discuss several possible causes of obesity.

3. Discuss the concept of optimal body weight. How is optimal body weight computed?

4. Explain the roles of resting metabolic rate and exercise metabolic rate in determining total caloric expenditure. Which is more important in total daily caloric expenditure in a sedentary individual?

5. Outline a simple method for computing your daily caloric expenditure. Give an example.

6. List the four major components of a weight loss program.

7. Discuss the weight loss myths concerning the following: spot reduction; grapefruit diet; eating before bedtime; cellulite reduction; and saunas, steam baths, and rubber suits.

8. Define the eating disorders anorexia nervosa and bulimia.

9. Discuss the role of behavior modification in weight loss.

10. Define the following terms:
energy balance theory of weight control
isocaloric balance
negative caloric balance
positive caloric balance

11. Explain the fat deficit concept of weight control.

12. Compare exercise metabolic rate with resting metabolic rate.

13. What is cellulite?

14. How does creeping obesity occur?

15. Discuss the process of combining diet and exercise to increase muscle mass.

Suggested Reading

AHA Dietary Guidelines. Revision 2000: A statement for healthcare professionals from the nutrition committee of the American Heart Association. *Circulation* 102:2284–2299, 2000.

Going, S., and R. Davis. Body composition. In *ACSM's Resource Manual for Guidelines for Exercise Testing and Prescription,* J. Roitman, ed. Philadelphia: Lippincott, Williams & Wilkins, 2001.

Kroll, S. Three tips to help your clients combat creeping obesity. *ACSM's Health and Fitness Journal* 5(3):22–24, 2001.

Leeds, M. *Nutrition for Healthy Living.* Boston: WCB-McGraw-Hill, 1998.

Manore, M. Low-carbohydrate diets for weight loss are back. *ACSM's Health and Fitness Journal* 3(5):41–43, 1999.

McInnis, K. Exercise for obese clients: Benefits, limitations, and guidelines. *ACSM's Health and Fitness Journal* 4(1): 25–31, 2000.

Powers, S., and E. Howley. *Exercise Physiology: Theory and Application to Fitness and Performance,* 4th ed. St. Louis: McGraw-Hill, 2001.

Ross, R., J. Freeman, and I. Janssen. Exercise alone is an effective strategy for reducing obesity and related co-morbidities. *Exercise and Sport Sciences Reviews* 28(4):165–170, 2000.

For links to the Web sites below visit Web Links at www.aw.com/fitness and choose Powers/Dodd Web Links from the drop-down menu.

American Dietetic Association

Contains articles about nutrition and fad diets.

Nutrition with Rick Hall

Provides links to over 700 health, weight loss, and nutrition-related websites.

References

1. Atkinson, R. Treatment of obesity. *Nutritional Reviews* 50:338–345, 1992.

1a. National Institutes of Health technology assessment conference statement: Methods for voluntary weight loss and control. *Nutrition Reviews* 50:340–345, 1992.

2. Wadden, T., J. Sternberg, K. Letizia, A. Stunkard, and G. Foster. Treatment for obesity by very low calorie diet, behavior therapy, and their combination: A five year prospective. *International Journal of Obesity* 13(Suppl. 2):39–46, 1989.

3. American College of Sports Medicine, L. Durstine, et al., eds. *Resource Manual for Guidelines for Exercise Testing and Prescription,* 2nd ed. Philadelphia: Lea and Febiger, 1993.

4. Bjorntorp, P., and B. Brodoff, eds. *Obesity.* Philadelphia: Lippincott, 1992.

5. Perri, M., A. Nezu, and B. Viegener. *Improving the Long-term Management and Treatment of Obesity.* New York: John Wiley and Sons, 1992.

6. Stefanik, M. Exercise and weight control. In *Exercise and Sport Science Reviews,* J. Holloszy, ed. Baltimore: Williams and Wilkins, 1993.

7. Stunkard, A., and T. Wadden, eds. *Obesity: Theory and Therapy.* New York: Raven Press, 1993.

8. Kuczmarski, R. Prevalence of overweight and weight gain in the United States. *American Journal of Clinical Nutrition* 55:495s–502s, 1992.

9. Bouchard, C., A. Tremblay, J. Despres, et al. The response to long-term overfeeding in identical twins. *New England Journal of Medicine* 322:1477–1482, 1990.

10. Stunkard, A., T. Sorensen, C. Hanis, et al. An adoption study of human obesity. *New England Journal of Medicine* 314:193–198, 1986.

11. Howley, E., and B. D. Franks. *Health Fitness: Instructors Handbook.* Champaign, IL: Human Kinetics, 1997.

12. Williams, M. *Lifetime Fitness and Wellness.* Dubuque, IA: Wm. C. Brown, 1996.

13. Van Itallie, T. Health implications of overweight and obesity in the United States. *Annals of Internal Medicine* 103:983–988, 1985.

14. Health implications of obesity: National Institutes of Health consensus development conference. *Annals of Internal Medicine* 103:977–1077, 1985.

15. Steppan, C. M., et al. The hormone resistin links obesity to diabetes. *Nature* 409:307–312, 2001.

16. Bouchard, C., R. Shepherd, T. Stephens, J. Sutton, and B. McPherson, eds. *Exercise, Fitness, and Health: A Consensus of Current Knowledge.* Champaign, IL: Human Kinetics, 1990.

17. Hockey, R. *Physical Fitness: The Pathway to Healthful Living,* 8th ed. St. Louis: Times Mirror/Mosby, 1996.

18. Getchell, B. *Physical Fitness: A Way of Life,* 5th ed. Needham Heights, MA: Allyn and Bacon, 1998.

19. Corbin, C., and R. Lindsey. *Concepts of Physical Fitness.* Dubuque, IA: Wm. C. Brown, 2000.

20. Pollock, M., and J. Wilmore. *Exercise in Health and Disease,* 3rd ed. Philadelphia: W. B. Saunders, 1999.

21. Powers, S., and E. Howley. *Exercise Physiology: Theory and Application to Fitness and Performance,* 4th ed. St. Louis: McGraw-Hill, 2001.

22. Changnon, Y. C., et al. Genomic scan for genes affecting body composition before and after training in Caucasions from HERITAGE. *Journal of Applied Physiology* 90:1777–1787, 2001.

23. Frubeck, G., J. Gomez-Amrosi, F. Muruzabal, and M. Burrell. The adipocyte: A model for integration of endocrine and metabolic signaling in energy metabolism regulation. *American Journal of Physiology* 280:E827–E847, 2001.

24. Bailey, J., R. Barker, and R. Beauchene. Age-related changes in rat adipose tissue cellularity are altered by dietary restriction and exercise. *Journal of Nutrition* 123: 52–58, 1993.

25. Blair, S. Evidence for success of exercise in weight loss control. *Annals of Internal Medicine* 119:702–706, 1993.

26. Poehlman, E. A review: Exercise and its influence on resting energy metabolism in man. *Medicine and Science in Sports and Exercise* 21:515–525, 1989.

27. Jequier, E. Body weight regulation in humans: The importance of nutrient balance. *News in Physiological Sciences* 8:273–276, 1993.

28. King, M., and F. Katch. Changes in body density, fatfolds, and girths at 2.3 kg increments of weight loss. *Human Biology* 58:709,1986.

29. Sizer, F., and E. Whitney. *Nutrition: Concepts and Controversies.* New York: West/Wadsworth, 1997.

30. AHA Dietary Guidelines. Revision 2000: A statement for healthcare professionals from the nutrition committee of the American Heart Association. *Circulation* 102:2284–2299, 2000.

31. Ross, R., J. Freeman, and I. Janssen. Exercise alone is an effective strategy for reducing obesity and related comorbidities. *Exercise and Sport Sciences Reviews* 28(4):165–170, 2000.

32. Coyle, E. Fat metabolism during exercise. *Sports Science Exchange* (Gatorade Sports Science Institute) 8:6, 1995.

33. Broeder, C., K. Burrhus, L. Svanevik, and J. Wilmore. The effects of either high intensity resistance or endurance training on resting metabolic rate. *American Journal of Clinical Nutrition* 55:802–810, 1992.

34. Bailey, C. *The New Fit or Fat.* Boston: Houghton Mifflin, 1991.

35. Romijn, J., E. Coyle, L. Sidossis, et al. Regulation of endogenous fat and carbohydrate metabolism in relation to exercise and duration. *American Journal of Physiology* 265:E380–E391, 1993.

36. Tremblay, A., S. Coveney, J. Despres, A. Nadeau, D. Prud'homme. Increased resting metabolic rate and lipid oxidation in exercise-trained individuals: Evidence for a role of beta-oxidation. *Canadian Journal of Physiology and Pharmacology* 70:1342–1347, 1992.

37. Mayer, J., N. Marshall, J. Vitale, J. Christensen, M. Mashayekhi, and F. Stare. Exercise, food intake, and body weight in normal rats and genetically obese adult mice. *American Journal of Physiology* 177:544–548, 1954.

38. Gwinup, G., R. Chelvam, and T. Steinberg. Thickness of subcutaneous fat and activity of underlying muscles. *Annals of Internal Medicine* 74:408–411, 1971.

39. Andersen, A. Anorexia nervosa and bulimia. *Journal of Adolescent Health Care* 4:15–21, 1983.

40. Borgen, J., and C. Corbin. Eating disorders among female athletes. *Physician and Sports Medicine* 15:89–95, 1987.

41. Leeds, M. *Nutrition for Healthy Living.* Boston: WCB-McGraw-Hill, 1998.

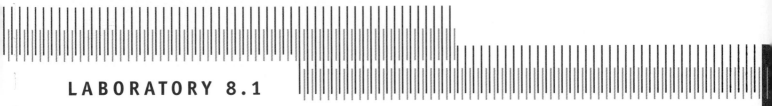

Determining Ideal Body Weight Using Percent Body Fat and the Body Mass Index

NAME _____ DATE _____

There are a number of different ways to compute an ideal body weight. In Chapter 2 we discussed percent body fat (estimated from skinfold measurements). Method A of this laboratory enables you to compute and record your ideal body weight using the percent body fat method. Method B enables you to calculate and record your ideal body weight using the body mass index procedure (Chapter 2). Choose one of these techniques and complete the appropriate section.

METHOD A: COMPUTATION OF IDEAL BODY WEIGHT USING PERCENT BODY FAT

STEP 1: CALCULATE FAT-FREE WEIGHT

100% − your percent body fat estimated from skinfold measurement = _____ % fat free weight. Therefore,

_____ % fat-free weight expressed as a decimal × your body weight in pounds = _____ pounds of fat-free weight.

STEP 2: CALCULATE OPTIMAL WEIGHT

Remember: Optimal body fat ranges are 10–20% for men and 15–25% for women.
Optimal weight = fat-free weight/(1.00 − optimal %fat), with optimal %fat expressed as a decimal. Therefore, the low and high optimal weight ranges for your gender are

For low %fat: Optimal weight = _____ pounds

For high %fat: Optimal weight = _____ pounds

(continued on next page)

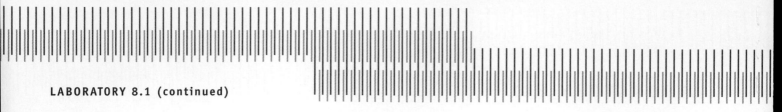

METHOD B: COMPUTATION OF IDEAL BODY WEIGHT USING BODY MASS INDEX (BMI)

The BMI uses the metric system. Therefore, you must express your weight in kilograms (1 kilogram = 2.2 pounds) and your height in meters (1 inch = 0.0254 meters).

STEP 1: COMPUTE YOUR BMI

BMI = body weight (kg)/(height in meters)^2

Your BMI = _____

STEP 2: CALCULATE YOUR IDEAL BODY WEIGHT BASED ON BMI*

The ideal BMI is 21.9 to 22.4 for men and 21.3 to 22.1 for women. The formula for computing ideal body weight using BMI is

ideal body weight (kilograms) = desired BMI $\times$ (height in meters)^2

Consider the following example as an illustration of the computation of ideal body weight. A woman who weighs 60 kilograms and is 1.5 meters tall computes her BMI to be 26.7. Her ideal BMI is between 21.9 and 22.4; therefore, her ideal body weight range is

ideal body weight = 21.9 $\times$ 2.25 = 49.3 kilograms
ideal body weight = 22.4 $\times$ 2.25 = 50.4 kilograms

Now complete this calculation using your values for BMI.

My ideal body weight range using the BMI method is _____ to _____ kilograms.

* Note: BMI may not be a good method to determine ideal body weight for a highly muscled individual.

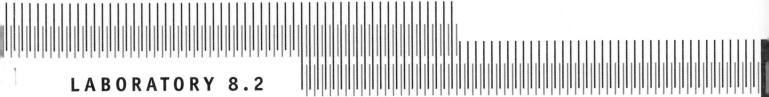

LABORATORY 8.2

Estimating Daily Caloric Expenditure and the Caloric Deficit Required to Lose 1 Pound of Fat Per Week

NAME _____ DATE _____

PART A. ESTIMATION OF YOUR DAILY CALORIC EXPENDITURE

Using Table 8.1, compute your estimated daily caloric expenditure.

Estimated daily caloric expenditure = _____ calories/day.

PART B. CALCULATION OF CALORIC INTAKE REQUIRED TO PROMOTE 1 POUND PER WEEK OF WEIGHT LOSS

Recall that 1 pound of fat contains approximately 3500 calories. Therefore, a negative caloric balance of 500 calories per day will result in a weight loss of 1 pound per week. Use the following formula to compute your daily caloric intake to result in a daily caloric deficit of 500 calories.

estimated daily caloric expenditure − 500 calories (deficit) = daily caloric intake needed to produce a 500-calorie deficit

In the space provided, compute your daily caloric intake needed to produce 1 pound per week of weight loss.

_____ (estimated caloric expenditure) −

___− 500_____ (caloric deficit)

= _____ target daily caloric intake

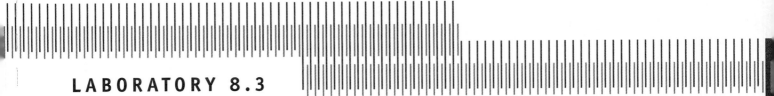

Weight Loss Goals and Progress Report

NAME _____ DATE _____

In the spaces provided, record your short-term and long-term weight loss goals. Then keep a record of your weight loss progress on the chart.

Ideal body weight (range): _____

Short-term weight loss goal: _____ (pounds/week)

Long-term weight loss goal: _____ pounds

Week No.	Body Weight	Date	Weight Loss
1			
2			
3			
4			
5			
6			
7			
8			
9			
10			
11			
12			
13			
14			
15			
16			
17			
18			
19			
20			
21			
22			
23			

(continued on next page)

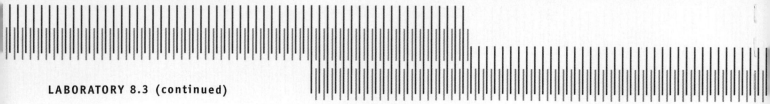

24 _____

25 _____

26 _____

27 _____

28 _____

29 _____

30 _____

31 _____

32 _____

33 _____

34 _____

35 _____

36 _____

37 _____

38 _____

39 _____

40 _____

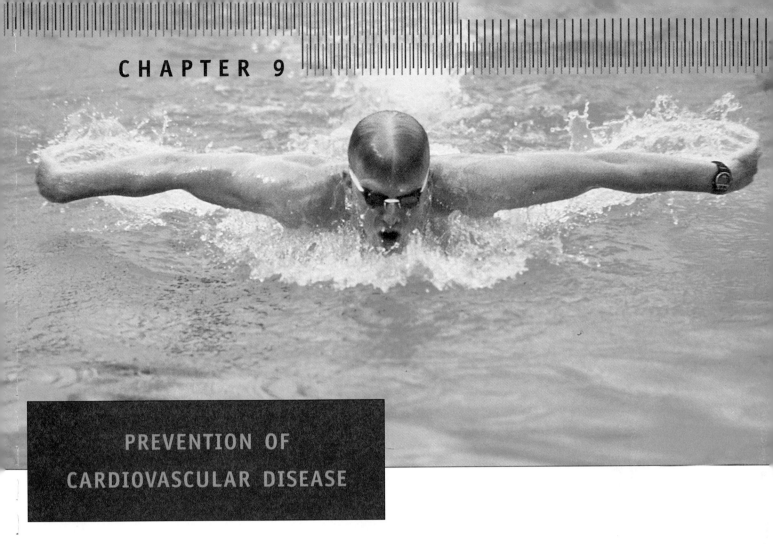

CHAPTER 9

PREVENTION OF CARDIOVASCULAR DISEASE

After studying this chapter, you should be able to:

1. Name the number one cause of death in the United States.

2. Identify four common cardiovascular diseases.

3. Discuss the major and contributory risk factors associated with the development of coronary heart disease.

4. Identify the coronary heart disease risk factors that can be modified by lifestyle alterations.

5. List the steps involved in reducing your risk of coronary heart disease.

6. Describe the link between dietary sodium and hypertension.

7. Identify the total blood cholesterol levels associated with low, moderate, and high risk of developing coronary heart disease.

8. Discuss the relationship between diet and elevated blood cholesterol levels.

Cardiovascular diseases are a major health problem around the world and account for millions of deaths each year. The incidence of cardiovascular disease is greatest in industrialized countries, and the United Stated has one of the world's highest death rates (1). Although it is impossible to place a dollar value on human life, the economic cost of cardiovascular disease in the United States is great (Figure 9.1). Estimates of lost wages and medical expenses exceed 95 billion dollars every year (1); therefore, developing a national strategy to reduce the risk of cardiovascular disease is a major heath priority. This chapter focuses on lifestyle changes (e.g., exercise and diet) that can reduce your risk of cardiovascular diseases. Let's begin our discussion with an overview of cardiovascular disease in the United States.

☀ Cardiovascular Disease in the United States

Although public awareness is currently more focused on diseases such as cancer and AIDS, **cardiovascular disease**—any disease that affects the heart or blood vessels—remains the number one cause of death in the United States, accounting for nearly one of every two deaths. Current data indicate that over 60 million adults have one or more forms of cardiovascular disease and that approximately 1 million people die annually from cardiovascular disorders (1). Equally alarming is the fact that cardiovascular disease is not restricted to the elderly. It is the leading cause of death in men between the ages of 35 and 44 (1). Although the death rate from cardiovascular disease has always been higher for men than for women, the incidence of cardiovascular disease in women has increased dramatically in recent years (1). (See Fitness and Wellness for All for a brief discussion of the segments of the population at greatest risk of cardiovascular disease.) Fortunately, it is possible to reduce your risk of developing cardiovascu-

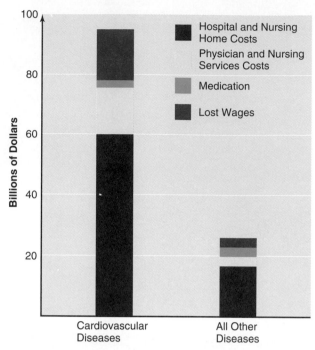

FIGURE 9.1
Annual economic costs of cardiovascular diseases and all other diseases in the United States.

lar disease, but before discussing how to do this, we will define the major types of cardiovascular disease.

☀ Cardiovascular Diseases

Although literally hundreds of diseases impair normal cardiovascular function, only four common cardiovascular diseases warrant discussion here.

ARTERIOSCLEROSIS

Arteriosclerosis is not a single disease but rather a group of diseases characterized by a narrowing or "hardening" of the arteries. The end result of any form of arteriosclerosis is that blood flow to vital organs may be impaired due to progressive blockage of the artery. **Atherosclerosis** is a special type of arteriosclerosis that results in arterial blockage due to buildup of a fatty deposit (called *atherosclerotic plaque*) inside the blood vessel. This plaque deposit is typically composed of cholesterol, cellular debris, fibrin (a clotting material in the blood), and calcium. Atherosclerosis is a progressive disease that begins in childhood, and symptoms appear later in life. Figure 9.2 illustrates the progression of arterial blockage caused by atherosclerosis. Note that atherosclerosis is not an "all or none" disease but occurs in varying degrees, with some arteries exhibiting little blockage and others exhibiting major obstruction. Development of severe atherosclerosis within arteries supplying blood to the heart is the cause of almost all heart attacks.

---

cardiovascular disease   Any disease that affects the heart or blood vessels.

arteriosclerosis   A group of diseases characterized by a narrowing or "hardening" of the arteries. The end result of any form of arteriosclerosis is that blood flow to vital organs may be impaired due to progressive blockage of the artery.

atherosclerosis   A special type of arteriosclerosis that results in arterial blockage due to buildup of a fatty deposit (called *atherosclerotic plaque*) inside the blood vessel.

FITNESS AND WELLNESS FOR ALL

Who Is at Greatest Risk of Cardiovascular Disease?

Ethnicity, gender, age, and socioeconomic status can all affect an individual's risk of developing cardiovascular disease, and these factors explain why cardiovascular disease is more prevalent in certain segments of the U.S. population. African Americans, for example, are at greater risk of developing hypertension (or high blood pressure, one form of cardiovascular disease) compared to the U.S. population as a whole. Similarly, Native Americans and people of Latino heritage have higher prevalences of diabetes, an important contributory risk factor for cardiovascular disease. Between the ages of 20 and 65, men are at greater risk than women for developing cardiovascular disease. Finally, individuals who earn low incomes experience higher incidences of both heart disease and obesity (a contributory risk factor for heart disease).

CORONARY HEART DISEASE

Coronary heart disease is the major disease of the cardiovascular system. **Coronary heart disease (CHD),** also called *coronary artery disease,* is the result of atherosclerotic plaque forming a blockage of one or more coronary arteries (the blood vessels supplying the heart; Figure 9.3). When the degree of blockage of a major coronary artery reaches 75%, the resulting lack of blood flow to the working heart muscle causes chest pain. This type of chest pain, called *angina pectoris,* occurs most frequently during exercise or emotional stress (2).

Severe blockage of coronary arteries may result in a blood clot forming around the layer of plaque. When this happens, a complete blockage of heart blood flow occurs, resulting in a **heart attack** (also called a **myocardial infarction**). Figure 9.4 illustrates what happens during a heart attack caused by complete blockage of the left coronary artery. The end result is the death of heart muscle cells in the left ventricle; the severity of the heart attack is judged by how many heart muscle cells are damaged. A "mild" heart attack may only damage a small portion of the heart, whereas a "major" heart attack may destroy a large number of heart muscle cells. Because the number of heart muscle cells destroyed during a heart attack determines the patient's chances of recovery, recognizing the symptoms of a heart attack and getting prompt medical attention are crucial (A Closer Look, p. 225).

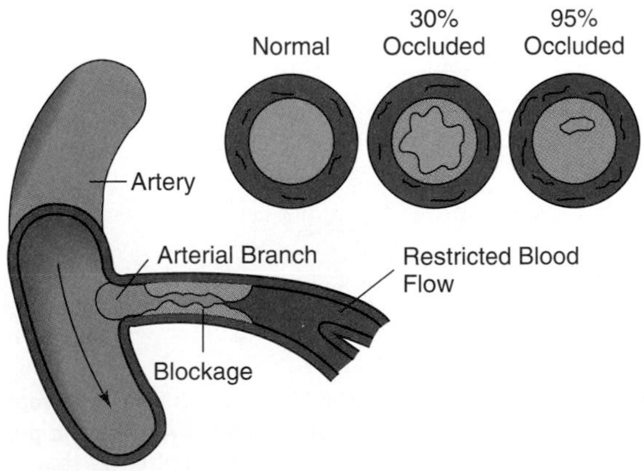

STROKE

It is estimated that each year 2 million Americans suffer a stroke (1). A **stroke** occurs when the blood supply to the brain is reduced for a prolonged period of time. A common cause of stroke is blockage (due to atherosclerosis) of arteries leading to the brain (Figure 9.5). However, strokes can also occur when a cerebral (brain) blood vessel ruptures and disturbs normal blood flow to that region of the brain.

Similar to a heart attack, which results in death of heart cells, a stroke results in death of brain cells. The severity of the stroke may vary from slight to severe, depending on the location and the number of brain cells

FIGURE 9.2
Progressive stages of atherosclerosis. The three cross-sections show (from left to right) a "normal" artery that has no blockage, and two arteries that have 30% and 95% blockages, respectively, due to the progressive buildup of atherosclerotic plaque within them.

coronary heart disease (CHD) Also called *coronary artery disease;* CHD is the result of atherosclerotic plaque forming a blockage of one or more coronary arteries (the blood vessels supplying the heart).
heart attack Stoppage of blood flow to the heart resulting in the death of heart cells; also called *myocardial infarction.*
stroke Brain damage that occurs when the blood supply to the brain is reduced for a prolonged period of time.

Heart and Coronary Arteries

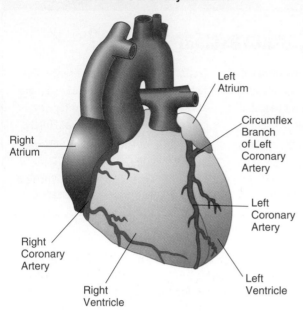

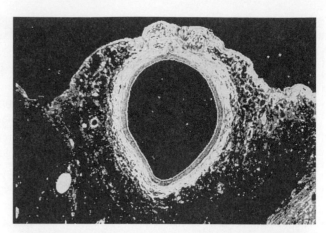

FIGURE 9.3
Locations of the coronary arteries, the vessels that carry blood to the working heart muscle. The photographs on the right show a normal coronary artery (top) and an atherosclerotic coronary artery (bottom). As plaque builds up in the walls of coronary arteries, the risk of heart attack increases.
(*Source:* From Melvin H. Williams, *Lifetime Fitness and Wellness,* 3rd ed. Copyright © 1993 Wm. C. Brown Communications, Inc. Reprinted by permission of Times Mirror Higher Education Group, Inc., Dubuque, Iowa. All rights reserved.)

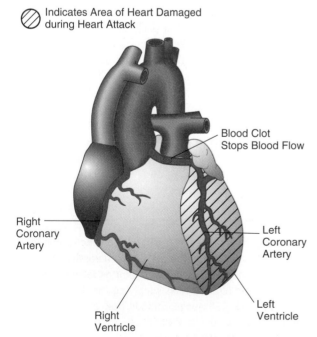

FIGURE 9.4
Effect of a myocardial infarction (heart attack). The cross-hatched area of the heart is damaged due to a stoppage of blood flow during the heart attack.

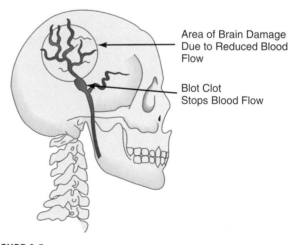

FIGURE 9.5
How blockage of an artery in the brain causes a stroke. Stoppage of blood flow through an artery supplying the brain produces damage to the portion of the brain supplied by that artery (indicated by the circle).

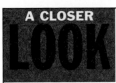

A CLOSER LOOK

Heart Attack: Recognition of Symptoms and Emergency Action

Recognition of heart attack symptoms and knowledge of the appropriate emergency action could save your life or that of someone else. First, here's how to recognize the symptoms of an ongoing heart attack.

WARNING SIGNALS OF A HEART ATTACK

Some of the most common symptoms of a heart attack (2) are

- Mild to moderate pain in your chest that may spread to the shoulders, neck, or arms

- Uncomfortable pressure or sensation of fullness in the chest

- Severe pain in the chest, dizziness, fainting, sweating, nausea, or shortness of breath

Note that not all of these symptoms occur in every heart attack. Therefore, if you or someone you're with experiences any one of these symptoms for 2 minutes or more, follow the emergency procedures described next.

Because 40% of heart attack victims die within the first hour, immediate medical attention is vital to a patient's survival.

WHAT TO DO IN THE CASE OF A HEART ATTACK

If you or someone near you experiences any of the aforementioned symptoms for 2 minutes or longer, call the emergency medical service or get to the nearest hospital that offers emergency cardiac care. If you are trained in cardiopulmonary resuscitation (CPR) and the patient is not breathing or does not have a pulse, call 911 or the emergency medical service in your area, and then start CPR immediately. In any cardiac emergency, rapid action may mean the difference between life and death.

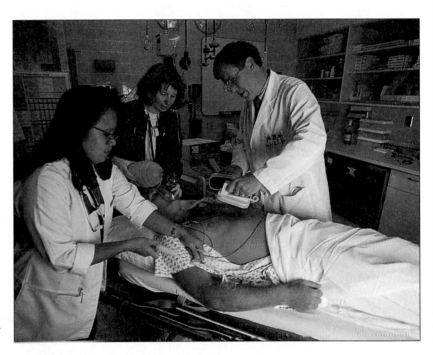

damaged. Minor strokes may involve a loss of memory, speech problems, disturbed vision, and/or mild paralysis in the extremities. In contrast, severe strokes may result in major paralysis or death.

HYPERTENSION

Hypertension is abnormally high blood pressure. Clinically, hypertension is generally defined as a resting blood pressure over 140 mm Hg systolic or 90 mm Hg diastolic (2). Approximately 10% of hypertension cases are caused by a specific disease (such as kidney disease). This type of hypertension is called *secondary hypertension,* because the hypertension is secondary to a primary disease. Nonetheless, in 90% of hypertension cases, the exact cause of the high blood pressure is unknown; this type of hypertension is called *essential hypertension.*

The prevalence of hypertension in the United States is remarkably high (Figure 9.6). The factors that increase your risk of hypertension include lack of exercise, a high-salt diet, obesity, chronic stress, family history of hypertension, gender (men have a greater risk than women), and race (blacks have a greater risk than whites).

Hypertension is a health problem for several reasons. First, high blood pressure increases the workload on the heart; this may eventually damage the heart muscle's ability to pump blood effectively throughout the body (2). Second, high blood pressure may damage the lining of arteries, resulting in the development of atherosclerosis and therefore increasing the risk of CHD and stroke (2).

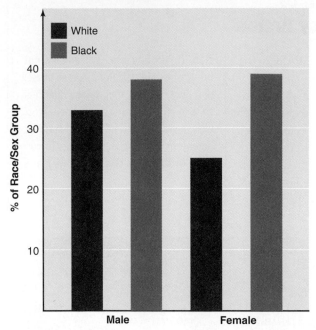

Hypertension in the United States (ages 18–74 years)

% of Race/Sex Group

- White
- Black

Male   Female

FIGURE 9.6
The prevalence of hypertension in selected groups in the United States.

Although exercise causes acute increases in blood pressure, this type of blood pressure elevation is transient and is not hypertension (i.e., hypertension is chronically elevated blood pressure). Further, the increase in blood pressure during exercise does not damage the heart or blood vessels.

The American Heart Association estimates that approximately one of every four people in the United States suffers from hypertension—that is, more than 62 million people (1). Unfortunately, because they lack symptoms, many people are not aware that they are hypertensive. Although severe hypertension may result in headaches and dizziness, these symptoms are often absent. Therefore, without annual medical checkups or blood pressure screenings, hypertension may go undiagnosed for many years. For this reason, hypertension is often called *the silent killer*.

---

major risk factors   Factors considered to be directly related to the development of CHD and stroke; also called *primary risk factors*.
contributory risk factors   Factors that increase the risk of CHD, but their direct contribution to the disease process has not been precisely determined; also called *secondary risk factors*.

☀ IN SUMMARY

- Cardiovascular disease remains the number one cause of death in the United States and in many other developed countries.
- The term *cardiovascular disease* refers to any disease that affects the heart or blood vessels.
- The four major cardiovascular diseases are arteriosclerosis, coronary artery disease, stroke, and hypertension.

☀ Risk Factors Associated with Coronary Heart Disease

In an effort to understand the causes and reduce the occurrence of CHD, researchers have identified a number of major and contributory risk factors that increase the chance of developing both CHD and stroke. **Major risk factors** (also called *primary risk factors*) are factors considered to be directly related to the development of CHD and stroke. In contrast, **contributory risk factors** (also called *secondary risk factors*) are those that increase the risk of CHD, but their direct contribution to the disease process has not been precisely determined.

MAJOR RISK FACTORS

Each year the American Heart Association publishes new information concerning the major risk factors associated with the development of CHD and stroke. The most recent list includes cigarette smoking, hypertension, high blood cholesterol levels, physical inactivity, heredity, gender, and increasing age (1) (Figure 9.7). The greater the number of CHD risk factors an individual has, the greater the likelihood that he or she will develop CHD (Figure 9.8). Let's discuss each of the major risk factors for CHD and stroke.

SMOKING   It is estimated that over 50 million people in the United States smoke (3). Many U.S. health care workers believe that cigarette smoking is the single largest cause of disease and premature death. Cigarette smoking has been linked to over 30 health problems, including cancer, lung disease, and cardiovascular disease (1–4). In regard to smoking and cardiovascular disease, a smoker's risk of developing CHD is more than twice that of a nonsmoker (1) (Figure 9.8). Smoking is also considered the biggest risk factor for sudden cardiac death (i.e., sudden death due to cardiac arrest, a heart attack, or irregular heartbeats). In addition, smoking promotes the development of atherosclerosis in peripheral blood vessels (arterial blockage in the arms or legs). Finally, smokers who have a heart attack are more likely to die suddenly (within an hour after the attack) than are nonsmokers.

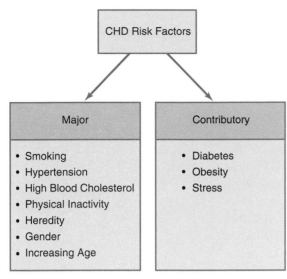

FIGURE 9.7
Coronary heart disease risk factors.

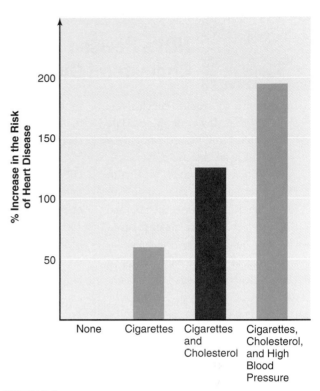

FIGURE 9.8
The effects of multiple risk factors for coronary heart disease. Your risk of developing CHD increases as the number of risk factors increases.

Is the risk of cardiovascular disease increased for nonsmokers who breathe in "secondhand" cigarette smoke? Unfortunately, the answer is "yes." Numerous studies have concluded that passive inhalation of cigarette smoke can increase the risk for both cardiovascular and lung disease (3). This has prompted the banning of smoking in many public places, including airplanes, restaurants, and shopping malls.

Cigarette smoking can influence your risk of cardiovascular disease in at least four ways. First, cigarette smoke contains the drug nicotine, which increases both heart rate and blood pressure (3). Second, smoking increases your blood's ability to clot; the elevated possibility of a blood clot forming raises your risk of heart attack (3). Third, nicotine also influences the way your heart functions, leading to irregular heart beats (called *arrhythmias*) (3). These arrhythmias can lead to sudden cardiac death. Finally, cigarette smoking increases your chance of developing atherosclerosis by elevating the amount of cholesterol in the blood and encouraging fat deposits in arterial walls (3).

When people stop smoking, their risk of heart disease rapidly declines. It is believed that within 10 years after quitting smoking, a person's risk of death from CHD is reduced to a level equal to that of someone who has never smoked (1). Strategies to stop smoking are discussed in Chapter 10.

HYPERTENSION Hypertension is a unique risk factor because it is both a disease and a risk factor for stroke and CHD. As mentioned earlier, hypertension is considered a disease because it forces the heart to work harder than normal, which can eventually damage the heart muscle. As a CHD risk factor, it contributes to the devel-

opment of CHD by accelerating the rate of atherosclerosis development (2, 5).

HIGH BLOOD CHOLESTEROL LEVELS As discussed in Chapter 7, cholesterol is a type of fat that can either be consumed in the diet or synthesized in the body, and it is a primary risk factor for CHD. Indeed, the risk of CHD increases as the blood cholesterol increases.

Because cholesterol is not soluble in blood, it is combined with proteins in the liver so it can be transported in the bloodstream. This combination of cholesterol and protein results in two major forms of cholesterol: **low-density lipoproteins (LDL)** and

---

low-density lipoproteins (LDL) A combination of protein, triglycerides, and cholesterol in the blood, composed of relatively large amounts of cholesterol. Promotes the fatty plaque accumulation in the coronary arteries that leads to heart disease. The association between elevated total blood cholesterol and the increased risk of CHD is due primarily to LDL. Research has shown that individuals with high blood LDL levels have an increased risk of CHD. Because of this relationship, LDL has been labeled "bad cholesterol."

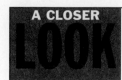

NIH's Revised Blood Cholesterol Guidelines

In response to studies conclusively showing that lowering blood LDL ("bad cholesterol") levels can reduce the risk of heart disease by 40% (6), the National Institutes of Health (NIH) has released new guidelines for optimal blood levels of LDL and HDL. Even though the major focus of the new guidelines is recommendations for the management of blood LDL levels, NIH included recommendations for blood levels of HDL ("good cholesterol") because HDL can carry cholesterol away from ar-

teries and back to the liver. The new guidelines are summarized in the table in this box.

In short, the guidelines consider LDL levels of 100 mg/dl or lower to be optimal for reducing the risk of developing CHD, whereas LDL levels above 190 mg/dl are considered indicative of a high risk for CHD. Because the presence of HDL can lower LDL levels, low blood levels of HDL can indicate an increased risk of developing CHD. Accordingly, the new guidelines consider blood HDL levels below 40

mg/dl to be low and undesirable in terms of CHD risk.

Cholesterol Concentration mg/dl	Classification
LDL	
< 100	Optimal
100–129	Near or above optimal
130–159	Borderline high
160–189	High
> 190	Very high
HDL	
< 40	Low (undesirable)
> 60	High (very desirable)

high-density lipoproteins (HDL). The association between elevated blood cholesterol and CHD is primarily due to LDL: Individuals with high blood LDL levels have an increased risk of CHD, whereas those with high levels of HDL have a decreased risk of CHD (1, 2, 6, 7). Because of these relationships, LDL has been called "bad cholesterol" while HDL has been called "good cholesterol."

Even though the risk of developing CHD is best predicted from LDL and HDL levels in the blood, measurement of total blood cholesterol (i.e., the sum of all types of cholesterol) also provides a good indication of CHD risk (1, 2, 7). As shown in Figure 9.9, a total blood cholesterol concentration that is less than 200 mg/dl (milligrams per deciliter) indicates a low risk of developing CHD, whereas a concentration that is greater than 240 mg/dl indicates a high CHD risk (2, 7). Unfortunately, because of high-fat diets and lack of exercise, over 21% of people in the United States have total blood cholesterol levels above 240 mg/dl (2).

The National Institutes of Health recently released new guidelines for assessing CHD risks using blood levels of LDL and HDL. For a brief overview of these guidelines, see A Closer Look above.

PHYSICAL INACTIVITY In 1992, the American Heart Association added physical inactivity (defined as a lack of regular exercise) to the list of major risk factors for the development of CHD. The addition of physical inactivity to the list of major risk factors for CHD is based on a large volume of research, which suggests that the incidence of CHD is much greater in people who do not engage in regular physical activity (7–11). Thus, exercise has gained new importance in the prevention of CHD.

Although it is known that exercise reduces the risk of CHD, whether exercise does so by reducing blood cholesterol levels remains the subject of much debate. Some studies have indicated that exercise induces a lowering of blood LDL levels, whereas other studies found that exercise has no effect on LDL levels (12, 13). In contrast, it is clear that regular endurance exercise (e.g., running or cycling) results in an elevation of HDL levels and reduce risk of CHD (12–14), even though the

high-density lipoproteins (HDL) A combination of protein, triglycerides, and cholesterol in the blood, composed of relatively large amounts of protein. Protects against the fatty plaque accumulation in the coronary arteries that leads to heart disease. Research has shown that individuals with high blood HDL levels have a decreased risk of CHD. Therefore, HDL is often called "good cholesterol."

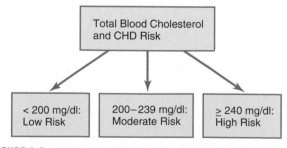

FIGURE 9.9
Total blood cholesterol levels and the CHD risks associated with each.

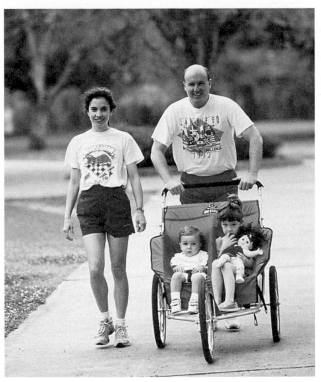

Even modest physical activity (walking for 20–30 minutes per day, three to five times per week) can reduce your risk of developing cardiovascular disease.

mechanism connecting exercise to increased HDL levels is unknown and remains an active area of research.

HEREDITY It is firmly established that inherited traits can increase your risk of CHD and stroke (1, 2). This means that children of parents with CHD are more likely to develop CHD than are children of parents who do not have CHD. Current evidence suggests that the familial risk for CHD may be linked to factors such as high blood cholesterol, hypertension, diabetes, and obesity (2).

Race is also a consideration, because African Americans develop hypertension two to three times more often than whites. Therefore, because hypertension increases the chances of developing CHD, African Americans have a greater risk for CHD than do whites. The reason for the high rate of hypertension among African Americans is unknown.

GENDER Men have a greater risk of developing CHD and stroke than do women. Much of the protection against CHD in women is linked to the female sex hormone estrogen, which may elevate HDL cholesterol. Although the risk of CHD increases in women after menopause, it never becomes as great as for men (2).

INCREASING AGE Advancing age increases the risk of developing CHD. The explanation for this observation is

that the buildup of arterial plaque is an ongoing process; the longer one lives, the greater the buildup. This is illustrated by the statistic that over 50% of all heart attack victims are 65 or older (1).

CONTRIBUTORY RISK FACTORS

Contributory risk factors are those that increase the risk of CHD, but their direct contribution to the disease process is unclear. You can think of contributory risk factors as those that increase your risk of developing a *major* risk factor. At present, the American Heart Association recognizes diabetes, obesity, and stress as contributory risk factors.

DIABETES As we saw in Chapter 1, diabetes is a disease that results in elevated blood sugar levels due to the body's inability to use blood sugar properly. Diabetes occurs most often in middle age and is common in people who are overweight. In addition to increasing your risk of kidney disease, blindness, and nerve damage, diabetes increases your risk of CHD and stroke. The link between diabetes and CHD is well established; more than 80% of all diabetics die from some form of cardiovascular disease. The role of diabetes in increasing your risk of CHD may be tied to the fact that diabetics often have elevated blood cholesterol levels, hypertension, and are inactive (9).

OBESITY Compared with individuals who maintain their ideal body weight, obese individuals are more likely to develop CHD, even if they have no other major risk factors (9). Further, obesity is often associated with elevated blood cholesterol levels and may contribute to hypertension (9).

Of particular interest is the fact that a person's fat distribution pattern affects the risk of CHD. As discussed in Chapter 2, waist-to-hip circumference ratios greater than 1.0 for men and 0.8 for women indicate a significant risk for development of CHD. The physiological reason for the link between CHD and regional fat distribution is not well established but may be due to the fact that people with high waist-to-hip circumference ratios often eat high-fat diets, which elevate blood cholesterol levels.

The fact that obesity is associated with a high incidence of hypertension is well established; however, the exact physiological link between obesity and hypertension is less clear. Possible causes of hypertension in obese individuals include a high-salt diet, which elevates blood pressure, and increased vascular resistance, which results in the need for higher pressure to pump blood to the tissues (2). The role of sodium in promoting hypertension is discussed in Nutritional Links to Health and Fitness, page 230.

Nutritional Links

High Sodium Intake Increases the Risk of Hypertension

A key factor in regulating blood pressure is dietary sodium. High sodium intake results in an elevated blood volume, which promotes higher blood pressure. Therefore, monitoring sodium intake is an important factor in preventing or controlling hypertension.

As mentioned in Chapter 7, sodium (contained in table salt) is a required micronutrient, but the daily requirement for most people is small (less than one-fourth teaspoon or 400 mg). Even athletes or laborers who lose large amounts of water and electrolytes via sweat rarely require more than 1.5 teaspoons (3000 mg) of salt per day. Currently, many U.S. citizens consume more than 6 teaspoons (12,000 mg) of salt per day; clearly, this level of sodium intake is unhealthy and can lead to hypertension.

What is the maximum amount of dietary sodium that the body can tolerate without developing hypertension? Even though a definitive answer to this question is not available, hypertension is rare in countries where sodium intake is less than 1 teaspoon per day.

The key to lowering your sodium intake is avoiding foods that are high in salt. The table in this box illustrates some common foods that are high in sodium. Take the time to learn which foods contain a lot of sodium and limit your intake of sodium to less than 1 teaspoon per day (14).

Food	Serving Size	Sodium Content (mg)
Bologna	2 oz	700
Cheese		
American	1 oz	305
Cheddar	1 oz	165
Parmesan	1 oz	525
Deviled crab	1	2085
Frankfurter	1	495
Hamburger patty	1 small	550
Pickles (dill)	1 medium	900
Pizza (cheese)	1 slice (14" diameter)	600
Potato chips	20	300
Pretzels	1 oz	890
Salami	3 oz	1047
Soup		
Chicken noodle	1 cup	1010
Vegetable beef	1 cup	1046
Soy sauce	1 tablespoon	1320

STRESS Stress increases the risk of CHD; however, the exact link between stress and CHD is unclear and continues to be studied. Nonetheless, it seems likely that stress contributes to the development of several major CHD risk factors. For example, stress may be linked to smoking habits. People under stress may start smoking in an effort to relax, or stress could influence smokers to smoke more than they normally would. Further, stress increases the risk of developing both hypertension and elevated blood cholesterol. The physiological connection between stress and hypertension appears to be the stress-induced release of "stress" hormones, which elevate blood pressure. Currently, it is unclear how stress is linked to high blood cholesterol.

☀ IN SUMMARY

- Researchers have identified several major and contributory risk factors that increase the chance of developing both coronary heart disease (CHD) and stroke.
- Major risk factors for CHD and stroke include smoking, hypertension, high blood cholesterol levels, physical inactivity, heredity, gender, and increasing age.
- Contributory risk factors for CHD and stroke include diabetes, obesity, and stress.

☀ Reducing Your Risk of Heart Disease

Although cardiovascular disease remains the number one killer in the United States, incidence of the disease has declined over the past 30 years (1). This drop is due primarily to people reducing their risk factors for CHD. Table 9.1 contains a list of the major and contributory CHD risk factors discussed earlier in the chapter. Note that four of the seven major risk factors and all three of the contributory factors can be modified by behavior. Therefore, 70% of the ten CHD risk factors presented in Table 9.1 can be modified to reduce your risk of developing cardiovascular disease.

How does one implement a CHD risk reduction program? The first step is the identification of your risk

TABLE 9.1
Major and Contributory Risk Factors for the Development of Coronary Heart Disease

Risk Factor	Risk Factor Classification	Is Behavior Modification Possible?	Behavior Modification to Reduce Risk
Smoking	Major	Yes	Smoking cessation
Hypertension	Major	Yes	Exercise and proper diet
High blood cholesterol	Major	Yes	Exercise and proper diet
Physical inactivity	Major	Yes	Exercise
Heredity	Major	No	
Gender	Major	No	
Increasing age	Major	No	
Diabetes	Contributory	Yes	Proper nutrition, exercise
Obesity	Contributory	Yes	Weight loss, proper nutrition, exercise
Stress	Contributory	Yes	Stress management, exercise

Data from Heart Facts, *American Heart Association, 1993.*

status. This can be done by completing Laboratory 9.1 on page 237 and by carefully examining Table 9.1. The next step is to implement a positive, healthy lifestyle to modify those CHD risk factors that can be altered.

MODIFICATION OF MAJOR RISK FACTORS

The four major CHD risk factors that can be modified are smoking, hypertension, high blood cholesterol, and physical inactivity. The risk of CHD decreases as soon as smokers quit. Clearly, smoking cessation is an important way of reducing CHD risk. The well-known fitness and wellness expert, Dr. Melvin Williams, offers the following advice on smoking (11): "If you don't smoke, don't start! If you smoke, quit!" Unfortunately, for most people, smoking is a difficult habit to break. Chapter 10 provides guidelines to assist in smoking cessation.

Hypertension can be reduced in several ways. In some instances, medication may be required to control high blood pressure. However, in many hypertension cases, exercise and a proper diet that features low sodium intake may assist in the reduction of blood pressure (Nutritional Links to Health and Fitness, p. 230).

High blood cholesterol may be lowered by diet, exercise, and drug treatment (including increasing your niacin intake) (2, 14). One of the simplest ways of reducing cholesterol is through diet. Decreasing your intake of saturated fats and cholesterol may significantly reduce your blood cholesterol levels (Nutritional Links to Health and Fitness, p. 232).

Further, new evidence suggests that a diet high in the antioxidant vitamins E and C may also reduce your risk of developing CHD (Nutritional Links to Health and Fitness, to the right).

Nutritional Links
TO HEALTH AND FITNESS

Antioxidant Vitamins May Reduce Your Risk of Coronary Heart Disease

New research suggests that antioxidant vitamins (i.e., vitamins E and C, and beta carotene) may reduce your risk of CHD. Specifically, several comprehensive studies have shown that diets high in antioxidant vitamins reduce the risk of arteriosclerosis. The mechanism that explains this observation is reduction by these antioxidants of the buildup of LDL (bad) cholesterol on arterial walls (15).

While it appears that a diet high in antioxidants may reduce your risk of CHD, the optimal intake of these antioxidant vitamins remains controversial. Most studies showing protective effects of antioxidants have used vitamin supplements at doses above the recommended dietary allowances (RDA). This has raised concern among many nutritionists, who argue that high doses of these vitamins may result in toxic side effects. Until additional research is performed, the best advice is to eat plenty of fresh fruits and vegetables to obtain as many antioxidants as possible from your diet (15).

Nutritional Links

Diet and Blood Cholesterol Levels

One of the easiest dietary means of reducing your blood cholesterol is to reduce your intake of saturated fat and cholesterol. Saturated fats stimulate cholesterol synthesis in the liver and therefore contribute to elevated blood cholesterol. Saturated fats are found mostly in meats and dairy products; avoiding high intake of these foods can reduce your blood cholesterol levels. The table in this box lists the cholesterol content of selected foods. See the Appendix for a more complete listing.

Food	Serving Size	Cholesterol (mg)	Saturated Fat (g)
Bacon	2 slices	30	0.7
Beef (lean)	8 oz	150	12
Butter	1 tablespoon	32	0.4
Cheese			
American	1 oz	27	5.4
Cheddar	1 oz	30	5.9
Egg	1 (boiled)	113	2.8
Frankfurter	1	30	5.2
Hamburger patty	1 small	68	5.9
Milk (whole)	1 cup	33	5
Milkshake	10 oz	54	8.2
Pizza (meat)	1 slice (14" diameter)	31	8
Sausage	3 oz	42	8.6

The addition of exercise to your daily routine is another simple way to reduce your CHD risk. Even modest levels of exercise (e.g., 20–30 minutes of walking performed three to five times per week) have been shown to reduce the risk of CHD development due to physical inactivity (1, 8–10). In addition, regular aerobic exercise has been shown to modify other CHD risk factors by positively influencing blood pressure, body composition, and blood cholesterol levels.

MODIFICATION OF CONTRIBUTORY CHD RISK FACTORS

The three contributory CHD risk factors that can be modified are obesity, diabetes, and stress. Body weight loss can be achieved by a combination of diet modification and exercise (Chapter 8). For example, a diet low in calories and fat coupled with an increase in physical activity will help reduce excess body fat. Regular exercise can reduce the risk of developing type II diabetes. Relaxation techniques (discussed in Chapter 10) can help in counteracting the effects of a stressful lifestyle and therefore reduce the risk for development of CHD.

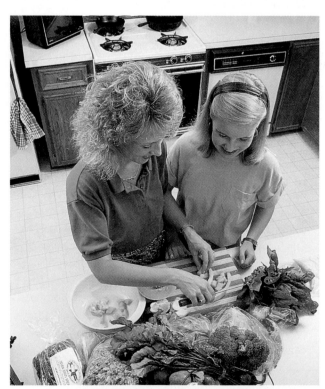

Parents should impress on their children the importance of good dietary habits in preventing cardiovascular disease.

☀ IN SUMMARY

- While heart disease remains the number one killer in the United States, the incidence of heart disease has declined during the past 30 years. This reduction in CHD has occurred because people have modified their behavior to reduce their risk factors for CHD.
- Four major CHD risk factors that can be modified are smoking, hypertension, high blood cholesterol, and inactivity.
- The contributory CHD risk factors that can be modified are obesity, diabetes, and stress.

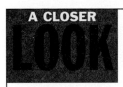

Frequently Asked Questions About Heart Disease, Diet, and Exercise

Question: Can dietary modifications or regular exercise slow the progression of atherosclerosis?

Answer: Several studies have concluded that a diet that is low in saturated fat can retard the development of atherosclerotic plaques in blood vessels, and regular endurance exercise has also been shown to prevent the progression of atherosclerosis. Clearly, then, a lifestyle that includes both regular exercise and a low-fat diet is a good strategy for slowing the buildup of atherosclerotic plaques.

Question: Some physicians are recommending that patients take aspirin daily to reduce the risk of heart attack. How does aspirin provide this benefit?

Answer: A heart attack occurs when part of the heart muscle is damaged by a stoppage of blood flow through arteries that supply that region of the heart. This often occurs when a blood clot forms and blocks an artery that has been narrowed by the buildup of atherosclerotic plaque. Extensive research indicates that daily doses of aspirin (80–325 mg/day) can prevent heart attacks by reducing the likelihood that blood platelets will stick together and precipitate a blood clot.

Despite these benefits, taking daily doses of aspirin is not for everyone (16). Aspirin may be contraindicated for people with bleeding disorders, liver disease, kidney disease, or peptic ulcers, or for individuals who are allergic to aspirin. Therefore, consult your physician before beginning a daily regimen of aspirin.

Question: I've read several newspaper accounts of several cases of sudden cardiac death in young athletes. How great is the risk of sudden cardiac death in young athletes?

Answer: Each year only 10–13 cases of sudden cardiac death are reported in the United States (17). Given that millions of young people participate in regular exercise or sports in the United States, the likelihood that a healthy young person will die from sudden cardiac death is extremely small.

Question: Can a medical exam identify people at risk for sudden cardiac death during exercise?

Answer: Yes. The combination of a medical history and a physical exam by a qualified physician can usually identify individuals with undetected heart disease that would place them at risk of sudden cardiac death during exercise.

⚙ Lowering Your Risk of Coronary Heart Disease: A Final Word

Regardless of your family history of cardiovascular disease, you can reduce your risk of disease by positively modifying your CHD risk factors. The more changes you make to lower your CHD risk, the better your chances are of preventing cardiovascular disease. Be prepared for occasional backsliding (e.g., eating a high-fat meal); however, when this occurs, quickly regain your focus and return to a healthy lifestyle. Proper CHD risk factor management can add both quality and years to your life. Take action today and lower your CHD risk. See A Closer Look above, for answers to some frequently asked questions about heart disease, diet, and exercise.

Summary

1. Heart disease is the number one cause of death in the United States. Almost one of every two deaths in the United States is due to heart disease.

2. Cardiovascular disease refers to any disease that affects the heart and blood vessels. Common cardiovascular diseases include arteriosclerosis, coronary artery disease, stroke, and hypertension.

3. Coronary risk factors are those that increase your risk for the development of coronary heart disease.

4. Coronary risk factors are classified as either major or contributory. Major risk factors are defined as those that directly increase the risk of coronary heart disease. Contributory risk factors may increase your chance of developing coronary heart disease by promoting the development of a major risk factor.

5. Major risk factors for the development of coronary heart disease include smoking, hypertension, high

blood cholesterol, physical inactivity, heredity, gender, and increasing age.

6. Contributory risk factors for the development of coronary heart disease include diabetes, obesity, and stress.

7. Your risk of developing coronary heart disease can be reduced by modification of the following risk factors: smoking, hypertension, high blood pressure, physical inactivity, obesity, and stress.

Study Questions

1. Identify the number one cause of death in the United States.

2. Define the following terms:
   cardiovascular disease
   coronary heart disease
   coronary artery disease
   hypertension

3. List the major and contributory risk factors for the development of coronary heart disease.

4. Discuss the difference between *major* and *contributory* risk factors for the development of coronary heart disease.

5. High-density and low-density lipoproteins have been labeled "good" and "bad" cholesterol, respectively. Explain.

6. Which major coronary heart disease risk factors can be modified?

7. Which contributory coronary heart disease risk factors can be modified?

8. How does a high-salt diet contribute to hypertension?

9. What is the link between diet and blood cholesterol?

10. How does smoking increase your risk of developing cardiovascular disease?

11. How are arteriosclerosis and atherosclerosis related?

Suggested Reading

AHA Dietary Guidelines. Revision 2000: A statement for healthcare professionals from the nutrition committee of the American Heart Association. *Circulation* 102:2284–2299, 2000.

American Heart Association. *Heart and Stroke Facts*. Dallas: American Heart Association, 2000.

Durstine, J. L., and R. Thompson. Exercise modulates blood lipids and exercise plan. *ACSM's Health and Fitness Journal* 4(4):44–46, 2000.

Manore, M. Dietary fat: How much fat do we need? *ACSM's Health and Fitness Journal* 4(1):44–46, 2000.

Peterson, J. A. Take ten: 10 ways to protect your heart. *ACSM's Health and Fitness Journal* 4(2):48, 2000.

Thomas, T., and T. LaFontaine. Exercise, nutritional strategies, and lipoproteins. In *ACSM's Resource Manual for Guidelines for Exercise Testing and Prescription*, 4th ed, J. Roitman, ed. Philadelphia: Lippincott Williams & Wilkins, 2001.

For links to the Web sites below visit Web Links at www.aw.com/fitness and choose Powers/Dodd Web Links from the drop-down menu.

Mayo Clinic Health

Contains wide-ranging information about diet, fitness, and health.

American Medical Association

Contains many sources of information about a wide variety of medical problems, including heart disease.

WebMD

Presents information about a wide variety of diseases and medical problems, including heart disease.

American Heart Association

Contains information about a variety of topics related to both heart disease and stroke.

References

1. American Heart Association. Heart and stroke facts. *Statistical Update*. Dallas: American Heart Association, 2000.

2. Barrow, M. *Heart Talk: Understanding Cardiovascular Diseases*. Gainesville, FL: Cor-Ed Publishing, 1992.

3. American Cancer Society. *Fifty Most Often Asked Questions About Smoking and Health and the Answers*. New York: The American Cancer Society, 1990.

4. American Cancer Society. *1996 Cancer Facts and Figures*. Atlanta: The American Cancer Society, 1993.

5. Pollack, M., and D. Schmidt. *Heart Disease and Rehabilitation*. Champaign, IL: Human Kinetics, 1995.

6. Third report of the National Cholesterol Education Program Expert Panel on Detection, Evaluation, and Treatment of High Blood Cholesterol in Adults. *Journal of the American Medical Association* 285(19):1–19, 2001.

7. Thomas, T., and T. LaFontaine. Exercise, nutritional strategies, and lipoproteins. In *ACSM's Resource Manual for Guidelines for Exercise Testing and Prescription*, 4th ed, J. Roitman, ed. Philadelphia: Lippincott Williams & Wilkins, 2001.

8. Blair, S. N., H. W. Kohl, R. S. Paffenbarger, D. G. Clark, K. H. Cooper, and L. W. Gibbons. Physical fitness and all-cause mortality: A prospective study of healthy men and women. *Journal of the American Medical Association* 262: 2395–2401, 1989.

9. Bouchard, C., R. Shephard, T. Stephens, J. Sutton, and B. McPherson. *Exercise, Fitness, and Health: A Consensus of Current Knowledge.* Champaign, IL: Human Kinetics, 1990.

10. Paffenbarger, R. S., R. T. Hyde, A. L. Wing, and C. C. Hsieh. Physical activity, all-cause mortality of college alumni. *New England Journal of Medicine* 314:605–613, 1986.

11. Kohl, H. Physical activity and cardiovascular disease: Evidence for a dose-response. *Medicine and Science in Sports and Exercise* 33(Suppl.):S472–S483, 2001.

12. Wood, P. Physical activity, diet, and health: Independent and interactive effects. *Medicine and Science in Sports and Exercise* 26:838–843, 1994.

13. Durstine, J., and W. Haskell. Effects of training on plasma lipids and lipoproteins. *Exercise and Sport Science Reviews* 22:477–521, 1994.

14. Durstine, J. L., and R. Thompson. Exercise modulates blood lipids and exercise plan. *ACSM's Health and Fitness Journal* 4(4):44–46, 2000.

15. Leeds, M. *Nutrition for Healthy Living.* Boston: WCB-McGraw-Hill, 1998.

16. American Heart Association. *Aspirin and Your Health.* Dallas: American Heart Association, 2000.

17. Rowland, T. Screening for risk of cardiac death in young athletes. *Sports Science Exchange* 12(3):1–5, 1999.

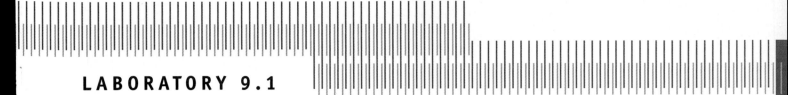

Assessment of Your Risk of Heart Disease

NAME _____ DATE _____

The following RISKO questionnaires were developed by the American Heart Association as a tool for evaluating your risk of developing coronary heart disease. RISKO scores are based on four of the most important modifiable factors that contribute to the development of heart disease: weight (obesity), hypertension, blood cholesterol levels, and smoking.

The RISKO score you compute for yourself estimates your risk of developing coronary heart disease over the next several years. Note that the RISKO heart appraisal is not a substitute for a thorough medical examination. Rather, it is designed to increase your awareness of heart disease risk and to assist you in reducing your risk.

DIRECTIONS

The purpose of this lab is to give you an estimate of your chances of suffering a heart attack.

RULES

Choose the table appropriate for your sex and then determine your score for each of the four risk factors. Enter your score for each factor. Total the four scores and enter the figure at the bottom of the table. This total—your score—will enable you to estimate your risk.

TO CALCULATE CHOLESTEROL

A cholesterol blood level is best. If you can't get one from your doctor, then estimate your total cholesterol as 200 (mg/100 ml) and your HDL as 40 (mg/100 ml).

TO CALCULATE BLOOD PRESSURE

If you have no recent reading but have passed an insurance or industrial examination, chances are you are 140 or less.

WHAT YOUR SCORE MEANS

Note: If you're diabetic, you have a greater risk of heart disease. Add 7 points to your total score.

0–2	You have a low risk of heart disease for a person of your age and sex.
3–4	You have a low-to-moderate risk of heart disease for a person of your age and sex. That's good, but there's room for improvement.
5–7	You have a moderate-to-high risk of heart disease for a person of your age and sex. There's considerable room for improvement in some areas.
8–15	You have a high risk of developing heart disease for a person of your age and sex. There's lots of room for improvement in all areas.
16 & Over	You have a very high risk of developing heart disease for a person of your age and sex. You should act now to reduce all your risk factors.

(Source: Reproduced with permission from RISKO, A Heart Health Appraisal, 1994. Copyright American Heart Association.)

(continued on next page)

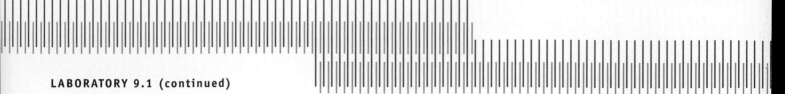

RISKO FOR WOMEN

NAME _____ DATE _____

1. *Systolic Blood Pressure*
If you **are not** taking anti-hypertensive
medications and your blood pressure is . . .

SCORE ☐

125 or less	0 points
between 126 and 136	2 points
between 137 and 148	4 points
between 149 and 160	6 points
between 161 and 171	8 points
between 172 and 183	10 points
between 184 and 194	12 points
between 195 and 206	14 points
between 207 and 218	16 points

If you **are** taking anti-hypertensive medications and your blood pressure is . . .

117 or less	0 points
between 118 and 123	2 points
between 124 and 129	4 points
between 130 and 136	6 points
between 137 and 144	8 points
between 145 and 154	10 points
between 155 and 168	12 points
between 169 and 206	14 points
between 207 and 218	16 points

2. *Blood Cholesterol*
Locate the number of points for your total
and HDL cholesterol in the table below.

SCORE ☐

HDL

		25	30	35	40	50	60	70	80
	140	2	1	0	0	0	0	0	0
	160	3	2	1	0	0	0	0	0
	180	4	3	2	1	0	0	0	0
	200	4	3	2	2	0	0	0	0
	220	5	4	3	2	1	0	0	0
Total	240	5	4	3	3	1	0	0	0
	260	5	4	4	3	2	1	0	0
	280	5	5	4	4	2	1	0	0
	300	6	5	4	4	3	2	1	0
	340	6	5	5	4	3	2	1	0
	4000	6	6	5	5	4	3	2	2

3. *Cigarette Smoking*

SCORE ☐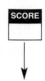

If you . . .	
do not smoke	0 points
smoke less than a pack a day	2 points
smoke a pack a day	5 points
smoke two or more packs a day	9 points

4. *Weight*
Locate your weight category in the table
below.
If you are in . . .

SCORE ☐

weight category A	0 points
weight category B	1 point
weight category C	2 points
weight category D	9 points

FT	IN	A	B	C	D
4	8	up to 139	140–161	162–184	185+
4	9	up to 140	141–162	163–185	186+
4	10	up to 141	142–163	164–187	188+
4	11	up to 143	144–166	167–190	191+
5	0	up to 145	146–168	169–193	194+
5	1	up to 147	148–171	172–196	197+
5	2	up to 149	150–173	174–198	199+
5	3	up to 152	153–176	177–201	202+
5	4	up to 154	155–178	179–204	205+
5	5	up to 157	158–182	183–209	210+
5	6	up to 160	161–186	187–213	214+
5	7	up to 165	166–191	192–219	220+
5	8	up to 169	170–196	197–225	226+
5	9	up to 173	174–201	202–231	232+
5	10	up to 178	179–206	207–238	239+
5	11	up to 182	183–212	213–242	243+
6	0	up to 187	188–217	218–248	249+
6	1	up to 191	192–222	223–254	255+

TOTAL SCORE ☐

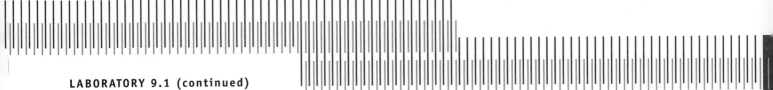

RISKO FOR MEN

NAME _____ DATE _____

1. *Systolic Blood Pressure*

SCORE ☐

If you **are not** taking anti-hypertensive medications and your blood pressure is . . .

124 or less	0 points
between 125 and 134	2 points
between 135 and 144	4 points
between 145 and 154	6 points
between 155 and 164	8 points
between 165 and 174	10 points
between 175 and 184	12 points
between 185 and 194	14 points
between 195 and 204	16 points
between 205 and 214	18 points
between 215 and 224	20 points

If you **are** taking anti-hypertensive medications and your blood pressure is . . .

120 or less	0 points
between 121 and 127	2 points
between 128 and 135	4 points
between 136 and 143	6 points
between 144 and 153	8 points
between 154 and 163	10 points
between 164 and 175	12 points
between 176 and 190	14 points
between 191 and 204	16 points
between 205 and 214	18 points
between 215 and 224	20 points

2. *Blood Cholesterol*

SCORE ☐

Locate the number of points for your total and HDL cholesterol in the table below.

			HDL					
	25	30	35	40	50	60	70	80
140	4	2	0	0	0	0	0	0
160	5	3	2	0	0	0	0	0
180	6	4	3	1	0	0	0	0
200	7	5	4	3	0	0	0	0
220	7	6	5	4	1	0	0	0
Total 240	8	7	5	4	2	0	0	0
260	8	7	6	5	3	1	0	0
280	9	8	7	6	4	2	0	0
300	9	8	7	6	4	3	1	0
340	9	9	8	7	6	4	2	1
400	10	9	9	8	7	5	4	3

3. *Cigarette Smoking*

SCORE ☐

If you . . .

do no smoke	0 points
smoke less than a pack a day	2 points
smoke a pack a day	5 points
smoke two or more packs a day	9 points

4. *Weight*

SCORE ☐

Locate your weight category in the table below. If you are in . . .

weight category A	0 points
weight category B	1 point
weight category C	2 points

FT	IN	A	B	C
5	1	up to 162	163–250	251+
5	2	up to 167	168–257	258+
5	3	up to 172	173–264	265+
5	4	up to 176	177–272	273+
5	5	up to 181	182–279	280+
5	6	up to 185	186–286	287+
5	7	up to 190	191–293	294+
5	8	up to 195	196–300	301+
5	9	up to 199	200–307	308+
5	10	up to 204	205–315	316+
5	11	up to 209	210–322	323+
6	0	up to 213	214–329	330+
6	1	up to 218	219–336	337+
6	2	up to 223	224–343	344+
6	3	up to 227	228–350	351+
6	4	up to 232	233–368	369+
6	5	up to 238	239–365	366+
6	6	up to 241	242–372	373+

TOTAL SCORE ☐

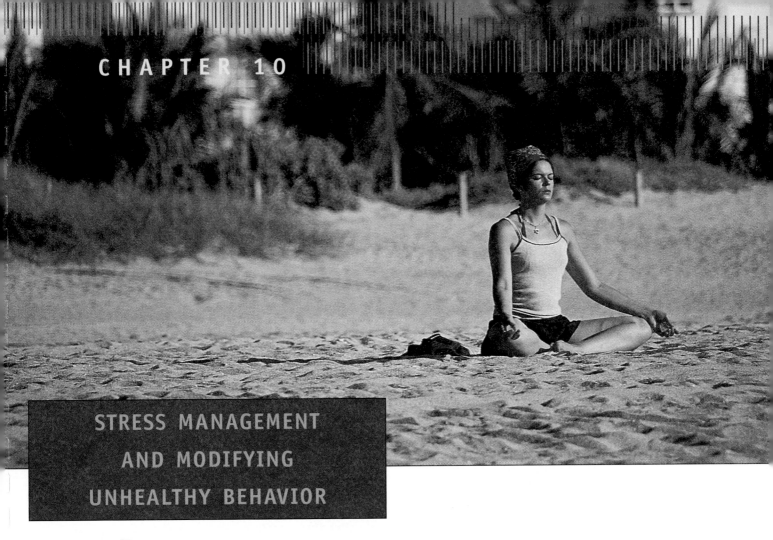

CHAPTER 10

STRESS MANAGEMENT AND MODIFYING UNHEALTHY BEHAVIOR

After studying this chapter, you should be able to:

1. Discuss the terms *stress* and *stressors*.

2. Outline the steps involved in stress management.

3. List several common relaxation techniques used to manage stress.

4. Outline the general model for behavior modification.

5. Provide an example of how behavior modification can be used to modify unhealthy behavior.

6. Identify the most common types of accidents.

7. Outline steps to reduce your risk of accidents.

Although many behaviors affect your health, the five that are most important for promotion of good health (1–4) are regular exercise, good nutrition, weight control, stress management, and modification of unhealthful behaviors that increase your risk of getting a disease or having an accident. Earlier chapters have focused on improving health through physical fitness, proper diet/weight control, and actively reducing the risk of cancer and heart disease. This chapter expands on these strategies by introducing the concepts of stress reduction and behavior modification aimed at reducing your risk of disease and accidents. Let's begin our discussion with an overview of stress management.

☼ Stress Management

Studies suggest that 10–15% of U.S. adults may be functioning at less than optimal levels because of stress-related anxiety and depression (4). Indeed, millions of people take medication for stress-related illnesses. Stress-related problems result in annual losses of billions of dollars to both businesses and government due to employee absenteeism and health care costs. Therefore, stress is a major health problem in the United States that affects individual lives and the economy as a whole. In the following sections we discuss several key aspects of stress management.

STRESS: AN OVERVIEW

Stress is a physiological and mental response to things in our environment that cause us to become uncomfortable. Any factor that produces stress is called a **stressor.**

Stressors can be physical in nature (such as an injury) or mental (such as emotional distress resulting from a personal relationship). Regardless of the nature of the stressor, the physiological and mental responses to stress usually include the feelings of strain, tension, and anxiety.

There are many sources of stress in everyday life. Driving in heavy traffic, being involved in an automobile accident, encountering emotional conflicts at work or school, and experiencing personal financial problems are just a few. Let's continue our discussion of stress by examining the link between stress and disease.

STRESS AND DISEASE

From a medical standpoint, stress can affect both emotional and physical health. Chronic (persistent) stress has been linked to elevated blood pressure, heart disease, hormonal imbalances, reduced resistance to disease, and emotional disorders (1–4) (Figure 10.1). The biologist Hans Selye was one of the first scientists to develop a scientific theory to explain the relationship between stress and disease. Selye proposed that humans adapt to stress in a response he termed the **general adaptation syndrome,** which involves three stages: an alarm stage, a resistance stage, and an exhaustion stage (5).

In the *alarm stage,* the body responds to stress by activating the sympathetic nervous system. This activation prompts many physiological changes, including the release of stress hormones (e.g., epinephrine, norepinephrine, and cortisol), increased muscle tension, and elevations in heart rate and blood pressure (5). During the alarm stage, an individual often experiences anxiety, headaches, and disrupted eating and sleeping

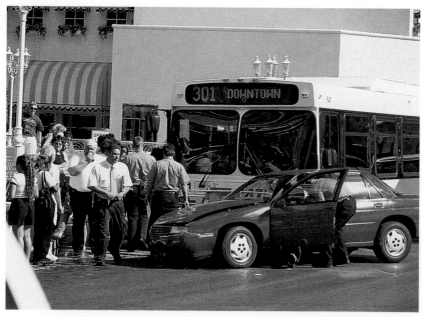

Automobile accidents are one of the many causes of stress in our society.

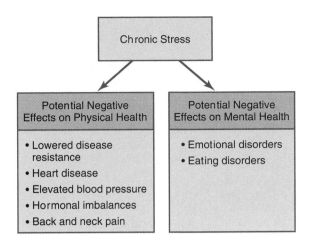

FIGURE 10.1
The health effects of chronic stress.

patterns, and the body becomes more susceptible to disease and more prone to accident.

With continued exposure to stress, the individual reaches the *resistance stage,* during which the body opposes the stress by activating mechanisms that resist disease effectively. In short, the resistance stage represents an improved ability to cope with stress (5).

If the stress persists, however, the individual reaches the *exhaustion stage.* Selye suggested that in this stage the body becomes very vulnerable to disease because it loses the ability to respond to stress due to the depletion of its resources. Note that "exhaustion" in this sense is not the fatigue associated with the conclusion of a hard exercise session or the end of a long day, but instead a life-threatening type of physical and psychological depletion that occurs after days or weeks of exposure to constant stress.

Although Selye's model of adaptation to stress is still viewed as an important contribution to our understanding of the response to stress, many newer research findings discount some aspects of the model. For example, it is no longer thought that the increase susceptibility to disease in the exhaustion stage is due to the body's *failure* to respond to stress; instead, current evidence indicates that the underlying cause of many stress-related diseases *is* the body's prolonged response to stress. Research into the relationships among the nervous system, the endocrine system (which produces hormones), and the immune system (which protects against disease) has shown that prolonged exposure to stress results in a continual release of stress hormones, including cortisol. High levels of cortisol in the blood impair the immune system's ability to fight infections, which increases the risk of contracting disease (6–8).

As previously mentioned, prolonged stress not only increases the chances of infection, but also increases

the risk for many other problems,. As a result, knowledge of stress management skills is an important tool in preventing stress-related conditions. Before we discuss stress management skills, let's begin with a discussion of how to assess your own level of stress.

ASSESSMENT OF STRESS

Stressors can be acute (such as the death of a loved one), cumulative (such as a series of events leading to a divorce), or chronic (such as daily job-related pressures). Although it is clear that chronic or extreme stress is unhealthy, some degree of stress is required to maximize performance. For instance, athletes and business professionals often perform better when faced with mild-to-moderate stress. A stress level that results in improved performance is called **eustress** or positive stress. Although some level of stress is desirable, each of us has a breaking point in terms of stress. This idea is illustrated in Figure 10.2. When we surpass the stress level needed to optimize performance (optimal stress), we reach our stress "break point," and distress (negative stress) results. Distress promotes a decline in performance, and chronic distress can increase the risk of disease.

Different people may react differently to the same stressful situation. For example, a violent movie may evoke anger in one person and no emotion at all in another. This difference in "stress perception" is due to personality differences. When it comes to stress, individuals can be classified into one of three personality categories: type A, type B, and type C (Figure 10.3). Type A individuals are highly motivated, time-conscious, hard driving, impatient, and sometimes hostile. They have a heightened response to stress. Because stress is a risk factor for heart disease, type A people exhibit this risk (4). In contrast, type B individuals are easygoing, non-aggressive, and patient. Type B personalities do not generally respond greatly to stress and are considered to be at low risk (from a stress perspective) for heart disease. People with type C personalities have many of the qualities of type A people. They are confident, highly motivated, and competitive. However, these unique individuals use their personality traits to their advantage by

---

stress   A physiological and mental response to something in the environment that causes people to become uncomfortable.
stressor   A factor that produces stress.
general adaptation syndrome   A pattern of responses to stress that consists of an alarm stage, a resistance stage, and an exhaustion stage.
eustress   A stress level that results in improved performance.

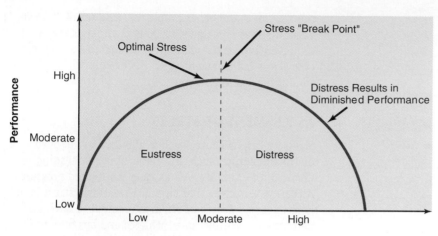

FIGURE 10.2
The concepts of eustress and distress.

maintaining a constant level of emotional control and channeling their ambition into creative directions. Interestingly, although type C personalities are highly driven, they experience the same low stress-related risk for heart disease as type B personalities.

The first step in learning to deal with stress is to examine your stress level. The most convenient way to do this is to complete a questionnaire designed to evaluate your stress level. Laboratory 10.1 on page 255 is designed to accomplish this goal. If the results suggest that you are under stress, you should begin implementing stress reduction techniques.

☼ IN SUMMARY

* Stress is a physiological and mental response to things in our environment (stressors) that cause us to be uncomfortable.
* Studies suggest that 10–15% of U.S. adults may be functioning at below optimal levels due to stress-related anxiety and/or depression.
* Hans Selye proposed that the body reacts to stress in a pattern of responses termed the general adap-

tation syndrome, which includes alarm, resistance, and exhaustion stages.
* Although chronic and/or extreme stress is unhealthy, some degree of stress is required to maximize performance. A stress level that results in improved performance is called eustress.

STEPS IN STRESS MANAGEMENT

Now that you have identified your stress level, it is time to deal with stress by using techniques known collectively as "stress management." Although there are no magic formulas or nutritional supplements capable of eliminating stress, there are two general steps to managing stress (4, 9): Reduce the amount of stress in your life, and learn to cope with stress by improving your ability to relax. Let's discuss each of these steps individually.

STRESS REDUCTION   Reducing sources of stress is the ideal means of lowering the impact of stress on your life. The first step in stress reduction is to recognize

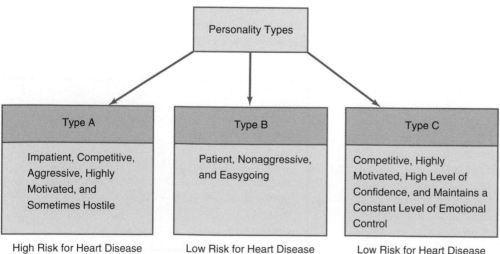

FIGURE 10.3
Personality types and their risks for heart disease.

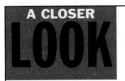

A CLOSER LOOK

Time Management Guidelines

Use the following guidelines to improve your time management skills and increase your productivity:

Establish goals. Establish a list of goals that you hope to accomplish. Identify your immediate and long-term goals, and rank your goals according to priority. By establishing goals and prioritizing them, you can focus your efforts on those projects that are the most important to you.

Use a daily planner. Plan your day by using a daily planner. Chart your daily schedule, hour by hour, and place priority on your most important goals.

Evaluate your time management skills regularly. At the completion of your day, take 5 to 10 minutes to evaluate your time management. Note the time that was wasted and make

plans to correct these mistakes for the following day.

Learn to say "no" to those activities that prevent you from achieving your goals. Before you accept a new responsibility, complete your current task or eliminate an unnecessary project. Although saying "no" is often difficult, it is critical in proper time management.

Delegate responsibility. Most of us like to feel in control, and this makes delegation of responsibilities to others difficult. Nonetheless, if you become overloaded when working on a group project, don't be afraid to ask for assistance. Delegating responsibility to others is an easy way to reduce your work load and lower stress.

Eliminate distractions. Interruptions and distractions can rob precious time from your day. Identify those factors that distract you and eliminate them if possible.

Schedule time for you. Find time each day to relax and do something you enjoy. Remember that taking an occasional break from your work is not wasting time and will improve your overall productivity by helping to energize yourself.

Reward yourself when you complete a goal. One of the simple pleasures in life is to reward yourself after you complete a goal. The reward can come in many forms: a new pair of shoes, a movie, a few days of relaxation, and so on. The importance of rewarding yourself cannot be overemphasized. People perform better when rewarded for a job well done, and a reward is an excellent means of providing encouragement (even for yourself) for future good work.

those factors that promote daily stress. After identifying these factors, you should eliminate activities that result in daily stress. While it may not be possible to avoid all sources of stress, many "unnecessary" forms of stress can be eliminated.

A classic example of stress that can often be avoided is overcommitment, a frequent cause of stress in college students. Plan your time carefully and prioritize your activities. It may not be possible to do everything that you want to do during a given day or week. Plan a daily schedule that allows you to do the things you need to accomplish without being overwhelmed with less important activities. A Closer Look above discusses the key elements of time management.

COPING WITH STRESS: RELAXATION TECHNIQUES

Because it is impossible to eliminate all forms of stress from daily life, it is necessary to use stress management techniques to reduce the potentially harmful effects of stress. Most of these techniques are designed to produce relaxation, which reduces the stress level. The following are some of the more common approaches used in stress management.

Progressive relaxation. Progressive relaxation is a stress reduction technique for reducing muscular ten-

sion using exercises designed to promote relaxation. In essence, the technique is practiced as follows. While sitting quietly or lying down, contract and then relax various muscle groups one at a time, beginning with your feet and then moving up the body to the hands and neck, until a complete state of muscle relaxation is achieved. The details of this technique are outlined in A Closer Look, page 246.

The proponents of progressive relaxation techniques for reducing stress argue that relaxing the muscles in this manner will also relax the mind and therefore relieve stress. The theory behind this concept is that an anxious (stressed) mind cannot exist in a relaxed body.

Breathing exercises. A simple way of achieving relaxation is by performing **breathing exercises.** A sample breathing exercise designed to reduce stress is performed as follows (4):

1. Assume a comfortable position, sitting or lying down, with eyes closed.

breathing exercises   A simple way of achieving relaxation.

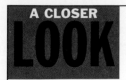

A CLOSER LOOK

Progressive Relaxation Training

There are many types of progressive relaxation training methods, and over 200 different exercises have been described. In essence, the technique involves contracting and relaxing muscle groups, starting in your lower body and moving toward your upper body. The following technique is one of the many forms that is easy to learn and use (4):

1. The first step is to assume a relaxed position (either sitting or lying down). Extend your legs, put your arms at your sides, and close your eyes. Let your muscles relax and your body go limp.

2. Take a few slow, deep breaths and concentrate on relaxing muscular tension.

3. Contract the following muscle groups in the order they are presented. For each muscle group, contract the muscle as hard as possible for 5 seconds. Release the contraction and take a deep breath. Repeat this procedure two

or more times until the muscle group is relaxed. Try to limit your contraction to the isolated body parts described here:

a. Curl the toes on your right foot. Repeat this action with your left foot.

b. Bend your right foot toward your head as far as possible. Repeat this action with your left foot.

c. Extend your right foot downward (point your toes) as far as possible. Repeat this action with your left foot.

d. Contract your upper leg (thigh). Repeat this action with your left leg.

e. Contract your stomach muscles by attempting to curl your upper body (like a sit-up without performing the sit-up).

f. Contract your shoulders by moving your shoulders as far forward as possible (keep your head and arms in place).

g. Contract your shoulders by moving your shoulders as far backward as possible (keep your head and arms in place).

h. Spread the fingers on your right hand as far as possible. Repeat this action with the left hand.

i. Contract the muscles in your forearm by making a fist with your right hand. Repeat this action with your left hand.

j. Contract the muscles in the front of your neck by bringing your head forward (chin to chest) as far as possible.

k. Contract the muscles in the back of your neck by moving your head backward (push your head toward your back).

l. Open your mouth as wide as possible.

m. Wrinkle your forehead.

With practice, you will improve your ability to isolate the muscle groups described, and your ability to relax using this technique will also improve. As you become more comfortable with progressive relaxation, feel free to incorporate your own exercises into this routine.

---

2. Begin inhaling and exhaling slowly. Count from one to three during each inhalation and each exhalation to maintain a slow and regular breathing pattern.

3. Now combine stretching and breathing to provide greater relaxation and stress reduction. For example, stretch your arms toward the ceiling as you inhale, then lower your arms during exhalation.

Try this exercise for 5 to 15 minutes in a quiet room. Although breathing exercises may not reduce all stress, they have been shown to be a simple means of stress reduction.

Rest and sleep. One of the most effective means of reducing stress and tension is to get an adequate amount of rest and sleep. How much sleep do you need? It appears that individual needs vary greatly; however, a good rule of thumb is 7 to 9 hours of restful sleep per night (A Closer Look, page 248). Further, because of the body's natural hormonal rhythms, it is rec-

ommended that you go to bed at approximately the same time every night.

In addition to a good night's sleep, 15 to 30 minutes of rest per day is useful in stress reduction. This can be achieved as simply as putting your feet up on a desk or table and closing your eyes. A well-rested body is the best protection against stress and fatigue.

Exercise. Although prolonged or high-intensity exercise can impose both mental and physical stress, research has shown that light-to-moderate exercise can reduce many types of stress. The recommended types of exercise for optimal stress reduction are low- to moderate-intensity aerobic exercises such as running, swimming, and cycling. The guidelines for this type of exercise prescription are presented in Chapter 4. Other popular types of exercise for reducing stress and achieving relaxation are yoga, tai-chi, and Pilates. Many gyms and health clubs offer classes in these forms of exercise.

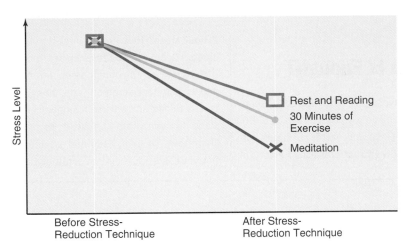

FIGURE 10.4
The effects of exercise and other activities on stress reduction.

How good is exercise at reducing stress? Studies have shown that exercise is a very effective form of stress reduction (10–12). Figure 10.4 compares the effects of a 30-minute session of light-to-moderate exercise (running) to three other common forms of stress reduction: rest, reading, and meditation. In this study, meditation provided the greatest stress reduction, with exercise finishing a close second (12).

Why does regular exercise reduce stress? Several possibilities exist. One theory is that exercise causes the brain to release several naturally produced tranquilizers, called *endorphins,* which reduce stress levels (13). Endorphins work by blocking the effects of stress-related chemicals in the brain. Another theory is that exercise may be a diversion that frees your mind from worry or other stressful thoughts. Another possibility is that regular exercise results in an improvement in physical fitness and self-image, which increases your resistance to stress. A final possibility is that all of these factors may be involved in the beneficial effects of exercise on stress management. The next time you feel stressed, try exercising; you will feel and look better as a result.

Meditation. Meditation has been practiced for ages in an effort to produce relaxation and achieve inner peace. There are many types of meditation, and there is no scientific evidence that one form is superior to another. Most types of meditation have the same common elements: sitting quietly for 15 to 20 minutes twice a day, concentrating on a single word or image, and breathing slowly and regularly. The goal of meditation is to reduce stress by achieving a complete state of physical and mental relaxation. Although beginning a successful program of meditation may require initial instruction from an experienced individual, the following is a brief overview of how meditation is practiced (4):

1. First, you must choose a word or sound, called a *mantra,* to be repeated during the meditation. The idea of using a mantra is that this word or sound should become your symbol of complete relaxation. Choose a mantra that has little emotional significance for you, such as the word *red.*

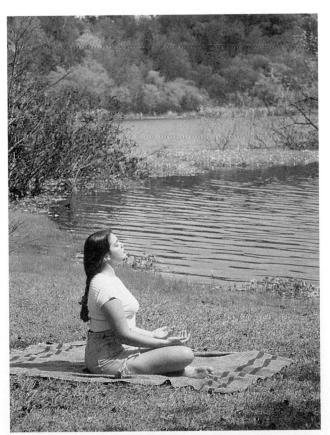

Assuming a relaxed position is important in progressive relaxation techniques.

meditation   A method of relaxation that has been practiced for ages in an effort to produce relaxation and achieve inner peace. No scientific evidence indicates that one form of meditation is superior to another.

2. To begin meditation, find a quiet area and sit comfortably with your eyes closed. Take several deep breaths and concentrate on relaxation; let your body go limp.

3. Concentrate on your mantra. This means that you should not hear or think about anything but your mantra. Repeat your mantra over and over again in your mind and relax. Avoid distracting thoughts and focus only on the mantra.

4. After 15 to 20 minutes of concentration on the mantra, open your eyes and begin to move your thoughts away from the mantra. End the session by making a fist with both hands and saying to yourself that you are alert and refreshed.

Visualization. Visualization (sometimes called imagery) uses mental pictures to reduce stress. The idea is to create an appealing mental image (such as a quiet mountain setting) that promotes relaxation and reduces stress. Visualization is similar to meditation except that instead of using a mantra, you substitute a relaxing scene.

To practice visualization, simply follow the instructions presented for meditation, substituting your relaxing scene for the mantra. If you fail to reach a complete state of relaxation after your first several sessions, don't be discouraged. Achieving complete relaxation with this technique may require numerous practice sessions.

In summary, there are many ways to successfully manage stress. The key is to find the technique that is best for you and stick with it. Regular exercise may be the only type of stress management you require. However, if exercise alone is not sufficient, try one of the other forms of stress management as well. Remember, regardless of your personality type or your lifestyle, you can successfully manage stress by applying one or more of the previously discussed techniques.

---

visualization A relaxation technique that uses appealing mental images to promote relaxation and reduce stress; also called *imagery*.

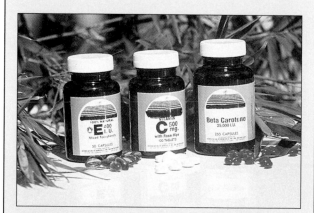
STRESS MANAGEMENT: CLOSING REMARKS

If you are one of the millions of Americans who suffer from one or more stress-related disorders, the first step in preventing or treating stress-related problems is

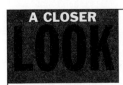

A Few Questions About Stress Management Issues

Question: How can anger best be managed to reduce stress?

Answer: The evidence suggests that anger, which is a normal human response to a perceived threat, can be controlled effectively by a variety of healthy methods (1–3). One approach is to suppress your anger by thinking about other things, and thinking peaceful thoughts can be especially calming. Perhaps even better is expressing your anger is a calm but assertive way, because simply talking about upsetting issues is often a good approach to controlling your anger and resolving conflict.

Question: What role does social support play in managing stress?

Answer: Having social support can be a very important factor in stress management. Research indicates that people with a strong social support network—that is, lots of friends—experience less distress during life's ups and downs than people who are more socially isolated (15). So taking the time to build a strong social network solidified by strong personal relationships is a great way to help you cope with life's many stresses.

---

recognizing that a problem exists. The way to begin is to assess your level of stress using an appropriate stress identification questionnaire such as the one in Laboratory 10.1 on page 255. Then, the next step is to select a stress management technique that is right for you—one that you enjoy, and, perhaps most importantly, one that you will practice regularly. For the answers to some questions about stress management, see A Closer Look above.

☼ IN SUMMARY

- The two general steps involved in stress management are reducing the sources of stress and using relaxation techniques to help you learn to cope with stress.
- The ideal way to lessen the effects of stress on your life is to reduce the sources of stress.
- Among the many relaxation techniques that can help you cope with stress are progressive relaxation, breathing exercises, getting more rest and sleep, exercise, meditation, and visualization.

☼ Modifying Unhealthy Behavior

A healthy lifestyle is achieved by eliminating unhealthful behavior; this requires behavior modification. Behavior modification is the process of changing an undesirable behavior to a more desirable behavior. In the next two sections we discuss behavior modification and provide specific examples of how unhealthful behavior can be eliminated.

MODEL FOR CHANGING BEHAVIOR

The general plan for modifying behavior is similar for all types of behavior modification (Table 10.1). A logical starting point in eliminating unhealthful behavior

is to analyze your current behavior and identify problem areas. Laboratory 10.1 on page 255 is designed to assist you.

The desire to change is the key point in any behavior modification plan. Without a genuine desire to make lifestyle changes, any behavior modification plan is doomed to fail.

After identifying the problem and establishing a desire to change a specific behavior, the next move is to analyze the history of the problem. The objective here is to learn what factors contribute to the development of the behavior to be modified. Learning the cause is useful when developing a strategy for change.

The next two steps in the behavior modification plan (steps 4 and 5 in Table 10.1) are the development

TABLE 10.1
General Steps in Behavior Modification

Step No.	Action
1	Identify the problem.
2	Desire change.
3	Analyze the past and current history of the problem.
4	Establish short-term written goals.
5	Establish long-term written goals.
6	Sign a contract (with friends).
7	Develop a strategy for change.
8	Implement the strategy and learn new coping skills to deal with the problem.
9	Evaluate your progress in making behavioral changes. Provide friends with progress reports.
10	Plan a long-term strategy for maintaining behavior changes.

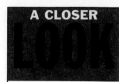

A CLOSER LOOK

Causes of Smoking Behavior

Before beginning a smoking cessation effort, it is useful to ask the question, "Why do I smoke?" Three explanations have been proposed to explain smoking behavior:

1. social learning theory
2. nicotine addiction theory
3. opponent process theory

The social learning theory of smoking argues that smokers develop the habit of smoking from peers and continue the habit be-cause of social reinforcement. Positive support from friends who smoke and the social interaction that centers around smoking make this habit difficult to break.

A second potential explanation for smoking behavior is that the smoker develops an addiction to nicotine. The evidence for this theory comes from smokers themselves, who attest to the sensation of a "smoker's high" and report that smoking cessation often leaves them with with-drawal symptoms and a physical craving for nicotine.

The theory of the *opponent process* argues that smoking results from two opposing processes, one pleasant and one unpleasant. Social reinforcement and the "smoker's high" interact to cause a pleasant emotion, whereas attempts to stop smoking result in unpleasant withdrawal symptoms that can be eliminated by smoking. Therefore, the pleasant sensation of smoking and the unpleasant sensation of not smoking combine to encourage regular smoking behavior.

---

of both short- and long-term goals for behavior change. Short-term goals establish the need for a rapid change in behavior. Long-term goals provide the incentive required to maintain behavior changes. The importance of goal setting in behavior modification cannot be overemphasized. A behavior modification plan without goals is like a race without a finish line.

The sixth stage in the behavior modification plan is to sign a behavior modification contract in the presence of friends (Laboratory 10.2). The purpose of signing a formal contract is to confirm in writing your commitment to a behavior change. Having friends present during the signing of the contract is important. They provide moral support and encouragement during the difficult early periods of behavior change.

The final four steps (steps 7–10) incorporate the development of a strategy for behavior change, the learning of new coping skills, evaluation of your progress, and the planning of long-term maintenance for behavior change.

Many people who have had previous difficulty in changing behavior develop the attitude that some bad habits cannot be changed. This is not true! Unhealthful behaviors are learned; therefore, they can be unlearned.

SPECIFIC BEHAVIOR MODIFICATION GOALS

Let's fill in the details of our behavior modification model by illustrating how these plans can be applied specifically to smoking cessation and weight loss.

SMOKING CESSATION As previously mentioned, cigarette smoking is a serious health risk that increases the risk of cancer and heart disease. Research shows that smoking is the largest avoidable cause of death in the United States (16). Although millions of people have quit smoking, the number of smokers has increased since the late 1960s because of an increase in young smokers, particularly young women.

The first step in smoking cessation is having the desire to stop. After expressing this desire and analyzing smoking behavior (A Closer Look, above), each individual can develop a three-phase plan to stop smoking that incorporates steps 4 through 10 of the general steps of the behavior modification model. Phase one is often termed the *preparation phase*. In this phase, smokers develop the confidence to stop smoking by establishing both short-term and long-term goals, signing a written contract, and developing a plan to stop smoking.

The second phase of smoking cessation is commonly termed *cessation*. On the cessation date established in the *stop smoking contract,* the individual stops smoking. Quitting smoking "cold turkey" has been shown to be more effective than a gradual slowdown (2). After a smoking cessation program has begun, it is important that the individual get strong peer support, especially during the first few days and weeks.

The final phase of smoking cessation is termed the *maintenance phase*. The obvious objective of the maintenance phase is to ensure that the individual does not start smoking again. Several strategies can assist in this process. Continued peer and family support for the individual's decision to stop smoking is critical, and its importance cannot be overemphasized. A second strategy is to avoid social circumstances that accept or encourage smoking. For example, if going to a bar encourages smoking, then the individual should avoid bars.

Finally, self-education about the health hazards of smoking provides a continual incentive to maintain a smokeless life.

WEIGHT CONTROL   In Chapter 8 we discussed the general principles of losing weight. Unfortunately, losing weight and maintaining weight loss are difficult for many people. Clearly, the application of behavior modification principles is essential in the weight loss process. Although no single weight loss program works for all people, the following eight components are common ingredients of most successful efforts:

1. The individual desires to lose weight.
2. The program begins with a 2-week dietary diary that includes the kind and amount of food eaten and the environmental and social circumstances involved.
3. Short- and long-term weight loss goals are established.
4. The individual signs a weight loss contract with friends.
5. The new dietary plan includes a balanced diet that results in a negative caloric balance and a fat deficit so that a loss of fat will result. Further, the addition of a regular exercise program is a key factor in any successful weight loss plan. (See Chapter 8 for details.)
6. New coping skills for overeating include avoiding those environments or social settings (such as parties) that promote it.
7. The individual evaluates weight loss progress on a weekly basis and gets positive feedback from a support group (such as a spouse, friends, or relatives).
8. After establishing weight loss goals, the individual makes a plan for long-term behavioral changes that maintain the desired weight.

In summary, weight control is a specific application of general behavior modification principles. Indeed, these eight components incorporate most of the general behavior modification principles outlined in Table 10.1. Remember: the key elements in a weight control program are the desire to lose weight, establishment of goals, development of a plan, and positive feedback from peer/family support.

ACCIDENT PREVENTION

In the United States, accidents are the number one killer of people under the age of 35, and they account for 50% of all childhood deaths (1, 2). Although accidents come in many forms, the most common types are automobile accidents, falls, poisonings, drownings, and fires. While most accidents may seem to be a matter of chance, this is not the case! By using behavior modification, you can reduce your risk of accident by gaining control over many risk factors. Let's examine the most common risk factors for accidents.

RISK FACTORS FOR ACCIDENTS   One of the most important accident risk factors is an unsafe attitude, which promotes risk-taking behaviors. For example, people who are overly confident in their driving skills may speed on a winding or wet road and increase their chances of having an automobile accident. Similarly, people who are overconfident in their job skills may take unnecessary risks at work.

Some people crave excitement or the sensation of danger (2). This type of thrill-seeking attitude increases the risk of accidents. These people often engage in high-risk physical activities such as skydiving, auto racing, or rock climbing, which increase their risk of injury due to accidents.

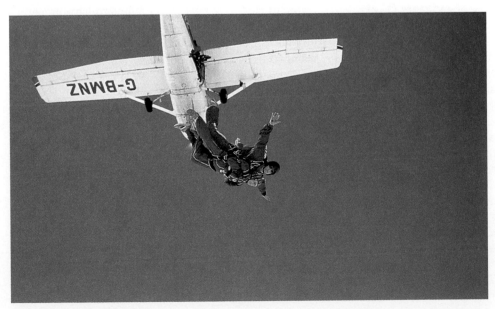

Skydiving is a high-risk activity.

TABLE 10.2
Reducing Your Risk of Injury

Bicycle or motorcycle accidents

- Always wear a helmet and use reflectors and protective clothing when riding.
- Ride with the traffic.
- Obey the rules of the road (e.g., use turn signals) and ride defensively.

Automobile accidents

- Never drive while or after using drugs or alcohol.
- Do not drive when you are overly tired or sleepy.
- Maintain your motor vehicle in good mechanical condition.
- Obey the rules of the road and drive defensively.
- If you need assistance, stay in your car and wait for help.
- Always wear your seat belt.
- Always drive within the legal speed limit.
- Do not drive when emotionally upset.

Falls

- Use handrails when going up and down stairs.
- Do not attempt to climb ladders or stairs when ill or physically impaired due to drug use.
- Maintain ladders and steps in good working condition.
- Never run up or down stairs.
- Make sure stairways are well lit.

Poisoning

- Properly label all drugs.
- Never take more of any drug than is recommended.
- Keep all drugs out of the reach of children.
- Use only nontoxic cleaning materials.
- Increase your knowledge of poisons.
- Do not take medication in the dark.
- Discard old or expired prescriptions.
- Do not combine drugs.
- Keep the poison control center's telephone number near your phone.

Fire

- Reduce the risk of fire in your home or workplace by storing combustible materials in a safe place.
- Maintain smoke detectors, fire extinguishers, and sprinkler systems in proper working condition.
- Know how to use a fire extinguisher properly.
- Practice safe evacuation procedures from your home and workplace.

Drowning

- Learn to swim, and learn proper water safety procedures.
- Do not swim alone or in the dark.
- Dive only in designated areas.
- Do not swim immediately after eating or when tired.
- Do not swim when using drugs of any kind.
- Avoid swimming in dangerous waters, such as rivers with strong currents.
- Learn cardiopulmonary resuscitation.

Stress also increases your risk of accidents (1, 2). During periods of emotional or physical stress, people tend to be less careful. If you find yourself having a series of small mishaps or "near misses" when performing routine activities such as yardwork, house cleaning, or sports activities, this may be an indication that you should reduce your stress level by resting and using stress management techniques.

As we have seen, alcohol and other drugs may increase your risk of accidents. Drug use does this by altering your judgment and by decreasing both reaction speed and motor coordination. Alcohol is involved in nearly one-half of all auto accidents and plays a major role in many boating accidents. Similarly, cocaine and marijuana use are associated with a wide range of accidents, including falls, drownings, fires, and automobile accidents.

A number of environmental factors can increase your risk of accident. For example, storing combustible materials close to a heater and failing to have properly operating smoke detectors both increase your risk of injury due to fire. Other factors, such as failing to properly maintain ladders or steps around your home or workplace, may also increase your risk of accidental injury.

REDUCING YOUR RISK OF ACCIDENTS There are a number of steps you can take to reduce your risk of injury. The key is to increase your awareness of the risk factors. Table 10.2 summarizes key steps that can reduce your risk of injury due to vehicular accidents, fire, falls, drowning, and poisoning. Take time to study each of these recommendations and to alter your lifestyle to reduce your injury risk.

☀ **IN SUMMARY**

- A healthy lifestyle can be achieved by eliminating unhealthful behaviors.

- Behavior modification is the process of changing an undesirable behavior to a more desirable behavior.
- The 10 general steps of behavior modification begin with the identification of a problem and the

desire to change. The process concludes with a long-term plan for maintaining the desired behavior change.

Summary

1. The five key behaviors that promote a healthy lifestyle are health-related physical fitness, good nutrition, weight control, stress management, and modification of unhealthful behaviors.

2. *Stress* is defined as a physiological and mental response to things in our environment that make us feel uncomfortable. Any factor that produces stress is called a *stressor*.

3. Two steps in stress management are to reduce stress in your life and to learn to cope with stress by improving your ability to relax.

4. Common relaxation techniques to reduce stress include progressive relaxation, visualization, meditation, breathing exercises, rest and sleep, and exercise.

5. Behavior modification is the process of changing an undesirable behavior to a more desirable behavior. The general model of behavior modification can be applied to achieve any desired health-related behavior.

6. The five most common types of accidents are automobile accidents, fires, drownings, poisonings, and falls.

7. Risk factors for accidents include unsafe attitudes, stress, drug use, and an unsafe environment.

Study Questions

1. Define *stress*. What is a *stressor?*

2. Why is stress management important to health?

3. List the steps in stress management. Identify some common stress management (relaxation) techniques.

4. Define *behavior modification.* What are the steps involved in behavior modification?

5. Outline a plan to use behavior modification to eliminate a specific unhealthful behavior.

6. Discuss the concept of eustress.

7. Explain how exercise is useful in reducing stress.

8. List the key guidelines for the development of a time management program.

9. List the steps to reduce your risks of injury due to automobile accidents, falls, fires, water accidents, and poisonings.

Suggested Reading

Benson, H. The Relaxation Response. New York: Avon, Wholecare, 2000.
Cowley, G. Stress-busters: What works. *Newsweek,* June 14, 1999, pp. 60–62.
Donatelle, R., and L. Davis. *Access to Health.* Needham Heights, MA: Allyn & Bacon, 2000.
Greenberg, J. *Comprehensive Stress Management,* 6th ed. Dubuque, IA: Brown and Benchmark, 1999.

For links to the Web sites below visit Web Links at www.aw.com/fitness and choose Powers/Dodd Web Links from drop-down menu.

Mayo Clinic Health

Contains wide-ranging information about stress, diet, fitness, and mental health.

American Medical Association

Includes many sources of information about a wide variety of medical problems, including stress-related disorders.

WebMD

Contains information about a wide variety of diseases and medical problems, including stress-related disorders.

American Psychological Association

Provides information on stress management and psychological disorders.

References

1. Donatelle, R., and L. Davis. *Access to Health.* Needham Heights, MA: Allyn and Bacon, 2000.

2. Hales, D. *An Invitation to Health,* 8th ed. San Francisco, CA: Benjamin Cummings, 1998.

3. Margen, S., et al., eds. *The Wellness Encyclopedia.* Boston: Houghton Mifflin, 1992.

4. Williams, M. *Lifetime Fitness and Wellness.* Dubuque, IA: Wm. C. Brown, 1996.

5. Selye, H. *The Stress of Life,* revised edition. New York: McGraw-Hill, 1978.

6. Anderson, B. L., et al. Stress and immune responses after surgical treatment for regional breast cancer. *Journal of the National Cancer Institute* 90:30–36, 1998.

7. Holroyd, K. A., et al. Management of chronic tension-type headache with tricyclic antidepressant medication, stress management therapy, and their combination: A randomized trial. *Journal of the American Medical Association* 285(17):2208–2215, 2001.

8. Sewitch, M., et al. Psychological distress, social support, and disease activity in patients with inflammatory bowel disease. *American Journal of Gastroenterology* 96(5):1470–1479, 2001.

9. Howley, E., and B. D. Franks. *Health Fitness: Instructors Handbook*. Champaign, IL: Human Kinetics, 1997.

10. Raglin, J., and W. Morgan. Influence of exercise and quiet rest on state anxiety and blood pressure. *Medicine and Science in Sports and Exercise* 19:456–463, 1987.

11. Berger, B., and D. Owen. Stress reduction and mood enhancement in four exercise modes: Swimming, body conditioning, hatha yoga, and fencing. *Research Quarterly for Exercise and Sport* 59:148–159, 1988.

12. Bahrke, M., and W. Morgan. Anxiety reduction following exercise and meditation. *Cognitive Therapy and Research* 2:323–333, 1978.

13. Farrell, P. Enkephalins, catecholamines, and psychological mood alterations: Effects of prolonged exercise. *Medicine and Science in Sports and Exercise* 19:347–353, 1987.

14. Clarkson, P. Vitamins and trace minerals. In *Ergonomics*, D. Lamb and M. Williams, eds. Madison, WI: Brown and Benchmark, 1991. 123–175.

15. Ystgaard, M. Life stress, social support, and psychological distress in late adolescence. *Social Psychiatry and Psychiatric Epidemiology* 32:277–283, 1997.

16. Fielding, J. Smoking: Health effects and controls. *New England Journal of Medicine* 313:491–497, 1985.

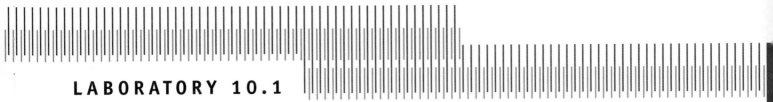

LABORATORY 10.1

Stress Index Questionnaire

NAME _____ **DATE** _____

DIRECTIONS

The purpose of this stress index questionnaire is to increase your awareness of stress in your life. Circle either "yes" or "no" to answer each of the following questions.

Yes No 1. I have frequent arguments.

Yes No 2. I often get upset at work.

Yes No 3. I often have neck and/or shoulder pains due to anxiety/stress.

Yes No 4. I often get upset when I stand in long lines.

Yes No 5. I often get angry when I listen to the local, national, or world news or read the newspaper.

Yes No 6. I do not have a sufficient amount of money for my needs.

Yes No 7. I often get upset when driving.

Yes No 8. At the end of a workday I often feel stress-related fatigue.

Yes No 9. I have at least one constant source of stress/anxiety in my life (e.g., conflict with boss, neighbor, mother-in-law, etc.).

Yes No 10. I often have stress-related headaches.

Yes No 11. I do not practice stress management techniques.

Yes No 12. I rarely take time for myself.

Yes No 13. I have difficulty in keeping my feelings of anger and hostility under control.

Yes No 14. I have difficulty in managing time wisely.

Yes No 15. I often have difficulty sleeping.

Yes No 16. I am generally in a hurry.

Yes No 17. I usually feel that there is not enough time in the day to accomplish what I need to do.

Yes No 18. I often feel that I am being mistreated by friends or associates.

Yes No 19. I do not regularly perform physical activity.

Yes No 20. I rarely get 7 to 9 hours of sleep per night.

SCORING AND INTERPRETATION

Answering "yes" to any of the questions means that you need to use some form of stress management techniques (see the text for details). Total your "yes" answers and use the following scale to evaluate the level of stress in your life.

Number of "Yes" Answers	Stress Category
6–20	High stress
3–5	Average stress
0–2	Low stress

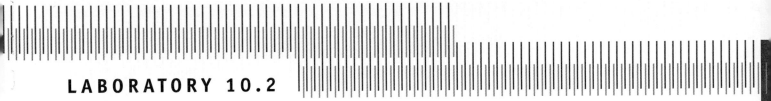

LABORATORY 10.2

Behavior Modification Contract

NAME _____ **DATE** _____

DIRECTIONS

Complete the following behavior modification contract, using friends or peers as witnesses. See the reverse of this sheet for an example of a completed contract.

BEHAVIOR MODIFICATION CONTRACT

1. I _____ (name) agree to make the following behavioral change(s):

   _____

   _____

   _____

   _____ beginning on _____ (date).

2. My short-term goal(s) are to

   _____

   _____ by _____ (date).

3. My long-term goal(s) are to

   _____

   _____

4. I will assess my progress on the desired behavioral change on a regular basis:

   _____ (note how often).

   Further, I will report my progress to at least two friends and/or peers on a regular basis.

   Signed: _____ Date: _____

   Witness: _____ Witness: _____

(continued on next page)

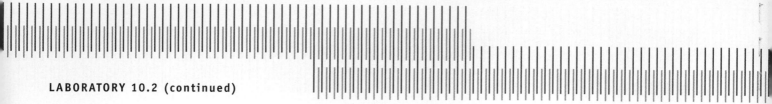

ILLUSTRATION OF BEHAVIOR MODIFICATION CONTRACT FOR SMOKING CESSATION

BEHAVIOR MODIFICATION CONTRACT

1. I ___*John Doe*___ agree to make the following behavioral change(s):

___*Stop smoking*___

_____

_____

_____

_____ beginning on *May 20, 2002* (date).

2. My short-term goal(s) are to

___*Stop smoking*___

_____ by *5/20/2002* (date).

3. My long-term goal(s) are to

Remain smoke free during the rest of my life _____

_____

4. I will assess my progress on the desired behavioral change on a regular basis:

_____*weekly*_____ (note how often).

Further, I will report my progress to at least two friends and/or peers on a regular basis.

Signed: ___*John Doe*___ Date: ___*April 1, 2002*___

Witness: ___*Roberto Jimenez*___ Witness: ___*William Jones*___

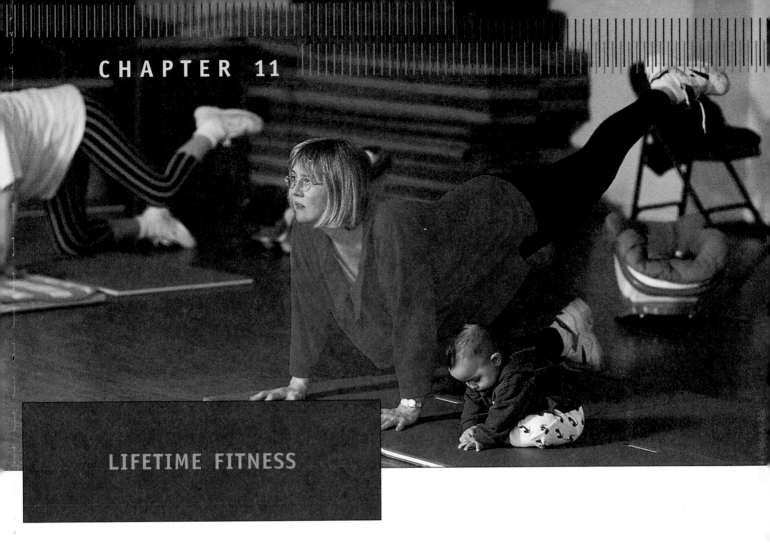

CHAPTER 11

LIFETIME FITNESS

After studying this chapter, you should be able to:

1. Identify several factors that will assist you in maintaining a regular exercise program over your lifetime.

2. List key considerations in choosing a fitness facility.

3. Discuss the term *fitness expert*.

4. Discuss several common exercise misconceptions.

5. Identify factors to consider when purchasing exercise equipment.

6. List several precautions for the use of hot tubs, saunas, and steambaths.

xercise must be performed regularly throughout your life to achieve the benefits of physical fitness, wellness, and disease prevention. Fitness cannot be stored! If you stop exercising, you begin to lose fitness.

This chapter suggests strategies for maintaining a lifetime fitness program. We also consider key factors in choosing an exercise facility or health club and discuss issues important to being an informed fitness consumer.

✸ Exercise Adherence: Lifetime Fitness

Studies have shown that over 60% of adults who start an exercise program quit within the first month (1). In contrast, people who start an exercise program and continue to exercise regularly for at least 6 months have an excellent chance of maintaining a regular exercise routine for years to come (1). Thus, the first 6 months of your exercise program are critical in determining your lifetime adherence to exercise. The significance of exercising regularly for several months is probably linked to the fact that 2 to 6 months of training are generally required to bring about significant improvements in both

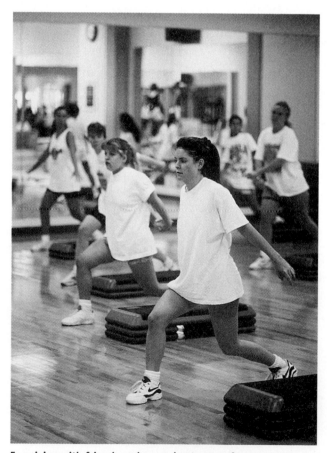

Exercising with friends makes workouts more fun.

fitness and body composition (i.e., fat loss). This positive feedback, once achieved, provides a strong incentive to continue exercising.

Beginning a lifetime exercise program requires a strong personal commitment to physical fitness and application of the principles of behavior modification to change from a sedentary lifestyle to an active lifestyle. In the next sections we discuss several factors that will assist you in maintaining a lifetime commitment to physical activity.

GOAL SETTING FOR ACTIVE LIFESTYLES

Although the first step in beginning a successful exercise program is desiring to be physically fit, the second step is establishing both short-term and long-term fitness goals (goal setting was introduced in Chapter 1 and discussed in detail in Chapter 3). Your goals should be based on your personal needs and desire for fitness, and they should be realistic. Goal setting provides a target to shoot for and adds an incentive to maintain regular exercise habits. Goals can be either maintenance goals or improvement goals. For example, a realistic short-term improvement goal for cardiorespiratory fitness might be to decrease your 1.5-mile run time from 15 minutes to 14 minutes during your first 6 months of training. In contrast, a short-term maintenance goal might be to average 20 miles of running per week during the first year of training. A key point to remember about fitness goals is that they should be modified from time to time to accommodate any changes in your fitness needs and to allow you to correct any unrealistic goals you may have set.

SELECTING ACTIVITIES

Exercise should be fun! You should choose exercise activities that you enjoy. However, not all enjoyable physical activities will promote improvement in health-related physical fitness. Which sports or activities provide the best training effect to improve physical fitness? Table 11.1 evaluates the fitness potential of a variety of popular sports and activities. Note that no one activity is rated as being excellent in promoting all aspects of fitness. To achieve total physical fitness, you should participate in several activities.

Another key consideration is the availability and convenience of the activity. Regardless of how much you enjoy a particular activity, if it is not convenient, your chances of regular participation are greatly reduced. For example, suppose you enjoy swimming but the pool closest to your home or school is 10 miles away, and to make matters worse, the pool hours of operation conflict with your daily schedule. In combination, these two factors decrease your chances of successfully using swimming as your primary mode of regular exercise. The solution to

TABLE 11.1
Fitness Evaluation of Various Activities and Sports

Sport/Activity	Cardiorespiratory Endurance	Upper Body Muscular Strength and Endurance	Lower Body Muscular Strength and Endurance	Flexibility	Caloric Expenditure (calories/min)
				Fitness Ranking	
Aerobic dance	Good	Good	Good	Fair	5–10
Badminton	Fair	Fair	Good	Fair	5–10
Baseball	Poor	Fair	Fair	Fair	4–6
Basketball	Good	Fair	Good	Fair	10–12
Bowling	Poor	Fair	Poor	Fair	3–4
Canoeing	Fair	Good	Poor	Fair	4–10
Football (flag/touch)	Fair	Fair	Good	Fair	5–10
Golf (walking)	Poor	Fair	Good/fair	Fair	2–4
Gymnastics	Poor	Excellent	Excellent	Excellent	3–4
Handball	Good	Good/fair	Good	Fair	7–12
Karate	Fair	Good	Good	Excellent	7–10
Racquetball	Good/fair	Good/fair	Good	Fair	6–12
Running	Excellent	Fair	Good	Fair	8–15
Skating (ice)	Good/fair	Poor	Good/fair	Good/fair	5–10
Skating (roller)	Good/fair	Poor	Good/fair	Fair	5–10
Skiing (alpine)	Fair	Fair	Good	Fair	5–10
Skiing (nordic)	Excellent/good	Good	Good	Fair	7–15
Soccer	Good	Fair	Good	Good/fair	7–17
Tennis	Good/fair	Good/fair	Good	Fair	5–12
Volleyball	Fair	Fair	Good/fair	Fair	4–8
Waterskiing	Poor	Good	Good	Fair	4–7
Weight training	Poor	Excellent	Excellent	Fair	4–6

Source: From Getchell, B. Physical Fitness: A Way of Life. Copyright © 1992. Reprinted by permission of Allyn and Bacon.

this problem is simple. Continue to swim when you have the opportunity, but choose another convenient activity that you enjoy as your regular exercise mode. Remember, selecting a convenient and enjoyable activity will greatly increase your chances of maintaining a regular exercise program.

PLANNING EXERCISE SESSIONS

Exercise sessions should be systematic and connected to your exercise goals (2, 3). This is particularly true during the first several weeks of an exercise program. To achieve your objectives, you must train on a regular basis.

Choosing a regular time to exercise helps to make it a habit. Some fitness instructors suggest that morning exercise is superior to exercise at other times of the day; however, there is no scientific evidence to support the notion that there is an optimal time of day to exercise. This is fortunate, because individual preferences for a daily exercise time vary. Some people prefer to exercise in the morning hours, whereas others may prefer a noon workout. Choose a time that works for you; the

key to exercising regularly is to choose a convenient time to work out and stick with it.

MONITORING PROGRESS

Monitoring your progress in achieving or maintaining physical fitness is an important factor in providing feedback and motivation to continue. You can monitor your progress in at least two ways. First, maintain a training log to provide feedback concerning the amount of exercise performed. For example, a daily training log can help you monitor the number of miles run, the amount of weight lifted, total calories expended during exercise, any changes in body weight, and so on. A number of commercially available training diaries and computer programs are available.

A second means of monitoring your fitness progress is through periodic fitness testing (Chapter 2). Fitness testing provides positive feedback when fitness levels are improving. This type of information is a useful motivational tool and should be a part of every fitness program.

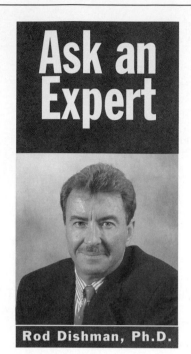

Ask an Expert

Rod Dishman, Ph.D.

Exercise Adherence

Dr. Dishman is professor of exercise science and Director of the Exercise Psychology Laboratory at the University of Georgia, Athens, GA. He is one of the world's leading experts in exercise psychology and issues related to exercise adherence. Dr. Dishman has published numerous scientific papers, books, and book chapters related to exercise adherence. In the following interview, Dr. Dishman addresses several questions related to adherence to regular exercise.

Q: What factors can help me stay motivated to maintain a regular exercise program?

A: Make exercise your top priority by actions, not just intentions. Schedule a time and pick a place to exercise. Many people find exercise at lunchtime or at the end of the day invigorating; however, most inactive people prefer relaxation. Also, strong intentions often weaken by day's end, and people may feel fatigued and want to rest, not exert. If the later scenario describes you, exercise early in the day.

If you lack the self-motivation to carry out exercise goals, pick other activities or rewards that are important to you and make a commitment not to indulge yourself until daily exercise goals are met. Also, keep a record to ensure that you don't conveniently forget or lie to yourself when you don't meet exercise goals.

Engineer your environment to make it hard to talk yourself out of exercising. Put exercise equipment near your bed at night, so you see it first thing in the morning. Keep exercise gear in your car or at work for availability whenever exercise opportunities arise.

Contrary to popular belief, there is little evidence that high level fitness is needed for health benefits. Moderate exertion seems effective too. Pick a type of exercise you most enjoy, a time that best fits your schedule, and an intensity that is pleasurable.

Don't judge the benefits of your exercise by fitness gains alone.

Research confirms that moderate exercise can have calming and mood elevating effects and may even improve sleep.

Q: How important is fitness goal setting as a motivating factor for beginning an exercise program?

A: Specific, long-term exercise goals are important to get an exercise program started. Goals don't have to be fully realistic. An idealized goal that you might not be able to reach can nevertheless be a good exercise incentive; however, you must plan a series of shorter term step-by-step goals that are attainable and can bring you closer to your ultimate objective. Distant goals should not change, but immediate daily goals can and often should be flexible. Avoid the abstainer's fallacy that there is only one rigid, unyielding plan that will work for you.

Q: Is it possible to develop a psychological dependence on exercise and, therefore, develop an addiction to exercise?

A: In the 1970s, William P. Morgan of the University of Wisconsin described eight cases of running addiction, when a commitment to running exceeded prior commitments to work, family, social relations, and medical advice. Similar cases have been labeled as positive addiction, runner's gluttony, fitness fanaticism, athlete's neurosis, obligatory running, and exercise abuse. Little is understood, however, about the origins, valid diagnosis, or the mental health impact of abusive exercise.

SOCIAL SUPPORT

Social support is another key factor in many successful exercise programs. Enjoying interaction with friends or colleagues during exercise or in the locker room before or after a workout is an important part of making exercise fun. See Fitness-Wellness Consumer for some tips on choosing a health club. Beginning an exercise program with a friend is an excellent way to start exercising on a regular basis, provided that both individuals share the same commitment to improving personal fitness.

PEERS AS ROLE MODELS

Your personal commitment to exercise can be positively influenced by peers who serve as good role models for the benefits of exercise. Most of us know individuals who exercise regularly and look terrific as a result of proper training and diet. These role models can be motivational to people who are beginning an exercise program.

CHANGING PHYSICAL ACTIVITY NEEDS

As we age, our needs for and interest in physical activity often change. It is thus important to modify your fitness program throughout your life. For instance,

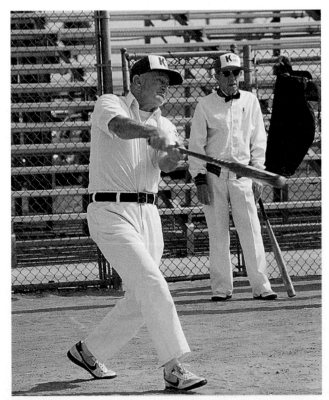

Aging may change your physical activity needs over the course of a lifetime.

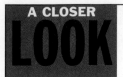

What Is a Fitness Expert?

Even though there is presently no standard definition of "fitness expert," anyone who has earned an advanced degree (such as an M.S. or a Ph.D.) in exercise science, kinesiology, or exercise physiology from a reputable university can generally be considered a fitness expert. Although individuals with bachelor's degrees in exercise science may have a sufficient background to answer many fitness-related questions, the more advanced the degree, the more knowledgeable the individual should be about exercise and fitness.

Exercise scientists who are actively conducting research in exercise physiology and are active in such professional organizations as the American Physiological Society or the American College of Sports Medicine are generally the best sources of valid information, especially concerning more technical matters. Additionally, physicians with postgraduate training in exercise physiology or a strong personal interest in preventive medicine are also good sources of scientifically based fitness information.

If you having difficulty finding a local fitness expert who can answer your questions, contact the American College of Sports Medicine (P.O. Box 1440, Indianapolis, IN 46206-1440) for the name of a fitness expert near you.

while some people engage in a single activity such as basketball over the course of several years, many people lose interest in repeating the same daily activity. When this occurs, it becomes important to find other activities that interest you. Many physical activity options exist, so individuals should remain flexible in their exercise habits and be willing to modify their programs as the need arises. Maintaining enthusiasm for exercise is the foundation of lifetime fitness. See A Closer Look below for some strategies that can help you adhere to a lifetime exercise program.

IN SUMMARY

- Over 60% of adults who start an exercise program quit within the first month.
- People who start an exercise program and exercise regularly for at least 6 months have an excellent chance of maintaining a regular exercise routine for years to come.

- Setting exercise goals, selecting enjoyable exercise activities, planning exercise sessions, monitoring fitness progress, exercising with friends, and adjusting your activity as you age are all important aspects of your lifetime adherence to exercise.

Diet and Fitness Products: Consumer Issues

The fitness boom in the United States has brought an explosion of fitness and diet books and magazines, as well as a huge number of companies that produce exercise equipment. Although some fitness books and magazines are written by experts, many are written by individuals with little formal training in exercise physiology. Unfortunately, books and articles written by nonexperts often convey misinformation, and some of these writings have created many exercise myths. Further,

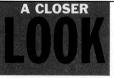

The Keys to Success in Exercise Adherence

Maintaining a regular program of exercise requires motivation and a lifetime commitment to exercise. The following positive steps (6, 7) are the keys to successfully adhering to a lifetime exercise program.

- Strive to maintain your desire and motivation to be physically fit.
- Establish both short-term and long-term fitness goals.
- Choose exercise activities that are fun.

- Select activities and/or places to work out that are convenient.
- Schedule time every day for a workout.
- Exercise with a friend.
- Associate with peers who are positive physical fitness role models.
- Adjust your exercise training routine as you age or as your exercise interests change.

Nutritional Links

Do Nutritional Ergogenic Aids Promote Physical Fitness?

The popular fitness literature is replete with claims that nutritional supplements improve physical fitness and build muscle mass. The following nutritional products are popular supplements that are often used by athletes or fitness enthusiasts:

Amino acids	Organ extracts
Bee pollen	Vitamin supplements
Gelatin	Wheat germ oil
Mineral supplements	Yeast

Do any of these supplements improve physical fitness or performance? The answer is "no" if you are eating a nutritionally balanced diet. Volumes of research clearly show that nutritional supplements do not improve physical fitness in well-fed, healthy individuals. (See reference 8 at the end of the chapter for a review.)

---

many exercise products are not useful in promoting physical fitness or weight loss. In the next several sections we discuss some key consumer issues related to exercise and weight loss.

COMMON MISCONCEPTIONS ABOUT PHYSICAL FITNESS

There are numerous misconceptions about exercise, weight loss, and physical fitness, and to thoroughly discuss them would require hundreds of pages of text. So, even though debunking all exercise myths is beyond the scope of this book, we can dispel some of the most common ones.

YOGA Supporters of yoga offer claims that practicing it regularly will improve fitness, assist in weight loss, and cure a host of diseases. Unfortunately, there is little evidence to support most of these claims (9). While yoga will improve flexibility and promote relaxation, many of the yoga positions may cause joint injury, particularly if performed improperly. In short, yoga is not a panacea and should not be the sole contributor to one's exercise prescription.

HAND WEIGHTS The popularity of handheld weights has increased rapidly in the past several years. Some manufacturers claim that using hand weights will greatly increase arm and shoulder strength. Although carrying hand weights will increase the energy expenditure during exercise, 1- to 3-pound hand weights do not promote significant strength gains (particularly in college-age individuals).

Further, there are some concerns about the use of hand weights. First, gripping them may increase blood pressure (10). Individuals with high blood pressure should seek a physician's advice about the use of hand weights during exercise (6, 8). Hand weights may also aggravate existing elbow or shoulder arthritis. Finally, some aerobics instructors have banned hand weights in large classes because of the potential danger of hitting someone with an outstretched hand.

RUBBER WAIST BELTS AND SPOT REDUCTION Recall that spot reduction of body fat is the concept of being able to lose body fat from a specific body location. Numerous myths exist concerning the spot reduction effects of such practices as wearing nylon suits or rubber waist bands, as well as exercise focused on a specific body area (e.g., sit-ups). The bottom line is that no method of spot reduction is effective in removing fat from a specific body area (Chapter 8). Although exercise can assist in creating a negative caloric balance and therefore promote fat loss, the loss of fat occurs throughout the body and is not localized to one particular area.

ERGOGENIC AIDS A drug or nutritional product that improves physical fitness and exercise performance is called an **ergogenic aid.** Numerous manufacturers market products that they claim promote strength and cardiovascular fitness. The popularity of these products usually stems from their reported use by champion athletes, but the key concern for the consumer is whether ergogenic aids promote fitness.

Only limited scientific evidence supports the notion that nutritional ergogenic aids promote fitness or increase athletic performance in humans (Nutritional Links to Health and Fitness). However, both anabolic steroids and the drug Clenbuterol have proved to increase muscle mass in animals (11, 12). Although this may seem to be good news for people who want to increase their muscle mass, the bad news is that both drugs have been shown to be harmful to health. Recent evidence has shown that prolonged use of both drugs may result in serious organ damage and, in some cases, death (13, 14). See references 15 and 16 at the end of the chapter for reviews on these topics.

---

ergogenic aid A drug or nutritional product that improves physical fitness and exercise performance.

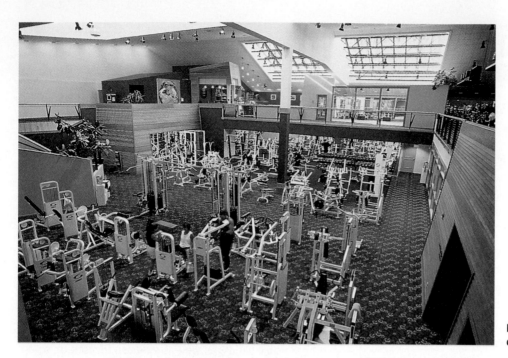

Examine the features of a health club carefully before joining.

EXERCISE EQUIPMENT   Many types of exercise equipment are available. Every week, magazine and television ads promote a "new" exercise device designed to trim waistlines and build huge muscles overnight. In truth, there are no "miracle" exercise devices capable of promoting such changes. In fact, there is really no need to buy *any* exercise devices to promote fitness. A well-rounded fitness program can be designed without exercise equipment. However, if you want to purchase exercise equipment for home use, buy from a reputable and well-established company (9). Beware of mail-order products, and examine the product before you buy (9). When in doubt about the usefulness of an exercise product, consult a fitness expert.

PASSIVE EXERCISE DEVICES   A **passive exercise** machine is a motor-driven device designed to move or vibrate the body without any muscular activity. Passive exercise devices come in many forms, including rolling machines, vibrating belts, pillows, and passive motion tables. Manufacturers claim that passive exercise devices improve physical fitness and assist in weight loss. Unfortunately, there is no such thing as effortless exercise. Passive exercise devices do not improve physical fitness or promote weight loss (17).

HOT TUBS, SAUNAS, AND STEAMBATHS   Hot tubs, saunas, and steambaths are popular attractions at many health clubs. Although they may improve mental attitudes by promoting relaxation, none promotes fat loss or improves physical fitness. While water loss due to perspiration will reduce your body weight temporarily, it does not result in fat loss. Further, the weight will return as soon as you replace the lost fluids by eating and drinking.

There are also potential dangers in the use of saunas, steambaths, and hot tubs. One of the major problems concerns the regulation of blood pressure. All of these forms of heat stress increase blood flow to the skin to promote cooling; this reduces blood return to the heart and may reduce blood flow to the brain, resulting in fainting. Therefore, when using a sauna, hot tub, or steambath, note the following precautions (9):

- Seek a physician's advice before using hot baths if you suffer from heart disease, hypertension, diabetes, kidney disease, or chronic skin problems, or if you are pregnant.
- Don't use hot bath facilities when you are alone; someone should be present to get emergency help if you develop a health problem, such as fainting.
- Don't wear jewelry in hot baths (the metal will absorb heat and may burn your skin).
- Don't drink alcohol prior to or while bathing because alcohol may increase your risk of fainting during heat exposure.

---

passive exercise   Movement performed on a motor-driven device designed to move or vibrate the body without any muscular activity. Passive exercise devices come in many forms, including rolling machines, vibrating belts, pillows, and passive motion tables, but they do not improve physical fitness or promote weight loss.

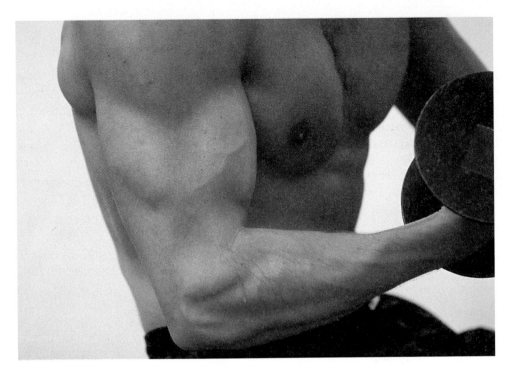

Having a championship physique does not make an individual a fitness expert.

- Don't exercise in a sauna, hot tub, or steam bath. The combination of exercise and a hot environment may result in overheating.

- Do not enter a sauna, hot tub, or steambath immediately following vigorous exercise. Entering a steambath without cooling down after exercise increases your risk of fainting.

- The duration of stay and recommended temperatures of saunas, steambaths, and hot tubs are as follows:
Sauna: Air temperature should not exceed 190°F (~88°C) and the stay in sauna should not exceed 15 minutes.
Steambath: Air temperature should not exceed 120°F (~38°C) and the stay in steambath should not exceed 10 minutes.
Hot tub (or whirlpool): Water temperature should not exceed 100°F (~38°C) and the stay in hot tub should not exceed 15 minutes.

FITNESS BOOKS AND MAGAZINES Book stores generally have numerous fitness-related publications on their shelves. Although many fitness books have been written by experts in the field of exercise science, oth-ers have been written by individuals with little or no formal training in exercise physiology. Dozens of fitness books and magazine articles have been written by models, movie stars, body builders, and even professional or Olympic athletes who have no academic training in exercise science. Clearly, having athletic talent or a good physique does not make an individual a fitness expert.

How do you evaluate the credibility of a fitness or weight control book? After reading and studying this book, you should be able to distinguish between fitness facts and fiction. For example, beware of texts that promise overnight results or quick, effortless weight loss. If you have doubts about the validity of a new fitness text, contact a local fitness expert for advice.

☀ IN SUMMARY

- Numerous misconceptions exist concerning physical fitness.

- Wearing rubber waist belts will not result in spot reduction of fat.

- Passive exercise devices do not improve physical fitness and will not promote weight loss.

- Although hot tubs, saunas, and steambaths are relaxing, they will not promote loss of body fat.

Summary

1. Exercise must be performed regularly throughout your life to achieve the benefits of physical fitness, wellness, and disease prevention.

2. Over 60% of the adults who start an exercise program quit within the first month. However, evidence exists that people who start an exercise program and continue to exercise for 6 months have an excellent chance of maintaining a regular fitness routine for years.

3. The following are important aspects of maintaining a lifetime commitment to physical activity: goal setting, activity selection, regularity of exercise sessions, monitoring your progress, social support, peers as role models, and modifying your physical activity program as a result of aging.

4. Before choosing a health club, you should consider the following factors: Check the club's reputation with the local Better Business Bureau before joining; investigate programs offered throughout your community before deciding to join a particular club; before joining any facility, examine the membership contract carefully; in general, avoid clubs that advertise "overnight" fitness or weight loss success; and arrange to make several trial visits to the facility before joining. Several visits to the facility will provide you with answers regarding whether the locker room facilities are well maintained and clean, the exercise machines are in good working order, the club employees are well trained and eager to answer your fitness-related questions, and the facility is not overcrowded during the hours that you plan to use the club.

5. There is no standard definition of a *fitness expert*. However, a fitness expert is, generally, someone who has earned an advanced degree in exercise science, kinesiology, or exercise physiology.

6. Numerous exercise misconceptions exist. After studying this book you should be able to distinguish between fact and fiction. If you have doubts about the validity of a new fitness product or textbook, contact a local fitness expert for advice.

Study Questions

1. Outline the key factors that play a role in maintaining a regular program of exercise.

2. List five points to consider when choosing a health club.

3. Give your definition of a *fitness expert*.

4. Numerous exercise misconceptions exist. Discuss the misconceptions associated with yoga, the use of hand weights, the use of rubber weight belts to lose body fat, and nutritional ergogenic aids.

5. What factors should be considered when purchasing exercise equipment?

6. List several precautions that should be considered when using hot tubs, saunas, or steambaths.

7. Do passive exercise devices promote physical fitness and weight loss? Explain your answer.

8. What percentage of people who start an exercise program quit within the first month?

9. Discuss the importance of activity selection in maintaining physical fitness.

10. List five activities that are considered to be good or excellent modes of promoting cardiorespiratory fitness.

Suggested Reading

ACSM's Guidelines for Exercise Testing and Prescription, 6th ed. Baltimore: Lippincott Williams & Wilkins, 2000.

Balady, G. Health clubs: Are they right for you? *Harvard Men's Health Watch,* November 6, 1998.

Franks, B., E. Howley, and Y. Iyriboz. *The Health Fitness Handbook.* Champaign, IL: Human Kinetics, 1999.

Health clubs: What to look for. *Consumer Reports,* February 1999.

Nieman, D. *Exercise Testing and Prescription: A Health-Related Approach.* Mountain View, CA: Mayfield, 1999.

Powers, S., and E. Howley, *Exercise Physiology: Theory and Application to Fitness and Performance,* 4th ed. St. Louis: McGraw-Hill, 2001.

For links to the Web sites below visit Web Links at www.aw.com/fitness and choose Powers/Dodd Web Links from the drop-down menu.

American College of Sports Medicine

Contains information about exercise, health, and fitness.

WebMD

Includes the latest information on a variety of health-related topics, including diet, exercise, and stress; also contains links to other sites on nutrition, fitness, and wellness topics.

American Council on Exercise

A nonprofit organization that provides information on a variety of topics related to exercise and fitness.

President's Council on Physical Fitness and Sports

Provides information concerning a wide range of subjects related to exercise and fitness.

References

1. Dishman, R., ed. *Exercise Adherence: Its Impact on Public Health.* Champaign, IL: Human Kinetics, 1988.

2. Getchell, B. *Physical Fitness: A Way of Life,* 5th ed. Needham Heights, MA: Allyn and Bacon, 1998.

3. Howley, E., and B. D. Franks. *Health Fitness: Instructors Handbook.* Champaign, IL: Human Kinetics, 1997.

4. Balady, G. Health clubs: Are they right for you? *Harvard Men's Health Watch,* November 6, 1998.

5. Health clubs: What to look for. *Consumer Reports,* February, 1999.

6. Dishman, R. *Advances in Exercise Adherence.* Champaign, IL: Human Kinetics, 1994.

7. Resnick, B. Testing a model of exercise behavior in older adults. *Research in Nursing and Health* 24:83–89, 2001.

8. Clarkson, P. Vitamins and trace minerals. In *Ergogenics,* D. Lamb and M. Williams, eds. Madison, WI: Brown and Benchmark, 1991.

9. Corbin, C., and R. Lindsey. *Concepts of Physical Fitness.* Dubuque, IA: Wm. C. Brown, 2000.

10. Graves, J., M. Pollock, S. Montain, A. Jackson, and J. O'Keefe. The effect of hand-held weights on the physiological response to walking exercise. *Medicine and Science in Sports and Exercise* 19:260–265, 1987.

11. Criswell, D., S. Powers, and R. Herb. Clenbuterol-induced fiber type transition in the soleus of adult rats. *European Journal of Applied Physiology* 74:391–396, 1996.

12. Heitzman, R. The effectiveness of anabolic agents in increasing rate of growth in farm animals: Report on experiments in cattle. In *Anabolic Agents in Animal Production,* F. Lu and J. Rendell, eds. Stuttgart, Germany: Georg Thieme, 1976.

13. Palmer, R., M. Delday, D. McMillan, B. Noble, P. Bain, and C. Maltin. Effects of the cyclo-oxygenase inhibitor, fenbufen, on clenbuterol-induced hypertrophy of cardiac and skeletal muscle of rats. *British Journal of Pharmacology* 101:835–838, 1990.

14. Taylor, W., S. Snowball, C. Dickson, and M. Lesna. Alterations in liver architecture in mice treated with anabolic androgens and dimethylnitrosamine. *NATO Advanced Study Institute Series, Series A* 52:279–288, 1982.

15. Powers, S., and E. Howley. *Exercise Physiology: Theory and Application to Fitness and Performance,* 4th ed. St. Louis: McGraw-Hill, 2001.

16. Lamb, D., and M. Williams. *Ergogenics: Enhancement of Performance in Exercise and Sport.* Vol. 4. Madison, WI: Brown and Benchmark, 1991.

17. Martin, A. D., and G. Kauwell. Continuous assistive-passive exercise and cycle ergometer training in sedentary women. *Medicine and Science in Sports and Exercise* 22: 523–527, 1990.

18. McArdle, W., F. Katch, and V. Katch. *Exercise Physiology.* Hagerstown, MD: Lippincott, Williams, and Williams, 2001.

19. McGlynn, G. *Dynamics of Fitness: A Practical Approach.* Dubuque, IA: Wm. C. Brown, 1998.

20. Pollock, M., and J. Wilmore. *Exercise in Health and Disease,* 3rd ed. Philadelphia: W. B. Saunders, 1999.

Healthy People 2010

Healthy People is a national health promotion and disease prevention initiative developed and coordinated by the U.S. Department of Health and Human Services, Office of Disease Prevention and Health Promotion. The goal of Healthy People 2010 is to improve the health of all Americans, eliminate disparities in health across populations, and increase the length and quality of life in the U.S. These goals can be achieved by meeting numerous health-related objectives. Selected Healthy People 2010 objectives include:

- Increase the proportion of people who engage in daily physical activity

- Reduce activity limitation due to chronic back conditions

- Reduce cigarette smoking among people

- Increase the consumption of fruits and vegetables

- Reduce the lung cancer death rate

- Reduce the melanoma death rate

- Reduce the number of college students that engage in heavy drinking of alcoholic beverages

- Reduce the number of people who experience adverse health effects from stress each year

- Reduce the number of overweight people of ages 20 and older

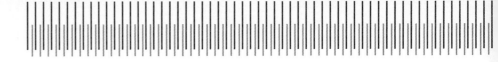

APPENDIX B

Nutritional Content of Common Foods and Beverages

This food composition table has been prepared for Benjamin Cummings and is copyrighted by DINE Systems, Inc., the developer and publisher of the DINE System family of nutrition software for personal computers. The values in this food composition table were derived from the USDA Nutrient Data Base for Standard Reference Release 10 and nutrient composition information from over 300 food companies. Nutrient values used for each food were determined by collapsing similar foods into one food, using the median nutrient values. In the food composition table, foods are listed within eight groups. The eight groups are, in order: fruits, vegetables, beverages, alcoholic beverages, grains, dairy, fats/sweets/other, and protein foods. Further information can be obtained from:

DINE Systems, Inc.
586 N. French Road
Amherst, NY 14228
(716) 688-2492
FAX (716) 688-2502

APPENDIX B
Nutritional Content of Common Foods
NOTE: Carbohydrate value does not include Added Sugar value.

Grains

Amount		Weight	Calories	Protein (g)	Total Fat (g)	Sat Fat (g)	Carb. (g)	Added Sugar (g)	Fiber (g)	Chol. (mg)	Sodium (mg)	Calcium (mg)	Iron (mg)
Bagel	1 bagel	68 g	175	7	10.22	0.22	32.5	2.25	1.5	0	325	20	1.8
Barley-cooked	1/2 cup	81 g	84	2.25	0.11	0	18.5	0	2.5	0	3	11	0.5
Biscuit	1 biscuit	30 g	100	2	3.78	1.22	13.5	0	0.5	2	262	47	0.7
Bread or roll-wheat	1 slice, 1 roll	27 g	65	2	0.89	0.22	10	2	1.4	0	106	20	0.7
Bread or roll-white	1 slice, 1 roll	28 g	70	2.75	1.11	0.33	11	2	0.5	0	132	20	0.7
Bread-mixed grain	1 slice	25 g	65	2	0.89	0.22	9.75	2.25	1.4	0	106	27	0.8
Bread-oatmeal	1 slice	37 g	90	4	1.78	0.33	10.5	4	1.5	0	140	40	1.1
Bread-pita, wheat	1 pita	57 g	145	5.5	0.89	0.22	28.5	0.5	4.1	0	360	50	1.4
Bread-pita, white	1 pita	57 g	160	6	1	0.22	30	1	1.1	0	300	80	0.7
Bread-raisin	1 slice	26 g	70	2	1	0.33	8.25	3	0.9	0	85	20	0.7
Bread-rye, pumpernickel	1 slice	30 g	80	2.75	0.89	0.11	13	1	1.1	0	185	22	1.1
Bread-wheat	1 slice	28 g	82	3	1	0.33	11.38	2	1.8	0	158.5	22.5	1
Bread-wheat, diet	1 slice	23 g	40	2.5	0.56	0.11	4.25	2	2	0	120	40	0.7
Bread-white	1 slice	27 g	67	2	1	0.22	11	1	0.7	0	135	21	0.7
Bread-white, diet	1 slice	23 g	40	3	0	0	6	1	2	0	110	40	0.7
Bread-whole wheat	1 slice	28 g	69	2.63	1.22	0.17	13	1.38	2	0	127	20	0.9
Breadsticks	1/3 large, 2 small	11 g	36	1.25	0.78	0.22	6	0.5	0.6	0	72	0	0.2
Bulgur	1/2 cup	67 g	113	4.25	0.22	0	23.5	0	3	0	3	13	3.7
Cake-nonfat	1 piece	56 g	140	3	0	0	32	15.5	1.2	0	170	0	0
Cereal-bran, fiber	1/3 cup	23 g	62	2	0.78	0.22	7.75	2.75	3.8	0	113	13	3
Cereal-granola	1/4 cup	28 g	130	3	4.89	0.89	13.5	4.5	1.7	0	55	19	0.9
Cereal-granola, fat free	1/4 cup	28 g	90	2	0	0	21	0.25	2.5	0	20	0	0.4
Cereal-oat flakes	1 cup	46 g	182	5	1.78	0.44	24.75	4.5	3.2	0	115	32	5.8
Cereal-other, cold	1 cup	29 g	110	2	0.22	0.11	19.5	3	0.6	0	226	4	1.8
Cereal-other, hot	2/3 cup	156 g	100	3	0	0	22	0	0.7	0	54	18	1.1
Cereal-sweetened	1 cup	29 g	120	1.25	1	0.44	13	13	0.5	0	210	0	4.5
Cereal-whole grain	3/4 cup	28 g	105	3	0.78	0.22	19	0	2.3	0	160	8	1.4
Cheese ravioli w/sauce	1 cup, 6 pieces	263 g	314	13	10.83	6.11	45.13	0.25	3.4	30	733	139	2
Cornbread, hushpuppies	1 square, 3 hushpuppies	51 g	166	3	5.33	1.78	25.75	0	1.6	42	421	87	0.8
Couscous	2/3 cup	108 g	120	4	0	0	26	0	4.3	0	5	0	0.7
Cracker sandwiches	2 large, 5 small	14 g	70	1.75	3.11	1.11	7.75	0.75	0.2	1	135	20	0.4
Crackers	5 crackers	14 g	60	1	2	0.44	8.75	0.75	0.4	0	120	0	0.5
Crackers-butter type	5 large, 10 small	14 g	70	1	3.56	1.11	8	0.25	0.2	1	193	4	0.4
Crackers-crispbread	1 large, 2 small	13 g	40	1	0.89	0.33	8.5	0	1.6	0	112	0	0.5
Crackers-lowfat	2 large, 5 small	14 g	60	2.25	2.33	0.33	10	0	0.6	0	100	0	0.4

Amount	Weight	Calories	Protein (g)	Total Fat (g)	Sat Fat (g)	Carb. (g)	Added Sugar (g)	Fiber (g)	Chol. (mg)	Sodium (mg)	Calcium (mg)	Iron (mg)
Crackers-wheat	4 crackers	18 g	70	1	2.22	0.44	8	0.5	1.5	0	75	0	0.4
Croissants	1 croissant	72 g	310	7	19	11.22	27	6	2	0	240	38	1.8
Croutons	4 tablespoons	10 g	46	1	1.78	0.44	6.25	0.25	0.3	0	124	6	0.3
English muffin	1 muffin	56 g	130	5	0.89	0.33	25	1.5	1.6	0	280	96	1.7
French toast	1 slice	59 g	151	4.25	7.33	1.89	16.25	3.5	0.5	48	277	48	1.1
Fried rice	1/2 cup	99 g	165	4	5.56	1	18.25	0.75	0.6	14	484	14	1.1
Grits	1/2 cup	124 g	73	1.5	0.11	0	16	0	0.3	0	136	0	0.8
Lasagna-meat	1 serving	308 g	350	27.5	23.11	6	31	1.5	2.6	73	1040	275	2.1
Lasagna-vegetable	1 serving	326 g	315	22	12	5.89	27	0.5	4.6	40	970	350	2.3
Macaroni	1/2 cup	66 g	95	3.25	0.33	0.11	19	0	0.9	0	4	5	0.9
Macaroni and cheese	1/2 cup	126 g	191	6	8.56	2.67	22.75	0	1.4	18	434	71	1.2
Macaroni-whole wheat	1 cup	150 g	202	8	1.11	0.22	39	0	7.4	0	10	20	4.5
Matzo or melba toast	1 matzo, 5 melba	19 g	100	3.25	0.56	0.11	22.25	0	0.9	0	6	4	0.9
Meat ravioli with sauce	1 cup, 6 pieces	227 g	324	13	8.33	2.89	46.75	0.75	3.1	20	878	54	2.1
Muffins	1 muffin	77 g	240	4.5	8.5	1.67	40	9	2	24.5	310	96.5	1.4
Muffins-fat free	1 muffin	66 g	165	3	0.17	0	38	10.63	1	2	175	60	0.7
Noodles-chow mein	1/2 cup	25 g	130	3	6.44	1.11	14.5	0	0.5	2	228	4	0.8
Noodles-egg	1/2 cup	160 g	106.5	3.75	1.17	0.22	19.88	0	0.9	26.5	69	9.5	1.3
Noodles-egg, macaroni	1 cup	145 g	190	7	0.56	0.11	37	0	1.1	0	30	14	2.1
Oatmeal-flavored	1 packet	38 g	140	4	2.22	0.44	18	8.25	2.4	0	181	100	4.5
Oatmeal-plain	2/3 cup cooked	176 g	109	4	1.78	0.33	18.25	0	3.3	0	1	15	1.9
Pancakes	1 pancake	38 g	73	2	1.22	0.44	11	1.25	0.5	7	239	50	0.6
Pasta w/parmesan cheese	1/2 cup	134 g	252	6.5	14.67	6.33	22.5	0	1.1	38	479	78	1.5
Rice cake	1 large cake	8 g	35	0.75	0	0	7.5	0	0.3	0	13	0	0
Rice-brown	1/2 cup	97 g	115	2.5	0.67	0.22	25	0	1.8	0	2	12	0.5
Rice-long grain & wild, mix	1/2 cup	88 g	137	3	2	0.56	23	2	0.9	0	579	11	1.1
Rice-seasoned	1/2 cup	107 g	150	3.5	3.78	1.67	23	1	1	5	700	13	1.2
Rice-white	1/2 cup	91 g	92	2	0	0	20.5	0	0.5	0	225	10	0.7
Roll-hamburger/hotdog, wheat	1 roll	43 g	114	4	1.11	0.22	21.25	0.75	2.5	0	242	46	1
Roll-hamburger/hotdog, white	1 roll	43 g	138	3.25	2.44	0.67	22.5	2	1.4	0	271	67	1.3
Roll-hoagie, sub	1 roll	135 g	400	11	7.11	1.78	68.5	4	1.8	0	684	100	3.8
Roll-wheat	1 roll	28 g	77	2.5	1.78	0.44	11.5	1.5	1.1	0	96	50	1
Roll-white	1 roll	34 g	105	3.25	1.67	0.44	16.25	1.75	0.6	0	148	28	1
Salad-pasta	1/2 cup	87 g	250	4	16	3.33	20.75	0	0.7	28	410	40	0.7
Spaghetti	1 cup	128 g	200	7.5	1	0.22	40.5	0	1.1	0	19	14	2
Spaghetti w/meatballs	1 cup	261 g	307	12	10.56	3.89	37	0	2.7	34	1220	53	3.3
Spaghetti-whole wheat	1 cup	144 g	200	9	1.11	0.22	39.5	0	5.8	0	10	20	2.7
Stuffing	1/2 cup	93 g	210	4.5	12.67	3	17.5	2.5	0.5	22	578	40	1.1
Taboule	1/2 cup	80 g	170	3	8.67	1.33	20	0	1.6	0	290	0	0.7
Taco shell	1 shell	11 g	50	0	2	1.11	8	0	0.2	0	5	0	0

Grains, continued

	Amount	Weight	Calories	Protein (g)	Total Fat (g)	Sat Fat (g)	Carb. (g)	Added Sugar (g)	Fiber (g)	Chol. (mg)	Sodium (mg)	Calcium (mg)	Iron (mg)
Tortilla	1 tortilla	30 g	65	2	1	0.11	12	0	0.9	0	1	42	0.6
Waffles	1 waffle	39 g	110	3	4.33	0.89	13	1.75	0.8	3	279	75	1.8
Vegetables													
Artichokes	1/2 cup, 1/2 vegetable	75 g	36	2	0.11	0	7.25	0	2.6	0	42	17	0.8
Asparagus	6 spears, 1/2 cup	90 g	24	1.75	0.33	0.11	3.75	0	1.5	0	4	22	0.6
Asparagus, canned	1/2 cup	122 g	21	1.5	0.33	0.11	2.75	0	1.9	0	425	17	1.5
Bamboo shoots	1/4 cup	30 g	4	0.25	0	0	0.5	0	0.3	0	1	4	0.1
Bamboo shoots-canned	1/4 cup	33 g	6	0.5	0.11	0	1	0	0.6	0	2	1	0.1
Bean sprouts	1/2 cup	59 g	16	1.25	0	0	2.75	0	2.2	0	3	7	0.5
Bean sprouts-canned	1/2 cup	62 g	8	0.75	0	0	1.25	0	2.3	0	149	9	0.3
Beets-canned	1/2 cup	123 g	36	0.75	0	0	8	0	2.9	0	324	17	0.8
Beets-pickled	1/2 cup	119 g	82	0.75	0	0	8.5	11.25	2.8	0	250	13	0.5
Beets-raw, cooked	1/2 cup	99 g	31	0.75	0	0	6.75	0	2.5	0	49	11	0.6
Bok choy-chinese cabbage	1/2 cup	35 g	5	0.25	0	0	0.75	0	0.6	0	23	37	0.3
Broccoli-cooked	1/2 cup, 2 spears	85 g	24	1.75	0.11	0	4.25	0	2.5	0	15	68	0.8
Broccoli-raw	1/2 cup	44 g	12	0.75	0.11	0	2	0	1.5	0	12	21	0.4
Brussels sprouts	1/2 cup, 4 sprouts	78 g	32	1.5	0.33	0.11	5.75	0	2.4	0	18	24	0.8
Cabbage-raw or cooked	1/4 cup cooked, 1/2 cup raw	36 g	9	0.25	0	0	1.75	0	1	0	7	13	0.2
Carrots-canned	1/2 cup	73 g	17	0.25	0.11	0	3.75	0	2.7	0	176	19	0.5
Carrots-raw or cooked	1/2 cup, 6 sticks	69 g	26	0.5	0	0	5.75	0	2.2	0	43	21	0.4
Cauliflower-raw or cooked	1/2 cup	67 g	15	0.75	0.11	0	2.5	0	1.3	0	7	15	0.3
Celery-raw or cooked	1/2 cup, 6 sticks	68 g	10	0.25	0	0	2.25	0	1.4	0	51	25	0.2
Chef salad	1 cup	137 g	25	2.5	0.17	0	4	0	2	0	23.5	30.5	0.5
Coleslaw	1/2 cup	92 g	154	0.5	14.44	2.67	4.25	1	1.5	7	287	32	0.4
Corn	1 ear, 1/2 cup	86 g	80	1.75	0.33	0	17.5	0	4.6	0	4	2	0.5
Corn-canned	1/2 cup	120 g	83	1.5	0.44	0.11	13	5.5	4.7	0	324	5	0.4
Cucumber	1/2 cup	52 g	7	0.25	0	0	1.5	0	0.7	0	1	7	0.1
Eggplant	1/2 cup	48 g	13	0.25	0.11	0	3	0	1	0	2	3	0.2
French fries	1 regular, 1-1/4 cups	85.1 g	241	3	12.72	3.89	29.5	0	2.8	0	129.5	0	1
Fried vegetables/onions	1/2 cup, 6 onion rings	68 g	180	2	10.78	2.67	15.5	0	1	0	150	12	0.7
Green beans-canned	1/2 cup	68 g	13	0.75	0	0	2.5	0	1.5	0	170	18	0.6
Green beans-raw or cooked	1/2 cup	68 g	20	1	0	0	4	0	1.8	0	3	30	0.7
Greens-collard & mustard	1/2 cup	73 g	16	1.75	0.22	0	3.75	0	1.4	0	15	64	0.7
Greens-mustard, turnip, cooked	1/2 cup	75 g	15	1	0.11	0	2.5	0	1.4	0	16	87	0.7
Greens-mustard, turnip, raw	1/2 cup	28 g	7	0.5	0	0	1.5	0	0.9	0	9	41	0.4
Greens-turnip, canned	1/2 cup	117 g	17	1	0.22	0.11	2.5	0	2.2	0	325	138	1.8
Kale-raw or cooked	1/2 cup	55 g	20	0.75	0.11	0	3	0	1.7	0	15	47	0.6
Lettuce-endive	1/2 cup	25 g	4	0.25	0	0	0.75	0	0.7	0	6	13	0.2
Lettuce-iceberg	1 cup	55 g	7	0.5	0.11	0	1.25	0	0.6	0	5	11	0.3

	Amount	Weight	Calories	Protein (g)	Total Fat (g)	Sat Fat (g)	Carb. (g)	Added Sugar (g)	Fiber (g)	Chol. (mg)	Sodium (mg)	Calcium (mg)	Iron (mg)
Mixed vegetables-canned	1/2 cup	82 g	39	1.25	0.11	0	8	0	3.5	0	122	22	0.9
Mixed vegetables-frozen	1/2 cup	81 g	22	0.75	0	0	4.5	0	2	0	22	27	0.6
Mushrooms-canned	1/2 cup	78 g	19	1	0.11	0	3.25	0	1.1	0	178	1	0.6
Mushrooms-fresh, cooked	1/2 cup	96 g	25	1.75	0.11	0	4.25	0	1.5	0	1	7	1.7
Mushrooms-raw	1/2 cup	35 g	9	0.5	0	0	1.5	0	0.6	0	1	2	0.4
Okra	1/2 cup	81 g	26	1	0.11	0	5.5	0	2.1	0	5	55	0.5
Onions	1/2 cup	71 g	29	0.5	0.11	0	6.25	0	1.4	0	8	20	0.3
Parsnips	1/2 cup, 1/2 vegetable	79 g	64	0.75	0.11	0	14.75	0	3.2	0	8	30	0.5
Peas-green	1/2 cup	85 g	63	3.75	0.11	0	11.5	0	3.5	0	70	19	1.2
Peas-green, canned	1/2 cup	85 g	59	3.25	0.11	0	8	2.75	5.3	0	186	17	0.8
Peas-snowpeas	1/2 cup	79 g	35	2.25	0.11	0	5.75	0	3.4	0	4	37	1.6
Peppers-hot	2 tablespoons	19 g	8	0.25	0	0	1.5	0	0.2	0	1	3	0.2
Peppers-sweet, green	1/2 cup, 1/2 vegetable	56 g	12	0.25	0.11	0	2.25	0	0.6	0	2	3	0.6
Peppers-sweet, red	1/2 cup	50 g	12	0.25	0.11	0	2.25	0	0.8	0	2	3	0.6
Potato skins-cheese, bacon	2 halves	96 g	302	11	15.89	7.44	27.5	0	1.4	34	267	225	4.5
Potato-baked/boiled	1/2 baked, 1/2 cup	78 g	73	1.5	0.11	0	16.75	0	1.4	0	4	6	0.3
Potatoes-mashed	1/2 cup	107 g	118	1.5	4.56	1.44	17	0	1.8	4	340	40	0.3
Radishes	2 radishes	9 g	2	0	0	0	0.25	0	0.1	0	2	2	0
Romaine lettuce	1 cup	53 g	9	1	0.11	0	1.25	0	1.3	0	4	19	0.6
Rutabaga	1/2 cup	103 g	35	0.75	0.11	0	7.5	0	2.1	0	19	43	0.5
Salad-potato	1/2 cup	121 g	153	3	7.78	1.89	15	1.5	1.9	47	512	19	0.5
Salad-three bean	1/2 cup	121 g	80	2	0	0	16.25	1.75	5	0	540	20	3.6
Salsa	1/4 cup	57 g	32	0.75	0	0	3	0	0.9	0	680	0	0
Sauerkraut	1/2 cup	118 g	22	0.75	0.11	0	4.5	0	4.1	0	780	36	1.7
Soup-vegetable	1 cup	251 g	81	2	1.56	0.44	11.25	2.25	0.5	2	892	16	1
Spaghetti sauce	1/2 cup	117 g	118	2	5	0.89	12.75	1.5	3.3	0	589	20	1.1
Spaghetti sauce w/meat	1/2 cup	104 g	80	2	3.11	0.67	12.5	2	3.3	2	630	20	1.1
Spinach-canned	1/2 cup	107 g	25	1.75	0.33	0.11	3.25	0	3.9	0	29	135	2.5
Spinach-fresh, cooked	1/2 cup	93 g	24	1.75	0.11	0	3.75	0	3	0	73	131	1.7
Spinach-raw	1/2 cup	28 g	6	0.5	0	0	0.75	0	1.1	0	22	28	0.8
Squash-summer	1/2 cup	96 g	18	0.5	0.11	0	3.75	0	1.5	0	3	22	0.4
Squash-winter	1/2 cup	109 g	41	0.75	0	0	9.5	0	3	0	4	23	0.6
Squash-zucchini-fresh, cooked	1 cup raw, 1/2 cup cooked	112 g	18	0.75	0	0	3.5	0	1.4	0	2	19	0.5
Sweet potato	1/2 cup	154 g	98	1.25	0	0	23	0	4	0	11	30	0.5
Sweet potato-candied	1/2 cup	114 g	190	1	0	0	26.5	20	4.4	0	60	20	0.7
Tomatoes-canned or stewed	1/2 cup	121 g	34	0.75	0.11	0	6.5	0.25	2.4	0	305	33	0.7
Tomatoes-raw	1/2 cup, 4 slices	86 g	17	0.5	0.11	0	3.5	0	1.3	0	8	6	0.5
Vegetable juice	3/4 cup	182 g	35	1	0	0	8	0	1	0	650	20	0.7
Waterchestnuts-canned	1/2 cup	70 g	34	0.25	0	0	8.25	0	1.5	0	3	3	0.3
Waterchestnuts-raw	1/2 cup	62 g	66	0.75	0	0	15.75	0	1.4	0	9	7	0.4

Vegetables, continued

	Amount	Weight	Calories	Protein (g)	Total Fat (g)	Sat Fat (g)	Carb. (g)	Added Sugar (g)	Fiber (g)	Chol. (mg)	Sodium (mg)	Calcium (mg)	Iron (mg)
Watercress-raw	1/2 cup	17 g	2	0.25	0	0	0.25	0	0.2	0	7	20	0
Wax beans	1/2 cup	68 g	18	1	0.11	0	4.25	0	1.5	0	6	27	0.6
Yams	1/2 cup	70 g	69	1.25	0.11	0	16.75	0	1.8	0	7	8	0.3
Fruits													
Apple cider	3/4 cup	186 g	94	0	0.11	0	17	6	0.1	0	6	7	0.4
Apples-sweetened	1/2 cup	102 g	68	0	0.11	0	12.5	3.25	2	0	4	4	0.3
Apples-unsweetened	1 fruit, 1/2 cup	133 g	77	0.25	0.44	0.11	20	0	2.1	0	0	8	0.2
Applesauce-sweetened	1/2 cup	128 g	97	0.25	0	0	3.75	10.75	1.1	0	3	8	0.4
Applesauce-unsweetened	1/2 cup	122 g	53	0.25	0	0	12.5	0	2.5	0	2	4	0.2
Apricots-sweetened	1 fruit	80 g	65	0.5	0	0	3.75	10.75	1.1	0	3	8	0.4
Apricots-unsweetened	1 fruit, 2 canned	35 g	17	0.5	0.11	0	4	0	0.8	0	0	5	0.2
Avocados	1/2 fruit, 1/2 cup	113 g	166	2	14.22	2.56	7.25	0	2.7	0	10	12	1
Banana	1 fruit, 1/2 cup	114 g	105	1	0.33	0.22	24	0	2.3	0	1	7	0.4
Blueberries-sweetened	1/2 cup	122 g	103	0.5	0.11	0	8.5	16.25	2.3	0	3	7	0.4
Blueberries-unsweetened	1/2 cup	75 g	41	0.5	0.22	0	9	0	1.7	0	2	5	0.2
Cherries-sweetened	1/2 cup	128 g	106	0.75	0	0	12.25	13	0.9	0	4	13	0.4
Cherries-unsweetened	10 fruits, 1/2 cup	93 g	44	0.75	0	0	10	0	0.9	0	2	12	0.4
Dates	5 fruits, 1/4 cup	43 g	118	0.75	0.22	0.11	28.5	0	3.7	0	1	14	0.5
Dried fruit	1/4 cup, 8 pieces	32 g	92	1	0	0	21.75	0	2.4	0	9	11	0.7
Figs, sweetened	2 fruit	57 g	45	0.25	0	0	7	3.75	1.3	0	1	15	0.2
Figs-unsweetened	4 fruit, 1/2 cup	67 g	144	1.63	0.61	0.11	37	0	6.4	0	4	74.5	1
Fruit cocktail	1/2 cup	125 g	56	0.5	0.11	0	14.5	2.5	1.4	0	6.5	8	0.4
Fruit cocktail-sweetened	1/2 cup	127 g	83	0.5	0	0	8.75	11	1.4	0	8	8	0.3
Fruit cocktail-unsweetened	1/2 cup	123 g	50	0.5	0	0	11.5	0	1.4	0	4	6	0.3
Grapefruit-sweetened	1/2 cup	127 g	76	0.5	0	0	10	8	0.5	0	2	18	0.5
Grapefruit-unsweetened	1/2 fruit, 1/2 cup	120 g	39	0.5	0	0	9	0	0.7	0	0	14	0.2
Grapes-sweetened	1/2 cup	128 g	94	0.5	0	0	10.5	12	0.5	0	7	12	1.2
Grapes-unsweetened	20 fruits, 1/2 cup	84 g	48	0.5	0	0	11.5	0	0.5	0	2	8	0.2
Guava	1 fruit	90 g	45	0.5	0.33	0.11	9.5	0	5	0	2	18	0.3
Juice-unsweetened	3/4 cup	186 g	90	0.5	0	0	22.5	0	0.2	0	8	16	0.5
Kiwi fruit	1 fruit	76 g	46	0.75	0.33	0.11	10	0	2.1	0	4	20	0.3
Mango	1/2 fruit, 1/2 cup	93 g	61	0.5	0.11	0	14.25	0	1.8	0	2	9	0.2
Melon	1/2 cup	97 g	30	0.5	0	0	7	0	0.7	0	9	8	0.2
Nectarines	1 fruit	137 g	68	1	0.56	0	14.5	0	3.3	0	0	6	0.3
Olives	3 olives	12 g	15	0.25	1.56	0.22	0.25	0	0.3	0	234	8	0.2
Orange	1 fruit, 1/2 cup	134 g	63	1	0	0	14	0	3.9	0	1	53	0.2
Papaya	1/2 fruit, 1/2 cup	146 g	56	0.75	0	0	12.75	0	1.8	0	4	35	0.2
Peaches-sweetened	1/2 cup	125 g	94	0.5	0	0	5.25	17	1.2	0	8	3	0.4
Peaches-unsweetened	1 fruit, 1/2 cup	113 g	44	0.5	0	0	10.75	0	1.3	0	3	5	0.1
Pears-sweetened	2 halves	158 g	103	0.5	0	0	6	18.5	3.2	0	8	8	0.4

	Amount	Weight	Calories	Protein (g)	Total Fat (g)	Sat Fat (g)	Carb. (g)	Added Sugar (g)	Fiber (g)	Chol. (mg)	Sodium (mg)	Calcium (mg)	Iron (mg)
Pears-unsweetened	1 fruit, 1/2 cup	136 g	98	0.75	0.67	0	25	0	4.3	0	0	18	0.4
Pineapple-sweetened	2 slices, 1/2 cup	120 g	93	0.5	0	0	7.5	15	0.9	0	2	15	0.4
Pineapple-unsweetened	2 slices, 1/2 cup	108 g	70	0.25	0	0	17.5	0	0.9	0	2	6	0.4
Plums-sweetened	2 plums	89 g	67	0.5	0.11	0	8	7.75	0.7	0	17	9	0.7
Plums-unsweetened	1 raw, 2 canned	69 g	37	0.5	0	0	8.25	0	0.9	0	1	5	0.2
Prunes-cooked	1/2 cup, 7 fruits	123 g	136	1.25	0.33	0	32	0	4.9	0	3	29	1.4
Prunes-dried	1/2 cup	74 g	209	2	0.44	0	49.25	0	6.8	0	4	45	2.1
Pumpkin-canned	1/2 cup	122 g	41	0.75	0.11	0.11	8.75	0	3.5	0	6	32	1.7
Raisins	1/4 cup	38 g	109	1	0	0	26	0	2.5	0	5	19	0.8
Raspberries-sweetened	1/2 cup	132 g	117	0.75	0.11	0	12	18.25	4.2	0	0	19	0.5
Raspberries-unsweetened	1/2 cup	62 g	30	0.5	0.22	0	6.5	0	3	0	0	14	0.3
Strawberries-sweetened	1/2 cup	133 g	100	0.5	0.11	0	9	15	2	0	4	14	0.6
Strawberries-unsweetened	1/2 cup	74 g	24	0.5	0.22	0	5.5	0	1.6	0	2	11	0.5
Tangerines-sweetened	1/2 cup	126 g	76	0.5	0	0	10	8.5	0.9	0	8	9	0.4
Tangerines-unsweetened	1 fruit, 1/2 cup	102 g	43	0.5	0	0	9.75	0	0.9	0	2	14	0.1
Watermelon	1/2 cup	80 g	25	0.5	0.22	0.22	5	0	0.3	0	2	6	0.2
Dairy													
Buttermilk	1 cup	245 g	99	8.75	2	1.33	11.25	0	0	9	257	285	0.1
Cheese spread	2 tablespoons	28 g	81	3.5	6.56	4.33	2	0	1	89	293	95	1
Cheese-American	1 ounce, 1 slice	28 g	106	6.75	8.22	5.44	0.5	0	0	27	406	174	0.1
Cheese-cheddar	1 ounce, 1 slice	28 g	113	7.5	8.67	5.89	0.5	0	0	30	177	203	0.2
Cheese-cottage	1/2 cup	109 g	113	14.5	4.78	3.11	3	0	0	17	440	65	0.2
Cheese-cottage, nonfat	1/2 cup	113 g	90	14	0	0	7	0	0	10	400	60	0
Cheese-cottage, lowfat	1/2 cup	113 g	96	15	1.22	0.78	4	0	0	5	440	74	0.2
Cheese-mozzarella	1 ounce, 1 slice	28 g	80	6	5.67	3.67	0.5	0	0	22	106	147	0.1
Cheese-mozzarella, light	1 ounce	28 g	72	7.25	4.11	2.78	0.75	0	0	16	150	183	0.1
Cheese-nonfat	1 ounce, 1 slice	28 g	40	8	0	0	1	0	0	5	290	210	0
Cheese-parmesan/romano	1 tablespoon	5 g	20	2	1.33	0.89	0.25	0	0	4	82	61	0
Cheese-provolone	1 ounce, 1 slice	28 g	100	7.75	7	4.78	0.5	0	0	20	248	214	0.2
Cheese-reduced fat	1 ounce, 1 slice	28 g	80	8	5	3	1	0	0	20	220	350	0
Cheese-ricotta	1/2 cup	124 g	216	15	14.89	10	3.75	0	0	63	104	257	0.5
Cheese-ricotta, part skim	1/2 cup	119 g	166	14.5	8.67	5.67	6.25	0	0	37	143	369	0.3
Cheese-Swiss	1 ounce	28 g	101	8	6.89	4.67	0.75	0	0	25	231	246	0.1
Hot cocoa prepared w/milk	1 cup	250 g	218	8	9	5.67	13.5	11.25	3	33	123	298	0.8
Ice cream	1/2 cup	70 g	148	2.5	7.44	4.67	4.5	11.75	0.2	30	58	88	0.3
Ice milk	1/2 cup	66 g	110	3	2.78	1.89	10	8	0.3	8	75	100	1
Lowfat chocolate milk	1 cup	258 g	175	8.5	3.78	2.33	12.25	16	1.3	12	150	294	0.7
Meal replacement drinks	1 cup	314 g	200	14	1	0.44	36	17	4	5	230	500	6.3
Milk-chocolate	1 cup	250 g	208	8.5	7.89	5.11	10.5	14.5	1.1	30	149	280	0.6
Milk-lowfat	1 cup	244 g	112	8.75	3.56	2.22	11.25	0	0	14	123	299	0.1

	Amount	Weight	Calories	Protein (g)	Total Fat (g)	Sat Fat (g)	Carb. (g)	Added Sugar (g)	Fiber (g)	Chol. (mg)	Sodium (mg)	Calcium (mg)	Iron (mg)
Dairy, continued													
Milk-skim	1 cup	245 g	86	9	0.44	0.33	11.5	0	0	4	126	302	0.1
Milk-whole	1 cup	244 g	150	8.5	7.67	5	11	0	0	33	120	291	0.1
Tofutti	1/2 cup	66 g	150	2.5	6.67	1.11	9	11	1.5	0	105	1	0.6
Yogurt-frozen	1/2 cup	96 g	100	3	1.78	1.11	8	10.25	0.1	7	59	100	1
Yogurt-lowfat w/fruit	1 container	227 g	240	9	3	2	27	16	0.3	10	120	330	1
Yogurt-nonfat w/fruit	1 container	96 g	95	3.5	0	0	8	12	0	0	70	150	1
Yogurt-plain, lowfat	1 container	227 g	142	11.25	3.67	2.44	15.75	0	0	15	160	422	0.6
Yogurt-plain, nonfat	1 container	227 g	110	11	0.22	0.22	16	0	0	4	160	430	1
Yogurt-plain, whole milk	1 container	198 g	145	8.75	6.89	4.56	11.5	0	0	32	123	312	0.6
Yogurt-w/fruit, artificial sweetener	1 container	184 g	90	7	0.67	0.44	14	0	0.5	5	110	250	1
Protein Foods													
Bacon substitute	1 strip	12 g	52	3	4.11	1.56	0	0	0	13	207	1	0.2
Beans-baked	1/2 cup	121 g	140	6	1.67	0.67	15	7.5	6	8	423	60	2.1
Beans-black	1/2 cup	86 g	113	6.5	0.33	0.11	20.75	0	4.4	0	1	24	1.8
Beans-kidney, pinto	1/2 cup	86 g	115	6.5	0.33	0.11	22.25	0	4.5	0	2	33	2.4
Beans-kidney, pinto, canned	1/2 cup	125 g	104	5.75	0.22	0	19.5	0	6.1	0	445	35	1.6
Beans-lima	1/2 cup	90 g	94	5.5	0.22	0.11	17.5	0	4.6	0	26	25	1.8
Beans-lima, canned	1/2 cup	124 g	93	4.75	0.22	0.11	17.5	0	5.8	0	309	35	2
Beans-navy, chickpeas	1/2 cup	87 g	132	6.75	1	0.22	23.75	0	4.8	0	4	52	2.4
Beans-navy, chickpeas, canned	1/2 cup	126 g	146	7	0.78	0.11	27.5	0	5	0	473	51	2
Beans-white, canned	1/2 cup	131 g	153	8.25	0.22	0.11	29.25	0	5	0	7	96	3.9
Beans-white, split peas	1/2 cup	93 g	125	7	0.22	0.11	23	0	5.3	0	2	66	2.6
Beef stew	1 cup	247 g	207	15.25	9	4.22	16.5	0.5	2.5	53	616	29	2.6
Beef-corned	3 ounces	85 g	182	18.25	12.11	5.22	0	0.25	0	65	768	11	1.5
Beef-mixed dish	1 cup	186 g	310	19.25	13.56	5.89	23.5	1.25	2.1	68	840	52	3.5
Biscuit w/egg, meat, cheese	1 biscuit	168 g	489	18.75	31.22	9.67	29	4	0.8	347	1240	151	2.9
Bologna sandwich	1 sandwich	106 g	311	11	18	6.56	22	3.75	1.7	32	845	60	2.5
Broadbeans-fava	1/2 cup	85 g	93	5.5	0.22	0	17	0	4.4	0	4	31	1.3
Broadbeans-fava, canned	1/2 cup	128 g	91	6	0.11	0	16.25	0	4.5	0	580	34	1.3
Burrito	1 burrito	230 g	213	8	7.22	3.56	29	0	3.2	33	558	53	2.3
Caviar	1 tablespoon	16 g	40	4.25	2.11	0.78	0.5	0	0	94	240	44	1.8
Cheeseburger (large) & roll	1 sandwich	280 g	711	32	43.33	16.78	33	4	1	113	1164	295	5
Cheeseburger (lowfat) & roll	1 sandwich	219 g	370	24	14	5	35	3.5	1.6	75	890	200	3.6
Cheeseburger (small) & roll	1 sandwich	172 g	461	29	27.56	13.67	25.25	3	0.8	95	906	245	3.3
Chicken breast sandwich	1 sandwich	195 g	509	26	26.89	4.78	34.75	1.75	1.7	83	1082	80	2.7
Chicken fingers/nuggets	4 fingers, 6 nuggets	98.5 g	275	15.75	14	3.11	15.25	0	0.4	49	558	7	0.8
Chicken salad	1/2 cup	84 g	179	14.75	12.22	2.89	0.75	0.75	0.3	118	329	21	0.9
Chicken wings	10 wings	257 g	617	39	46.56	13.56	15	1	0.4	198	1581	36	1.8
Chicken w/skin	3 ounces	85 g	189	22.25	9.22	2.56	0	0	0	70	60	12	1

Amount	Weight	Calories	Protein (g)	Total Fat (g)	Sat Fat (g)	Carb. (g)	Added Sugar (g)	Fiber (g)	Chol. (mg)	Sodium (mg)	Calcium (mg)	Iron (mg)
Chicken w/out skin	3 ounces	85 g	147	24.5	3.89	1.11	0	0	0	72	63	12	0.9
Chicken-fried, no skin	4 ounces	113 g	107	19.25	4.22	1.33	0.25	0	0	50	46	9	0.8
Chicken-fried, w/skin	3 ounces	85 g	155	15.75	8.44	2.44	4.75	0	0.2	52	149	11	0.8
Chicken-mixed dish	1 cup	216 g	365	15.25	17.78	5.56	13.5	0	1	103	600	30	2.2
Chickpeas	1/2 cup	101 g	138	6.5	1.67	0.11	24.75	0	4.8	9	183	39	2
Chili con carne	1 cup	247 g	286	15.75	12.44	5.78	28.5	0	6.5	43	964	86	3
Chili-vegetarian	1 cup	226 g	240	18	12	1.78	13	2	16.4	0	860	6	3.2
Chimichanga	1 chimichanga	182 g	425	18.5	17.11	8.33	41.25	0	5.2	30	933	145	4
Chop suey	1 cup	250 g	300	26	16	4.33	13	0	1.5	68	1053	60	4.8
Chow mein-beef or chicken	3/4 cup	165 g	65	6.5	1.44	0.56	5.25	0.75	1.4	26	845	80	1.3
Clams, oyster, shrimp-fried	4 pieces	43 g	103	5.25	6.11	1.11	6	0	0.1	23	183	20	0.6
Clams, oysters, shrimp	1/2 cup, 3 ounces	90 g	71	12.25	1.22	0.33	2.5	0	0	62	108	41	6
Coconut-shredded	2 tablespoons	10 g	44	0.25	3	2.67	2.25	2.25	0.4	0	24	1	0.2
Crabmeat	3 ounces	85 g	86	12.5	1	0.22	4.5	0	0	26	713	25	0.4
Egg salad	1/2 cup	103 g	267	11	22.89	5.78	1	3	0.3	418	513	43	1.8
Egg-boiled, poached	1 egg	50 g	79	6.5	5.56	2.11	0.5	0	0	274	69	28	1
Egg-fried, scrambled	1 egg	55 g	89	6.25	6.78	3	1	0	0	281	150	37	0.9
Egg-omelet	1 omelet (3 eggs)	228 g	382.5	24.13	25.17	7.33	6	0	0.4	675	625	171.5	2.6
Egg-substitute	1/4 cup	56 g	43	5.5	1.56	0.22	1.5	0	0	0	115	30	0.8
Eggroll	1 eggroll	85 g	173	6.75	4.56	0.89	25	3	0.8	7	471	20	1.1
Enchilada	1 enchilada	178 g	322	10.5	16.89	9.67	30	0	5.8	42	1052	276	2.2
Fish casserole	1 cup	259 g	407	18.5	23.78	7.56	26.25	0.75	1.8	70	1314	182	2.3
Fish sandwich	1 sandwich	177 g	488	19	26.56	5.89	39.25	3.75	1.5	70	928	46	2
Fish sticks	3 pieces	57 g	150	6.75	8.22	2.22	12	0.75	0.7	15	280	0	0.5
Fish-fried	3 ounces	85 g	209	8.75	11.56	2.67	16.25	1.25	0.7	39	350	0	0.5
Fish-not fried	3 ounces	85 g	81	17	1	0.33	7.5	0	0	45	57	13	0.4
Fish-smoked, pickled	1 ounce	28 g	56	6.25	2.33	0.67	0	0	0	14	235	5	0.3
Grilled cheese sandwich	1 sandwich	120 g	442	17	30.67	13.78	23	2.25	1.7	53	1200	402	1.8
Ground beef-lean	3 ounces, 3/4 cup	85 g	228	22.5	13.94	5.44	0	0	0	76.5	62.5	8	2.1
Ground beef-regular	3 ounces, 3/4 cup	85 g	246	20.75	17.56	6.89	0	0	0	80	71	9	2.1
Ham	3 ounces	85 g	124	15.75	6.56	2.33	0	0	0	41	1064	6	0.8
Ham sandwich	1 sandwich	140 g	343	23.5	15.89	7.67	23	2	1.7	60	1577	229	2.5
Hamburger (large) & roll	1 sandwich	228 g	594	27.5	33	12.67	33.25	2	0.9	101	688	87	4.8
Hamburger (lowfat) & roll	1 sandwich	206 g	320	22	10	4	35	3.5	1.6	60	670	150	3.6
Hamburger (small) & roll	1 sandwich	137 g	355	22	19.33	8.22	22.25	3	1.7	95	556	71	3.2
Hot dog	1 hot dog	50 g	144	5.75	12.89	5.22	0.25	1.25	0	30	547	20	0.7
Hot dog and roll	1 sandwich	105 g	298	9.25	17.56	6.67	20	2.5	0.7	29	880	60	2.2
Julienne salad	2 cup	483 g	489	47.5	29	13.89	7.5	0	3.5	281	1340	360	3.4
Lamb	3 ounces	85 g	169	19.75	11.11	5.33	0	0	0	68	49	8	1.5
Lentils	1/2 cup	99 g	115	7.75	0.22	0	20.25	0	2.8	0	2	19	3.3
Liver	3 ounces	85 g	127	17.75	4.56	2	2.5	0	0	258	52	8	5.8
Luncheon meat-beef, pork	2 slice	56 g	152	8.5	12.22	5.11	0	1	0	36	696	6	0.8

Protein Foods, continued

	Amount	Weight	Calories	Protein (g)	Total Fat (g)	Sat Fat (g)	Carb. (g)	Added Sugar (g)	Fiber (g)	Chol. (mg)	Sodium (mg)	Calcium (mg)	Iron (mg)
Luncheon meat-chicken, turkey	2 slice	56 g	64	11.5	1.33	0.44	0	0	0	24	716	6	0.6
Luncheon meat-lean	2 slice	56 g	90	8	4	3.11	3	1.5	0	30	586	0	0.8
Meatloaf	3 ounces	85 g	204	16	12	4.44	7	0.25	0.7	104	303	18	2
Miso	1/2 cup	138 g	284	14.25	7.33	1.11	39.25	0	7.4	0	5032	92	3.8
Nuts-mixed	3 tablespoons, 26 nuts	28 g	170	4.25	13.56	2.22	6.25	0	1.6	0	170	20	1.1
Pate	1 tablespoon	13 g	41	2	3.67	1.44	0	0	0	51	91	9	0.7
Peanut butter	2 tablespoons	32 g	190	9	14.56	2.78	4.5	0	2.4	0	150	11	0.6
Peanut butter & jelly sandwich	1 sandwich	101 g	371	12.25	17.89	3.56	26.5	17.75	3.8	0	426	66	2.2
Peanuts	3 tablespoons, 32 nuts	28 g	164	6.25	12.33	1.78	5.25	0	2.5	0	110	7	0.5
Peas-black eyed	1/2 cup	86 g	100	5.75	0.33	0.11	18.25	0	8.3	0	3	21	2.2
Peas-black eyed, canned	1/2 cup	120 g	92	5	0.33	0.11	16.5	0	8.2	0	359	24	1.2
Pepperoni	3 ounces	85 g	440	16.5	41.56	14.56	2.25	2	0	72	1589	5	0.6
Pizza-cheese & vegetable	1 slice	130 g	249	12.5	9.22	5.11	30	0.5	4	15	518	195	2.3
Pizza-cheese topping	1 slice	65 g	199	11.5	8.44	4.44	28.25	0.5	2	17	456	250	1.2
Pizza-cheese, meat & vegetable	1 slice	120 g	270	16	12.44	6	26.5	0.5	3.5	27	682	230	2.5
Pizza-French bread	1 slice	164 g	410	17.5	19.22	8	39	2	2	35	1030	200	2.7
Pizza-meat topping	1 slice	106 g	271	11.5	13	5.33	27	0.5	1.2	20	733	132	1.8
Pork and beans	1/2 cup	126 g	134	6.5	1.89	0.67	17	8	6.6	9	521	71	2.1
Pork chop	3 ounces	85 g	217	23.5	12.89	4.89	0	0	0	70	48	21	0.8
Pork chop-lean cut	3 ounces	85 g	177	0	8	0	0	0	0	0	0	0	0
Pork feet	8 ounces	227 g	138	14.5	8.78	3.22	0	0	0	71	597	32	1.1
Pork rinds	3 ounces	113 g	458	51.75	26	10	0	0	0	80	2275	19	0.5
Pork roast	3 ounces	85 g	232	23	15	5.56	0	0	0	78	53	16	1
Pork roast-lean cut	3 ounces	85 g	180	24	8.33	3.11	0	0	0	78	55	14	1.2
Pork spareribs	3 ounces	113 g	132	10.25	9.89	3.89	0	0	0	41	31	16	0.6
Pork-fresh, fried	3 ounces	114 g	144	11	11.22	4.22	0	0	0	41	25	4	0.4
Pork-fresh, roasted	4 ounces	114 g	164	15.75	10.22	3.89	0	0	0	54	37	4	0.6
Refried beans	1/2 cup	113 g	135	6	1.33	0.56	18	0	6	0	400	40	2.2
Roast beef sandwich	1 sandwich	164 g	353	27.25	14.89	7.33	30.25	2.25	1.7	49	766	87	4.1
Roast beef-lean cut	3 ounces	85 g	156	24.75	5.67	1.89	0	0	0	69	54	4	2.7
Roast beef-regular	3 ounces	85 g	222.5	22.75	13.5	5.11	0	0	0	69.5	53	5	2.4
Sausage	3 ounces	85 g	264	12	22.33	8.67	0	1.5	0	42	774	12	1.2
Seafood or fish salad	1/2 cup	104 g	160	13.5	9.78	2.33	1.75	0.25	0.4	142	250	31	0.9
Sloppy Joe sandwich	1 sandwich	146 g	302	18.5	13.78	6	23.75	2.5	1.4	63	509	31	0.9
Soybeans-roasted	1/4 cup	44 g	205	14.25	10.22	1.56	13.5	0	1.9	0	1	89	2
Steak	3 ounces	85 g	191	24	9.33	3.44	0	0	0	71	54	7	2.7
Steak-lean cut	3 ounces	85 g	176	24.5	7.89	3	0	0	0	69	56	5	2.4
Submarine/hoagy	1 submarine	401 g	934	34.5	51.22	12.67	73.25	3.75	3.1	87	1538	294	5.7
Sweet & sour chicken, pork	1 cup	258 g	426	17.5	13.89	3.33	23.5	31.75	1.3	83	1209	27	1.9

Amount	Weight	Calories	Protein (g)	Total Fat (g)	Sat Fat (g)	Carb. (g)	Added Sugar (g)	Fiber (g)	Chol. (mg)	Sodium (mg)	Calcium (mg)	Iron (mg)
Taco	1 taco	171 g	370	21	18.44	11.11	26.5	0	3.4	57	802	221	2.4
Taco salad	1-1/2 cup	198 g	279	13.5	13.33	6.67	24	0	4.3	44	763	192	2.3
Tahini	1 tablespoon	16 g	92	2.5	7.33	1.11	3.75	0	1.5	0	10	109	2.2
Tofu	3 ounces	85 g	65	6.75	2.33	0.33	2.25	0	1	0	8	68	1.1
Tostada	1 tostada	198 g	325	13.75	13.89	9.67	28	0	7.5	40	834	214	2.2
Tripe	4 ounces	114 g	61	12.5	1.11	0.67	0	0	0	58	44	77	0.3
Tuna casserole	1 cup, 18 chips	231 g	248	16	10.44	3.33	26.75	0	0.7	36	1072	120	1.4
Tuna in oil	1/2 cup	74 g	142	22	5.44	1.11	0	0	0	18	275	7	0.8
Tuna in water	1/2 cup	74 g	90	19.25	1.44	0.44	0	0	0	28	400	0	0.7
Tuna salad	1/2 cup	102 g	183	14	9.44	1.89	2.25	0	0.4	13	412	23	0.8
Tuna sandwich	1 sandwich	120 g	364.5	16.25	23	4.11	24.13	2.25	1.7	25	599	53	2
Turkey hot dog	1 hot dog	45.4 g	102	6.5	8	3.11	0.25	1.5	1.7	51	641	51	0.9
Turkey sandwich	1 sandwich	194 g	355	30.25	14.67	2.67	23.5	2.25	1.7	76	385	75	3.3
Turkey w/skin	3 ounces	85 g	168	24	7.89	2.11	0	0	0	70	57	20	1.5
Turkey w/out skin	3 ounces	85 g	137	25.5	3.22	1	0	0	0	72	64	19	1.5
Veal	3 ounces	85 g	195	25.63	10.17	4	0	0	0	95.5	69.5	16.5	1
Veal-lean cut	3 ounces	85 g	167	27	5.33	1.67	0	0	0	98	76	20	1
Veal-mixed dish	1 serving	168 g	327	28.25	17.78	9.78	9.5	0.75	1.7	137	634	138	3.7
Venison	3 ounces	85 g	147	25.75	3.11	1.22	0	0	0	95	280	6	3.8
Beverages												
Beer-nonalcoholic	12 fluid ounces, 1-1/2 cups	359 g	55	0.75	0	0	11	0	0	0	19	25	0.1
Coffee	1 cup	237 g	5	0.25	0	0	1	0	0	0	7	6	0.6
Coffee-decaffeinated	1 cup	239 g	3	0.25	0	0	0.75	0	0	0	8	8	0.1
Cola	12 fluid ounces	366 g	150	0	0	0	0	37	0	0	70	0	0
Cola diet	12 fluid ounces	360 g	2	0.25	0	0	0.25	0	0	0	70	0	0
Cola-diet, no caffeine	12 fluid ounces	358 g	2	0	0	0	0	0	0	0	70	0	0
Cola-no caffeine	12 fluid ounces	363 g	155	0	0	0	0	38.75	0	0	73	0	0
Juice drink	3/4 cup, 1 juice box	190 g	106	0	0	0	6.5	19.5	0	0	7	1	1
Mellow Yellow, Mountain Dew	12 fluid ounces	371 g	177	0	0	0	0	44	0	0	30	0	0
Noncola-diet, no caffeine	12 fluid ounces	342 g	4	0	0	0	0.5	0	0	0	42	0	0
Noncola-no caffeine	12 fluid ounces	364 g	157	0	0	0	0	37.75	0	0	46	2	0.1
Postum	1 teaspoon	3 g	12	0	0	0	3	0	1.3	0	0	0	0
Tea-herbal, no caffeine	1 cup	240 g	4	0	0	0	0.75	0	0	0	3	5	0.2
Tea-plain	1 cup	239 g	3	0	0	0	0.5	0	0	0	0	0	0
Wine-nonalcoholic	5 fluid ounces	136 g	42	0.5	0	0	9.75	0	0	0	7	12	0.6
Beverages-Alcoholic												
Beer	12 fluid ounces, 1-1/2 cups	360 g	145	1	0	0	13.25	0	0	0	8	12	0
Beer-light	12 fluid ounces, 1-1/2 cups	355 g	110	1	0	0	7	0	0	0	8	15	0
Chianti	5 fluid ounces	148 g	106	0.25	0	0	2.5	0	0	0	8	12	0.6
Cocktail-mixed drink	1 cocktail	134 g	139	0	0	0	1	1.5	0	0	6	4	0.1

© 2002, DINE Systems, Inc., 586 N. French Rd., Amherst, NY 14228

Beverages-Alcoholic, continued

Amount	Weight	Calories	Protein (g)	Total Fat (g)	Sat Fat (g)	Carb. (g)	Added Sugar (g)	Fiber (g)	Chol. (mg)	Sodium (mg)	Calcium (mg)	Iron (mg)
Liqueur	1 glass, 1-1/2 ounces	50 g	167	0	0.11	0	8.5	9.5	0	0	4	1	0
Liquor	1 jigger, 1-1/2 fluid ounces	42 g	110	0	0	0	0	0	0	0	0	0	0
Vermouth	5 fluid ounces	148 g	100	0.25	0	0	1	0	0	0	8	12	0.4
Wine	5 fluid ounces	148 g	104	0.25	0	0	2.5	0	0	0	12	12	0.4
Wine cooler	12 fluid ounces, 1-1/2 cups	360 g	173	0.75	0	0	7.75	9.75	0	0	25	32	1.4
Wine-light	5 fluid ounces	148 g	73	0.5	0	0	1	0	0	0	10	13	0.6

Fats/Sweets/Other

Amount	Weight	Calories	Protein (g)	Total Fat (g)	Sat Fat (g)	Carb. (g)	Added Sugar (g)	Fiber (g)	Chol. (mg)	Sodium (mg)	Calcium (mg)	Iron (mg)
Bacon	1 slice	9.25 g	37	2.35	3.11	1.16	0.09	0.05	0	8	160.5	0.88	0.2
Bacon bits	1-1/2 tablespoons	7 g	21	2.5	1.11	0.33	0	0	0	6	181	1	0.1
Breakfast milk powder	1 packet	36 g	130	6	0	0	0	26.25	0.4	0	185	80	4.5
Brownie	1 square	38 g	150	2	6.22	1.67	6.5	15	0.9	10	105	1	0.7
Butter	1 teaspoon, 1 pat	5 g	34.7	0	3.81	2.41	0	0	0	10.7	39.7	0.7	0.3
Cake	1 piece	98 g	280	4	11.33	3	15.25	22.25	0.5	56	285	57	1
Candy-chewy	1 ounce	28 g	109	0	1	0.56	1.5	20.5	0	0	32	1	0
Candy-chocolate & peanut butter	1 package, 1-1/2 ounces	47 g	237	6	13.78	5.89	4	22	2.5	3	90	34	0.7
Candy-chocolate	1 ounce	28 g	150	2	8.22	4.78	2.25	15	0.8	6	24	50	0.3
Candy-chocolate covered	1 ounce	28 g	132	1.25	5.56	2.11	3	13.25	1.5	3	43	33	0.4
Candy-fudge	1 cube	28.4 g	119	1	4.06	1.06	1.7	17.93	0.4	2.7	54.1	27	0.3
Candy-hard	5 pieces	28 g	110	0	0	0	2.75	27.5	0	0	7	3	0.1
Catsup	1 tablespoon	15 g	17	0	0	0	2.75	1.5	0.2	0	168	3	0.1
Cheese puffs	1 cup	28 g	160	2	9.78	1.78	16	0	0.3	0	330	0	0.4
Cheese sauce	1/4 cup	70 g	71	3.5	3.56	1.89	6.5	0	0	10	412	139	0.1
Chili sauce	1 tablespoon	15 g	17	0.25	0	0	2.75	1.25	0.9	0	196	2	0.1
Chip dip	1/4 cup	60 g	120	2	10	6	4	0.5	0	40	360	80	0
Coffee whitener	1 tablespoon	11 g	22	0	2.11	1.33	2.25	1	0	0	12	1	1
Cookies-fig bars	2 bars	28 g	100	1	1.78	0.44	10.5	10.5	1.2	1	90	20	0.7
Cookies-nonfat	2 cookies	23 g	75	1	0	0	17.5	6.5	0.6	0	115	0	0.2
Cookies-oatmeal raisin	3 cookies	40 g	195	2.25	8.11	1.89	13.5	13.5	1.4	1	150	0	0.8
Cookies-others	3 cookies	42 g	180	1.5	8.11	2.89	10	15	0.3	3	131	1	0.7
Corn chips	1 cup	28 g	152	2	9.44	1.33	16	0	1.3	0	205	36	0.2
Cream cheese	2 tablespoons	30 g	106	2.5	10.22	6.67	1	0	0	34	90	24	0.4
Cream cheese-light	2 tablespoons	28 g	80	3	7	4	1	0	0	25	115	20	1
Cream-coffee, half & half	1 tablespoon	15 g	25	0.5	2.22	1.44	0.5	0	0	8	6	15	0
Cream-whipped	1 tablespoon	5 g	15	0.25	1.33	1.11	0.25	0.25	0	2	4	3	1
Cupcakes	1 cupcake	39 g	140	1.25	4.56	1.89	8.5	15	0.7	12	121	24	0.6
Danish	1 danish	71 g	252	4.5	11.67	3.67	10.25	19	0.7	14	249	36	1.1
Danish-nonfat	1 danish	33 g	90	2	0	0	20	9.75	0.2	0	85	20	1
Dessert topping-no sugar	1 tablespoon	5 g	5	0	0.56	0.44	0	0	1	4	5	2	1

Food	Amount	Weight	Calories	Protein (g)	Total Fat (g)	Sat Fat (g)	Carb. (g)	Added Sugar (g)	Fiber (g)	Chol. (mg)	Sodium (mg)	Calcium (mg)	Iron (mg)
Diet bar	1 bar	31 g	120	2	4	1.44	19	9.5	3	1	30	150	2.7
Doughnut or sweet roll	1 doughnut, 1 sweet roll	60 g	220	3.75	9.89	3.33	29.5	18	1	5	230	22	1.1
Frozen desserts-nonfat	1/2 cup	68 g	100	2	0.22	0.11	23.5	9.5	0.4	1	48	100	0.2
Frozen yogurt cone-lowfat	1 serving	85 g	105	4	1	0.56	22	13	0.1	3	80	112	0.2
Frozen yogurt sundae-lowfat	1 sundae	171 g	240	6	3	2.33	50.5	43	0.8	6	170	190	0.1
Gelatin	1/2 cup	127 g	105	2	1	1	23	22	0	0	57	0	0
Gelatin-sugar free	1/2 cup	121 g	8	1.5	0	0	0	0	0	0	31	0	0
Granola bars	1 bar	28 g	133	2	6	2	18.25	13	0.6	0	70	20	0.5
Gravy	1/4 cup	60 g	30	1	1.44	0.56	2.25	0.5	0.1	1	260	3	0.4
Hollandaise sauce	1/4 cup	64 g	230	2.25	23.44	8.44	2.5	0	0	140	316	50	1
Honey	2 teaspoons	14 g	42	0	0	0	0	10.5	0	0	1	1	0.1
Hot cocoa mix	1 envelope	26 g	110	1.5	2.78	1.56	3.5	16	1.1	2	165	40	0.7
Ice cream bar	1 bar	57 g	172	2	11.78	7.11	6	11.5	0.3	17	50	80	0
Jam or jelly	2 teaspoons	13 g	35	0	0	0	1	7.5	0.1	0	1	1	1
Lard	1 tablespoon	13 g	115	0	12.22	5	0	0	0	12	0	0	0
Margarine-stick	1 teaspoon, 1 pat	5 g	33.7	0	3.52	0.67	0	0	0	0	44.3	1.3	0
Margarine-stick, light	1 teaspoon, 1 pat	5 g	20	0	2.22	0.33	0	0	0	0	36.7	0.33	0.3
Margarine-tub	1 tablespoon	14 g	101	0	8.89	2	0	0	0	0	152	4	0
Margarine-tub, light	1 tablespoon	14 g	50	0	5.89	1	0	0	0.1	0	110	1	1
Marshmallows	2 pieces	14 g	47	0.25	0	0	0	11.75	0	0	7	2	0.1
Mayonnaise	1 tablespoon	14 g	100	0.25	11	1.89	0.25	0.25	0	8	74	1	1
Mayonnaise-light	1 tablespoon	14 g	48	0.25	4.56	1	0.75	1	0	5	95	1	1
Mayonnaise-nonfat	1 tablespoon	16 g	12	0	0	0	3	3	0	0	190	0	0
Meal replacement bar	1 serving	48 g	270	11	14	5	24	22.5	0	0	330	250	4.5
Milkshake	10 fluid ounces, 1-1/4 cups	290 g	368	10	12.78	8.22	26.5	19.25	0.5	54	243	375	0.5
Milkshake-lowfat	1 serving	293 g	320	10.75	1.33	0.56	66	44.75	0	10	170	327	0.1
Miracle Whip	1 tablespoon	14 g	64	0	5.89	0.89	2.5	0.5	0	5	95	2	1
Miracle Whip-nonfat	1 tablespoon	16 g	20	0	0	0	5	5	0	0	210	0	0
Molasses	1 tablespoon	20 g	55	0	1.44	0	0	14.5	0	0	11	75	1.8
Mustard	1 teaspoon	5 g	6	0.25	0.33	0	0.25	0	0	0	60	0	0
Noncola-diet	12 fluid ounces, 1-1/2 cups	369 g	2	0	0	0	0.5	0	0	0	8	0	0
Nutrasweet-Equal	1 packet	1 g	4	0.5	0	0	0.5	0.5	0	0	0	0	0
Oil	1 tablespoon	14 g	120	0	12.78	1.89	0	0	0	0	0	0	0.1
Pickles-dill	2 spears	61 g	7	0	0.11	0	1	0.75	0.9	0	584	9	0.4
Pickles-sweet	1 pickle, 3 slices	18 g	18	0	0	0	0.5	4	0.3	0	107	2	0.2
Pie-custard or cream	1 slice	152 g	346	6.75	13.11	6.22	20.75	25.75	1	125	375	122	0.8
Pie-fruit	1 slice	158 g	405	4	16.22	5.33	54.75	25.25	4	6	423	17	1.6
Pie-pecan	1/6 of 9" pie	138 g	575	7	29.67	5.67	33	37.25	2.2	100	305	65	4.6
Popcorn	1 cup	11 g	32	0.75	1.44	0.44	5.5	0	0.8	0	68	0	0.2
Popsicle	1 popsicle	69 g	50	0	0	0	0	13	0	0	10	0	0
Potato chips	1 cup, 20 chips	28 g	150	2	9.67	2	15	0	1.4	0	190	0	0.4
Pretzels	2/3 cup	28 g	110	2.75	0.89	0.22	21.75	1	0.9	0	610	9	1.4

Fats/Sweets/Other, continued

	Amount	Weight	Calories	Protein (g)	Total Fat (g)	Sat Fat (g)	Carb. (g)	Added Sugar (g)	Fiber (g)	Chol. (mg)	Sodium (mg)	Calcium (mg)	Iron (mg)
Pudding	1/2 cup	147 g	150	4.5	2.22	1.44	10	18	0	9	443	152	0
Pudding-diet	1/2 cup	132 g	90	4	2.44	1.57	13	0	0.4	9	423	152	0.1
Relish	2 tablespoon	28 g	35	0	0	0	1.25	7.5	0.2	0	243	6	0.2
Saccharin	1 packet	1 g	2	0	0	0	0	0	0	0	2	0	0
Salad dressing	1 tablespoon	16 g	80	0	8.22	1.33	0.25	0.25	1	0	146	2	1
Salad dressing-light	1 tablespoon	15 g	16	0.25	0.33	0.11	0.75	0.5	0.3	0	137	1	1
Salad dressing-no oil	1 tablespoon	17 g	12	0	0	0	2.5	0	0.7	0	0	1	1
Salad dressing-nonfat	1 tablespoon	15 g	16	0	0	0	3	3	0	0	143	0	0
Salt	4 shakes	0 g	0	0	0	0	0	0	0	0	64	0	0
Sherbet	1/2 cup	97 g	136	1	1.89	1.22	6	23.5	0	7	44	52	0.2
Soft drinks	12 fluid ounces, 1-1/2 cup	369 g	156	0	0	0	0	39.5	0	0	22	0	0
Soup-beef or chicken	1 cup	266 g	74	4.25	2.22	0.67	8.5	0	1	7	910	17	0.9
Soup-bouillon, broth	1 cube, packet(s), 1 cup	5 g	9	0.75	0.22	0.11	0.25	1	0	1	965	1	0.1
Soup-broth based, no salt	1 cup	241 g	135	5.75	3.89	0.78	16.5	0	2.8	0	115	47	1.8
Soup-cream, chowder	1 cup	246 g	140	5.5	6.11	2.89	14	0	0.9	22	1010	150	0.6
Soup-low salt	1 cup	246 g	110	4	3	1	12	0	0.5	2	100	17	1.3
Soup-miso	1 cup	199 g	152	4.5	6.44	0.89	19	0	3	0	490	20	1.3
Sour cream	2 tablespoons	24 g	52	0.5	5.11	3.11	1	0	0	10	34	28	0
Sour cream-imitation	2 tablespoons	26 g	50	1.5	4.67	4	1.5	0	0	2	20	14	0
Sour cream-nonfat	2 tablespoons	28 g	16	2	0	0	2	0	0	0	20	40	0
Soy sauce	1 tablespoon	18 g	10	1.25	0	0	1.25	0	0	0	1015	3	0.4
Steak/Worcestershire sauce	1 tablespoon	15 g	11	0	0	0	1	1.75	0	0	143	0	0
Sugar	1 teaspoon	4 g	15	0	0	0	0	3.75	0	0	0	0	0
Sunflower seeds	2 tablespoons	19 g	116	3.75	10.78	1.11	4	0	1.7	0	1	11	1.3
Syrup-pancake, table	2 tablespoons	40 g	110	0	0	0	0	27.5	0	0	21	1	1
Tortilla chips	1 cup, 10 chips	19 g	95	1.25	4.67	1.33	12	0	0.9	0	123	23	0.3
White sauce	1/4 cup	63 g	99	2.5	5.67	2.22	6	0	0.1	8	222	73	0.2

© 2002, DINE Systems, Inc., 586 N. French Rd., Amherst, NY 14228

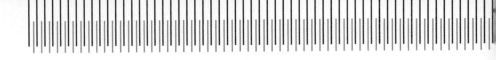

Nutritional Content of Fast Foods*

ARBY'S

BURGER KING

JACK IN THE BOX

KFC

MCDONALD'S

PIZZA HUT

TACO BELL

* Source: CyberSoft, Inc. the *NutriBase Nutrition Facts Desk Reference,* 2nd ed. Avery, a member of Penguin Putnam, Inc. © 2001 by Cybersoft, Inc.

APPENDIX C
Nutritional Content of Fast Foods

Name	Serving Size	Gram weight	Calories	Protein (g)	Carb. (g)	Total Fat (g)	Sat Fat. (g)	% Calories from Fat	Chol. (mg)	Sodium (mg)	Fiber (g)	Sugar (g)	Calcium (mg)	Iron (mg)	Vit. A (IU)	Vit. C (mg)
Arby's																
Arby's – Breakfast																
Egg, Scrambled	1.8 Oz	50	70	6	0	5	2	65.22	220	70	0	0	20	0.72	*	0
French Toastix w/o Powdered Sugar or Syrup (5 Oz)	3 Hotcakes	124	370	7	48	17	4	41.02	0	440	4	*	70	1.80	*	0
Sausage Patty	1.4 Oz	39.70	200	7	1	19	7	84.24	60	290	0	0	0	0.72	*	0
Arby's – Sides																
French Fries, Cheddar Curly	6 Oz	170	450	7.50	52	25	6	48.60	5	1420	0	*	80	2.70	*	12
French Fries, Curly, Medium	4.5 Oz	128	380	5	49	19	4.50	44.19	0	1100	0	*	0	1.80	*	12
French Fries, Homestyle, Medium	5 Oz	142	420	5	57	19	3	40.81	0	830	4	*	0	1.44	*	21
Jalapeno Bites	3.9 Oz	110	330	7	29	21	9	56.76	40	670	2	*	40	0.72	*	1.20
Mozzarella Sticks	4.8 Oz	137	470	18	34	29	14	55.65	60	1330	2	*	400	0.72	*	1.20
Onion Petals	4 Oz	113.40	410	4	43	24	3	53.47	0	300	2	*	20	0.72	*	0
Potato Cakes	2 Cakes	85.10	220	2	21	14	3	57.80	0	460	3	*	0	1.08	*	6
Potato, Baked Broccoli 'n Cheddar	13.6 Oz	384	550	14	71	25	13	39.82	50	730	7	*	250	3.96	*	63.60
Arby's – Poultry and Seafood																
Chicken Finger Meal	10.7 Oz	303	880	35	81	47	8	47.69	60	2240	0	*	0	1.80	*	9
Chicken Finger Snack	7.4 Oz	208	610	20	62	32	6	46.75	30	1610	0	*	0	1.80	*	9
Fish Fillet Sandwich	7.9 Oz	223	540	23	51	27	7	45.08	40	880	2	*	80	3.60	*	1.20
Roast Turkey Deluxe, Lowfat	6.9 Oz	196	230	19	33	5	1.50	17.79	25	870	4	*	60	2.70	*	9
Arby's – Sandwiches																
Barbecue Sandwich, Arby-Q	6.6 Oz	186	380	19	42	15	5	35.62	30	990	3	*	100	3.60	*	4.80
Chicken Bacon 'N Swiss Sandwich	7.8 Oz	222	610	37	52	30	9	43.13	75	1620	5	*	200	2.70	*	2.40
Chicken Breast Fillet Sandwich	7.6 Oz	216	560	30	49	28	6	44.37	55	1080	6	*	80	2.70	*	1.20
French Dip Sub	7.1 Oz	200	490	30	43	22	8	40.41	56	1440	3	*	120	6.30	*	1.20
Grilled Chicken Deluxe Sandwich	8.7 Oz	247	420	30	42	16	4	33.33	60	930	3	*	80	2.70	*	12
Grilled Chicken Sandwich, Lowfat	6.3 Oz	179	280	30	33	5	1.50	15.15	50	920	4	*	50	2.52	*	4.80
Italian Sub	10.3 Oz	291	800	28	49	54	16	61.21	85	2610	2	*	350	4.50	*	9

* Values Unavailable.

Name	Serving Size	Gram weight	Calories	Protein (g)	Carb. (g)	Total Fat (g)	Sat Fat. (g)	% Calories from Fat	Chol. (mg)	Sodium (mg)	Fiber (g)	Sugar (g)	Calcium (mg)	Iron (mg)	Vit. A (IU)	Vit. C (mg)
Roast Beef Sandwich, Regular	5.6 Oz	158	400	23	36	20	7	43.27	40	1030	3	*	50	4.50	*	0
Roast Chicken Club	8.4 Oz	239	540	37	39	29	8	46.19	70	1590	3	*	200	2.70	*	2.40
Roast Chicken Deluxe, Lowfat	7 Oz	196	260	23	32	5	1.50	16.98	40	950	4	*	60	2.70	*	9
Turkey Sub	10.7 Oz	303	670	29	49	39	10	52.94	60	2130	2	*	350	4.50	*	9
Arby's – Beverages and Shakes																
Milk	8 Oz	227	120	8	12	5	3	36	20	120	0	*	300	0.36	*	2.40
Orange Juice	10 Oz	283	140	1	34	0	0	0	0	0	0	*	0	0	*	78
Shake, Chocolate	10.3 Oz	292	390	8	69	9	6	20.82	10	270	0	*	250	0.90	*	*
Shake, Jamocha	10.3 Oz	292	380	8	66	9	6	21.49	10	300	0	*	250	0.90	*	*
Shake, Strawberry	10.3 Oz	292	380	8	67	9	6	21.26	10	270	0	*	250	0.90	*	*
Shake, Vanilla	10.3 Oz	292	380	8	67	9	6	21.26	12	270	0	*	250	0.90	*	0
Arby's – Salads																
Salad, Garden, w/ 1 Crouton Packet and 2 Saltine Crackers	10.2 Oz	290	110	9	16	3	0	21.26	0	150	1	*	200	0.36	*	72
Salad, Grilled Chicken, Lowfat	14.2 Oz	401	190	25	16	4	0.50	18	40	530	1	*	200	0.36	*	75
Salad, Roast Chicken, Lowfat	14.2 Oz	401	200	25	16	5	0.50	21.53	40	800	1	*	200	0.36	*	75
Arby's – Breads																
Biscuit w/Margarine	2.8 Oz	78.50	270	5	26	16	3	53.73	0	750	0	*	0	0	*	0
Croissant	2.2 Oz	62	260	6	28	16	10	51.43	20	300	0	*	0	2.70	*	0
Arby's –Dessert and Snacks																
Turnover, Iced Apple	3.4 Oz	96.10	360	4	54	14	3	35.20	0	180	6	*	0	1.44	*	1.20
Turnover, Iced Cherry	3.5 Oz	97.80	350	4	53	14	3	35.59	0	190	0	*	0	1.44	*	4.80

* Values Unavailable.

Source: CyberSoft, Inc. *The NutriBase Nutrition Facts Desk Reference.* 2nd ed. Avery, a member of Perguin Putnam, Inc. © 2001 by CyberSoft.

Burger King

Name	Serving Size	Gram weight	Calories	Protein (g)	Carb. (g)	Total Fat (g)	Sat Fat (g)	% Calories from Fat	Chol. (mg)	Sodium (mg)	Fiber (g)	Sugar (g)	Calcium (mg)	Iron (mg)	Vit. A (IU)	Vit. C (mg)
Burger King – Breakfast																
Biscuit w/Egg	1 Sandwich	132	380	11	37	21	5	49.61	140	1010	1	3	60	2.70	200	0
Biscuit w/Sausage	1 Sandwich	130	490	13	36	33	10	60.24	35	1240	1	3	40	2.70	0	0
Biscuit w/Sausage, Egg & Cheese	1 Sandwich	188	620	20	37	43	14	62.93	185	1650	1	4	150	2.70	500	0
French Toast Sticks	5 Sticks	113	440	7	51	23	5	47.15	2	490	3	12	60	1.80	0	0
Burger King – Sides																
French Fries, Medium, Salted	1 Serving	116	400	3	50	21	8	47.13	0	820	4	0	0	0.72	0	0
French Fries, Unsalted, Medium	1 Serving	116	400	3	50	21	8	47.13	0	760	4	0	0	0.72	0	0
Hash Brown Rounds, Large	1 Serving	128	410	3	42	26	10	56.52	0	750	4	0	0	1.08	0	0
Onion Rings, Medium	1 Serving	94	380	5	46	19	4	45.60	2	550	4	4	100	0.72	0	0
Cini-Minis, w/o Vanilla Icing	4 Rolls	108	440	6	51	23	6	47.59	25	710	1	20	60	2.70	1000	1.20
Burger King – Chicken																
Chicken Tenders, 5 Piece	5 Pieces	77	230	14	11	14	4	55.75	40	590	0	0	0	0.36	0	0
Patty, BK Broiler Chicken Breast	1 Serving	99	140	21	4	4	1	26.47	90	570	*	*	*	*	*	*
Burger King – Burgers																
Cheeseburger	1 Serving	133	360	21	27	19	9	47.11	60	760	1	4	150	2.70	300	0
Cheeseburger, Bacon	1 Serving	140	400	24	27	22	10	49.25	70	940	1	4	150	2.70	300	0
Cheeseburger, Double Patty	1 Serving	198	580	38	27	36	17	55.48	120	1060	1	5	250	4.50	400	0
Cheeseburger, Double Whopper	1 Serving	374	1010	55	47	67	26	59.64	180	1460	3	8	300	7.20	750	9
Cheeseburger, Whopper	1 Serving	295	760	35	47	48	17	56.84	110	1380	3	8	250	4.50	750	9
Hamburger	1 Serving	120	320	19	27	15	6	42.32	50	520	1	4	80	2.70	100	0
Hamburger, Double Whopper	1 Serving	349	920	49	47	59	21	58.03	155	980	3	8	150	7.20	500	9
Hamburger, Whopper	1 Serving	270	660	29	47	40	12	54.22	85	900	3	8	100	4.50	500	9
Burger King – Sandwiches																
Chick 'n Crisp Sandwich	1 Sandwich	139	460	16	37	27	6	53.41	35	890	3	3	40	1.80	0	0
Chicken Sandwich	1 Sandwich	229	710	26	54	43	9	54.74	60	1400	2	4	100	3.60	0	0
Croissan'wich w/ Sausage & Cheese	1 Sandwich	106	450	13	21	35	12	69.84	45	940	1	3	100	1.80	200	0
Fish Sandwich, BK Big	1 Sandwich	252	720	23	59	43	9	54.13	80	1180	3	4	80	3.60	100	0

* Values Unavailable.

Name	Serving Size	Gram weight	Calories	Protein (g)	Carb. (g)	Total Fat (g)	Sat Fat. (g)	% Calories from Fat	Chol. (mg)	Sodium (mg)	Fiber (g)	Sugar (g)	Calcium (mg)	Iron (mg)	Vit. A (IU)	Vit. C (mg)
Burger King – Beverages and Shakes																
Chocolate Shake, Medium	1 Serving	397	440	12	75	10	6	20.55	30	330	4	67	300	2.70	400	0
Coca Cola Classic®, Medium	22 Fl Oz	660	280	0	70	0	0	0	0		0	70	0	0	0	0
Diet Coke®, Medium	22 Fl Oz	660	1	0	0	0	0	0	0		0	0	0	0	0	0
Sprite®, Medium	22 Fl Oz	682	260	0	66	0	0	0	0		0	66	0	0	0	0
Vanilla Shake, Medium	1 Medium	397	430	13	73	9	5	19.06	30	330	2	66	400	0	400	6
Burger King – Dessert																
Pie, Dutch Apple	1 Serving	113	300	3	39	15	3	44.55	0	230	2	22	0	1.44	0	6

Source: CyberSoft, Inc. *The NutriBase Nutrition Facts Desk Reference.* 2nd ed. Avery, a member of Penguin Putnam, Inc. © 2001 by CyberSoft.

Name	Serving Size	Gram weight	Calories	Protein (g)	Carb. (g)	Total Fat (g)	Sat Fat. (g)	% Calories from Fat	Chol. (mg)	Sodium (mg)	Fiber (g)	Sugar (g)	Calcium (mg)	Iron (mg)	Vit. A (IU)	Vit. C (mg)
Jack In The Box – Breakfast																
Breakfast Jack Sandwich	1 Sandwich	126	280	17	28	12	5	37.50	190	750	1	3	150	3.60	400	3.60
Breakfast Sandwich, Ultimate	1 Sandwich	243	600	34	39	34	10	51.17	400	1470	2	7	300	3.60	750	6
French Toast Sticks w/Bacon	1 Serving	131	470	12	53	23	4	44.33	30	700	2	10	100	0.72	0	0
Pancake w/Bacon	1 Serving	157	370	12	59	9	2	22.19	30	1020	3	14	80	2.70	0	0
Jack In The Box – Sides																
Egg Rolls	3 Egg Rolls	170	440	15	40	24	6	49.54	35	1020	4	5	80	4.50	750	12
French Fries, Curly Chili Cheese	1 Serving	230	650	14	60	41	12	55.49	25	1760	4	3	150	2.70	750	0
French Fries, Curly Seasoned	1 Serving	125	410	6	45	23	5	50.36	0	1010	4	0	40	1.80	300	0
French Fries, Regular	1 Serving	113	350	4	46	16	4	41.86	0	710	3	0	10	0.72	0	6
Hash Browns	1 Serving	57	170	1	14	12	2	64.29	0	250	1	0	10	0.18	0	0
Stuffed Jalapenos	7 Jalapenos	168	530	14	46	31	12	53.76	60	1730	3	5	300	1.44	1000	21
Onion Rings	1 Serving	125	410	6	45	23	5	50.36	0	1010	4	0	40	2.70	200	18
Potato, Bacon Cheddar Wedges	1 Serving	265	800	20	49	58	16	65.41	55	1470	4	2	350	1.44	500	9
Jack In The Box – Chicken and Seafood																
Chicken Breast Pieces	5 Pieces	150	360	27	24	17	3	42.86	80	970	1	0	20	1.80	200	1.20
Chicken Teriyaki Bowl	1 Serving	502	670	26	128	4	1	5.52	15	1730	3	27	100	4.50	6500	24
Fish & Chips	1 Serving	281	780	19	86	39	9	45.53	45	1740	6	2	20	2.70	100	15
Jack In The Box – Burgers																
Cheeseburger	1 Burger	115	320	14	30	16	6	45	40	720	2	5	150	3.60	300	1.20
Cheeseburger, Bacon Ultimate	1 Burger	302	1020	58	37	71	26	62.71	210	1740	1	7	300	7.20	750	0.60
Cheeseburger, Double Patty	1 Burger	165	460	24	32	27	12	52.03	80	1090	2	5	200	4.50	500	2.40
Cheeseburger, Jumbo Jack	1 Burger	282	680	31	39	45	16	59.12	115	1130	2	9	250	4.50	1000	9
Hamburger	1 Burger	103	280	12	30	12	4	39.13	30	490	2	5	100	3.60	100	1.20
Hamburger, Jumbo Jack	1 Burger	267	590	27	39	37	11	55.78	90	670	2	10	150	4.50	500	9
Hamburger, Sourdough Jack	1 Burger	233	690	34	37	45	15	58.78	105	1180	2	3	200	4.50	750	9

Name	Serving Size	Gram weight	Calories	Protein (g)	Carb. (g)	Total Fat (g)	Sat Fat. (g)	% Calories from Fat	Chol. (mg)	Sodium (mg)	Fiber (g)	Sugar (g)	Calcium (mg)	Iron (mg)	Vit. A (IU)	Vit. C (mg)
Jack In The Box – Sandwiches																
Chicken Fajita Pita Sandwich	1 Sandwich	187	280	24	25	9	4	29.24	75	840	3	5	150	2.70	1250	0
Chicken Sandwich	1 Sandwich	184	420	16	39	23	4	48.48	40	950	2	4	100	2.70	200	4.80
Croissant, Sausage	1 Sandwich	187	700	21	38	51	20	66.04	240	1000	0	6	100	1.80	400	0.60
Grilled Chicken Fillet Sandwich	1 Sandwich	242	480	27	39	24	6	45	65	1110	4	6	200	4.50	400	9
Philly Cheesesteak Sandwich	1 Sandwich	234	580	33	56	16	8	28.80	80	1860	1	3	200	2.70	400	3.60
Jack In The Box – Deserts And Snacks																
Iced Tea, Regular	20 Fl Oz	600	0	0	0	0	0	0	0	0	0	0	0	0	0	0
Minute Maid® Lemonade, Regular,	20 Fl Oz	560	190	0	65	0	0	0	0	100	0	65	0	0	0	0
Barq's® Root Beer, Regular,	20 Fl Oz	627	180	0	50	0	0	0	0	40	0	50	0	0	0	0
Strawberry Ice Cream, Regular	16 Fl Oz	473	640	10	35	28	15	39.87	85	300	0	67	350	0	750	0
Jack In The Box – Mexican																
Taco	1 Serving	82	170	7	12	10	4	54.22	20	460	2	1	100	1.08	300	1.20
Taco, Monster	1 Serving	125	270	12	19	17	6	55.23	30	670	4	2	200	1.44	400	1.20
Jack In The Box – Salads																
Salad, Chicken Garden	1 Salad	253	200	23	8	9	4	39.51	65	420	3	4	200	0.72	3500	12
Jack In The Box – Desserts and Snacks																
Cake, Carrot	1 Serving	99	370	3	54	16	3	38.71	40	340	2	28	20	1.44	5350	0.60
Cake, Double Fudge	1 Serving	85	300	3	50	10	2	29.80	50	320	1	25	40	1.98	300	0.60
Cheesecake	1 Serving	103	320	7	32	18	10	50.94	65	220	1	22	50	0.18	700	3
Turnover, Hot Apple	1 Serving	107	340	4	41	18	4	47.37	0	510	2	12	10	1.80	100	10.20

Source: CyberSoft, Inc. *The NutriBase Nutrition Facts Desk Reference.* 2nd ed. Avery, a member of Penguin Putnam, Inc. © 2001 by CyberSoft.

KFC

KFC – Sides

Name	Serving Size	Gram weight	Calories	Protein (g)	Carb. (g)	Total Fat (g)	Sat Fat. (g)	% Calories from Fat	Chol. (mg)	Sodium (mg)	Fiber (g)	Sugar (g)	Calcium (mg)	Iron (mg)	Vit. A (IU)	Vit. C (mg)
Barbecue Baked Beans	5.5 Oz	156	190	6	33	3	1	14.75	5	760	6	13	80	1.80	400	**
Cole Slaw	5 Oz	142	232	2	26	13.50	2	52.03	8	284	3	20	30	**	450	34.20
Corn On The Cob	5.7 Oz	162	150	5	35	1.50	0	7.78	0	20	2	8	**	**	100	3.60
Macaroni & Cheese	5.4 Oz	153	180	7	21	8	3	39.13	10	860	2	2	150	**	1000	**
Potato Salad	5.6 Oz	160	230	4	23	14	2	53.85	15	540	3	9	20	2.70	500	**
Potato Wedges	4.8 Oz	135	280	5	28	13	4	46.99	5	750	5	1	20	1.80	**	1.20
Potato, Mashed w/Gravy	4.8 Oz	136	120	1	17	6	1	42.86	1	440	2	0	**	0.36	**	**

KFC – Chicken

Name	Serving Size	Gram weight	Calories	Protein (g)	Carb. (g)	Total Fat (g)	Sat Fat. (g)	% Calories from Fat	Chol. (mg)	Sodium (mg)	Fiber (g)	Sugar (g)	Calcium (mg)	Iron (mg)	Vit. A (IU)	Vit. C (mg)
Chicken Wing, Honey Barbecue	6 Pieces	189	607	33	33	38	10	56.44	193	1145	1	18	40	1.44	400	4.80
Chicken Wing, Hot	6 Pieces	135	471	27	18	33	8	62.26	150	1230	2	0	40	1.44	**	**
Chicken, Breast, Extra Crispy	1 Breast	168	470	39	17	28	8	52.94	160	874	1	0	20	1.08	**	**
Chicken, Breast, Original Recipe	1 Breast	153	400	29	16	24	6	54.55	135	1116	1	0	40	1.08	**	**
Chicken, Drumstick, Extra Crispy	1 Drumstick	67	195	15	7	12	3	55.10	77	375	1	0	**	0.72	**	**
Chicken, Drumstick, Original Recipe	1 Drumstick	61	140	13	4	9	2	54.36	75	422	0	0	**	0.72	**	**
Chicken, Popcorn, Larger	6.0 Oz	170	620	30	36	40	10	57.69	73	1046	0	0	20	0.72	0	0
Chicken, Thigh, Extra Crispy	1 Thigh	118	380	21	14	27	7	63.45	118	625	1	0	20	1.08	**	**
Chicken, Thigh, Original Recipe	1 Thigh	91	250	16	6	18	4.50	64.80	95	747	1	0	20	0.72	**	**
Chicken, Whole Wing, Extra Crispy	1 Wing	55	220	10	10	15	4	62.79	55	415	1	0	**	0.36	**	**
Chicken, Whole Wing, Original	1 Wing	47	140	9	5	10	2.50	61.64	55	414	0	0	**	0.36	**	**
Crispy Chicken Strips	3 Strips	115	300	26	18	16	4	45	56	1165	1	1	**	1.08	100	**
Pot Pie, Chunky Chicken	13 Oz	368	770	29	69	42	13	49.09	70	2160	5	8	100	1.80	4000	1.20

KFC – Sandwiches

Name	Serving Size	Gram weight	Calories	Protein (g)	Carb. (g)	Total Fat (g)	Sat Fat. (g)	% Calories from Fat	Chol. (mg)	Sodium (mg)	Fiber (g)	Sugar (g)	Calcium (mg)	Iron (mg)	Vit. A (IU)	Vit. C (mg)
Chicken Sandwich, Tender Roast w/o Sauce	1 Sandwich	177	270	31	26	5	1.50	16.48	65	690	1	1	40	1.80	**	**
Chicken Sandwich, Triple Crunch w/o Sauce	1 Sandwich	176	390	25	39	15	4.50	34.53	50	650	2	0	40	2.70	**	**

** Contains less than 2 % of the Daily Value of these nutrients.

Name	Serving Size	Gram weight	Calories	Protein (g)	Carb. (g)	Total Fat (g)	Sat Fat. (g)	% Calories from Fat	Chol. (mg)	Sodium (mg)	Fiber (g)	Sugar (g)	Calcium (mg)	Iron (mg)	Vit. A (IU)	Vit. C (mg)
KFC – Bread																
Biscuit	1 Biscuit	56	180	4	20	10	2.50	48.39	0	560	0	2	20	1.08	**	**
KFC – Desserts and Snacks																
Cake, Double Chocolate Chip	1 Serving	76	320	4	41	16	4	44.44	55	230	1	28	40	1.80	0	0
Little Bucket Parfait, Chocolate Creme	1 Serving	113	290	3	37	15	11	45.76	15	330	2	25	40	1.08	**	0
Little Bucket Parfait, Fudge Brownie	1 Serving	99	280	3	44	10	3.50	32.37	145	190	1	35	20	1.08	100	0
Little Bucket Parfait, Lemon Creme	1 Serving	127	410	7	62	14	8	31.34	20	290	4	50	200	0.72	100	2.40
Pie, Apple	1 Slice	113	310	2	44	14	3	40.65	0	280	0	23	0	1.08	0	0
Pie, Pecan	1 Slice	113	490	5	66	23	5	42.16	65	510	2	31	20	1.44	200	0
Pie, Strawberry Creme	1 Slice	78	280	4	32	15	8	48.39	15	130	2	22	0	0.72	100	2.40

** Contains less than 2 % of the Daily Value of these nutrients.

Source: CyberSoft, Inc. *The NutriBase Nutrition Facts Desk Reference.* 2nd ed. Avery, a member of Penguin Putnam, Inc. © 2001 by CyberSoft

McDonald's

Name	Serving Size	Gram weight	Calories	Protein (g)	Carb. (g)	Total Fat (g)	Sat Fat. (g)	% Calories from Fat	Chol. (mg)	Sodium (mg)	Fiber (g)	Sugar (g)	Calcium (mg)	Iron (mg)	Vit. A (IU)	Vit. C (mg)
McDonald's – Breakfast																
Biscuit, Bacon Egg & Cheese	1 Sandwich	168	540	21	36	34	10	57.30	250	1550	1	4	200	2.70	500	*
Biscuit, Sausage w/Egg	1 Sandwich	178	550	18	35	37	10	61.10	245	1160	1	3	100	2.70	300	*
Burrito, Breakfast	1 Serving	117	320	13	21	20	7	56.96	195	660	1	2	150	1.80	500	9
Egg McMuffin	1 Sandwich	136	290	17	27	12	4.50	38.03	235	790	1	3	200	2.70	500	1.20
Hotcakes w/ Margarine & Syrup	1 Serving	228	600	9	104	17	3	25.29	20	770	3	40	100	4.50	400	*
Hotcakes, Plain	1 Serving	156	340	9	58	8	1.50	21.18	20	630	3	9	100	4.50	*	*
Hash Browns	1 Serving	53	130	1	14	8	1.50	54.55	0	330	1	0	*	0.36	*	2.40
Sausage w/Egg McMuffin®	1 Sandwich	162	440	19	27	28	10	57.80	255	890	1	3	250	2.70	500	*
Spanish Omelette Bagel	1 Sandwich	258	690	27	59	38	14	49.85	275	1560	10	10	250	4.50	750	15
Ham, Egg & Cheese Bagel	1 Sandwich	218	550	26	58	23	8	38.12	255	1490	9	10	200	4.50	750	*
Steak, Egg & Cheese Bagel	1 Sandwich	245	660	36	57	31	11	42.86	285	1300	9	9	200	5.40	750	*
McDonald's – Chicken																
Chicken McNuggets®	6 Piece	108	290	15	20	17	3.50	52.22	55	540	2	0	20	0.72	*	*
McDonald's – Sandwiches																
Crispy Chicken Sandwich	1 Sandwich	234	550	23	54	27	4.50	44.10	50	1180	2	7	200	3.60	300	6
Filet-O-Fish Sandwich	1 Sandwich	156	470	15	45	26	5	49.37	50	890	1	5	200	1.80	200	*
McDonald's – Beverages And Shakes																
McFlurry, Oreo®	1 Serving	337	570	15	82	20	12	31.69	70	280	0	69	450	1.08	1250	2.40
Milkshake, Chocolate, Large	22 Fl Oz	458	582	15.57	93.89	16.95	10.59	25.64	59.54	444	3.66	81	518	1.42	425.94	1.83
Milkshake, Vanilla, Large	22 Fl Oz	458	508	16.03	81.98	13.74	8.51	23.78	50.38	375	1.83	80	558	0.41	595.40	3.66
McDonald's – Burgers																
Cheeseburger	1 Burger	121	320	16	35	13	6	36.45	40	830	2	7	250	2.70	300	2.40
Cheeseburger, Quarter Pounder	1 Burger	200	530	28	38	30	13	50.56	95	1310	2	9	350	4.50	500	2.40
Hamburger	1 Burger	107	270	13	35	8	3.50	27.27	30	600	2	7	200	2.70	500	2.40
Hamburger, Big Mac	1 Burger	216	570	26	45	32	10	50.35	85	1100	3	8	250	4.50	300	3.60
Hamburger, Quarter Pounder	1 Burger	172	430	23	37	21	8	44.06	70	840	2	8	200	4.50	100	2.40
French Fries, Medium	1 Serving	147	450	6	57	22	4	44	0	290	5	0	20	1.08	*	18

* Values Unavailable.

Source: CyberSoft, Inc. *The NutriBase Nutrition Facts Desk Reference.* 2nd ed. Avery, a member of Penguin Putnam, Inc. © 2001 by CyberSoft.

Name	Serving Size	Gram weight	Calories	Protein (g)	Carb. (g)	Total Fat (g)	Sat Fat. (g)	% Calories from Fat	Chol. (mg)	Sodium (mg)	Fiber (g)	Sugar (g)	Calcium (mg)	Iron (mg)	Vit. A (IU)	Vit. C (mg)
McDonald's – Salads																
Salad, Shaker, Chef	1 Salad	206	150	17	5	8	3.50	45	95	740	2	2	150	1.44	1500	15
Salad, Shaker, Garden	1 Salad	149	100	7	4	6	3	55.10	75	120	2	1	150	1.08	1500	15
Salad, Shaker, Grilled Chicken Caesar	1 Salad	163	100	17	3	2.50	1.50	21.95	40	240	2	1	100	1.08	1250	12
McDonald's – Desserts And Snacks																
Cinnamon Roll	1 Serving	95	390	6	50	18	5	41.97	65	310	2	24	60	1.44	400	*
Cookie, Chocolate Chip	1 Serving	35	170	2	22	10	6	48.39	20	120	1	13	20	1.08	200	*
Danish, Cheese	1 Serving	105	400	7	45	21	5	47.61	40	400	2	16	80	1.44	300	*
Ice Cream Cone, Vanilla, Lower Fat	1 Serving	90	150	4	23	4.50	3	27.27	20	75	0	17	100	0.36	300	1.20
Pie, Baked Apple	1 Serving	77	260	3	34	13	3.50	44.15	0	200	0	13	20	1.08	*	24
Sundae, Hot Fudge	1 Serving	179	340	8	52	12	9	31.03	30	170	1	47	250	0.72	500	1.20
Sundae, Strawberry	1 Serving	178	290	7	50	7	5	21.65	30	95	0	46	200	0.36	500	1.20

* Values Unavailable.

Source: CyberSoft, Inc. *The NutriBase Nutrition Facts Desk Reference*. 2nd ed. Avery, a member of Penguin Putnam, Inc. © 2001 by CyberSoft

Name	Serving Size	Gram weight	Calories	Protein (g)	Carb. (g)	Total Fat (g)	Sat Fat. (g)	% Calories from Fat	Chol. (mg)	Sodium (mg)	Fiber (g)	Sugar (g)	Calcium (mg)	Iron (mg)	Vit. A (IU)	Vit. C (mg)
Pizza Hut																
Pizza Hut – Pasta																
Cavatini Pasta	1 Serving	357	480	21	66	14	6	26.58	8	1170	9	12	150	3.60	1250	*
Cavatini Supreme Pasta	1 Serving	396	560	24	73	19	8	30.59	10	1400	10	11	150	4.50	1500	*
Spaghetti w/ Marinara Sauce	1 Serving	473	490	18	91	6	1	11.02	0	730	8	10	150	3.60	1000	*
Spaghetti w/ Meat Sauce	1 Serving	467	600	23	98	13	5	19.47	8	910	9	10	100	3.60	1750	*
Pizza Hut – Pizza																
Cheese, Hand Tossed, Med.	1 Slice	103	309	14	43	9	4.80	26.21	11	848	3.40	8	190	1.26	450	2.40
Cheese, Pan, Med.	1 Slice	111	361	13	44	15	5.70	37.19	11	678	3.30	1	200	2.52	500	2.40
Cheese, Thin & Crispy, Med.	1 Slice	79	243	11	27	10	4.90	37.19	11	653	2.40	1	190	1.26	450	2.40
Chicken Supreme, Hand Tossed, Med.	1 Slice	116	291	15	44	6	3	18.62	17	841	3.50	9	120	1.26	400	6
Chicken Supreme, Pan, Med.	1 Slice	125	343	15	45	12	3.90	31.03	16	671	3.40	2	150	2.70	400	6
Chicken Supreme, Thin & Crispy, Med.	1 Slice	102	232	13	29	7	3.20	27.27	19	681	2.50	2	120	1.44	400	7.20
Meat Lover's, Thin & Crispy, Med.	1 Slice	107	339	15	28	19	7.80	49.85	35	970	2.60	1	140	1.80	450	2.40
Meat Lover's, Hand Tossed, Med.	1 Slice	121	376	17	44	15	6.40	35.62	30	1077	3.60	8	140	1.62	400	2.40
Meat Lover's, Pan, Med.	1 Slice	129	428	16	45	21	7.30	43.65	29	607	3.40	1	140	2.88	450	2.40
Pepperoni, Hand Tossed, Med.	1 Slice	100	301	13	43	8	4	24.32	15	867	3.20	8	120	1.26	350	2.40
Pepperoni, Pan, Med.	1 Slice	106	353	12	44	14	4.80	36	14	697	3.10	1	130	2.52	350	2.40
Pepperoni, Thin & Crispy, Med.	1 Slice	74	235	10	27	10	4.10	37.82	14	672	2.10	1	120	1.26	350	2.40
Supreme, Hand Tossed, Med.	1 Slice	123	333	15	44	11	4.90	29.55	18	927	3.70	9	130	1.62	400	6
Supreme, Pan, Med.	1 Slice	130	385	14	45	17	5.70	39.33	18	757	3.60	1	140	2.88	400	6
Supreme Pizza, Thin & Crispy, Med.	1 Slice	110	284	13	29	13	5.50	41.05	20	784	2.80	2	130	1.62	400	16.80
Veggie Lover's, Hand Tossed, Med.	1 Slice	120	281	12	45	6	3	19.15	7	771	3.80	9	130	1.44	450	9.60
Veggie Lover's, Pan, Med.	1 Slice	125	333	11	46	12	3.90	32.14	7	601	3.60	2	130	2.88	450	9.60
Pizza Hut – Desserts and Snacks																
Apple Dessert Pizza	1 Slice	81	250	3	48	4.50	1	16.56	0	230	2	25	*	1.08	*	*
Cherry Dessert Pizza	1 Slice	81	250	3	47	4.50	1	16.84	0	220	3	24	*	1.44	450	*
Pizza Hut – Bread																
Bread Stick	1 Serving	38	130	3	20	4	1	28.13	0	170	1	1	*	1.08	*	*
Bread, Garlic	1 Slice	37	150	3	16	8	1.50	48.65	0	240	1	1	40	1.44	500	*

* Values Unavailable.

Source: CyberSoft, Inc. *The NutriBase Nutrition Facts Desk Reference.* 2nd ed. Avery, a member of Penguin Putnam, Inc. © 2001 by CyberSoft

Taco Bell

Taco Bell – Mexican

Name	Serving Size	Gram weight	Calories	Protein (g)	Carb. (g)	Total Fat (g)	Sat Fat. (g)	% Calories from Fat	Chol. (mg)	Sodium (mg)	Fiber (g)	Sugar (g)	Calcium (mg)	Iron (mg)	Vit. A (IU)	Vit. C (mg)
Bean Burrito, 7 Oz	1 Burrito	198	370	13	54	12	3.50	28.72	10	1080	12	3	150	2.70	2250	0
Burrito Supreme, Beef, 8.75 Oz	1 Burrito	248	430	17	50	18	7	37.67	40	1210	9	4	150	2.70	2500	4.80
Burrito Supreme, Chicken, 8.75 Oz	1 Burrito	248	410	20	49	16	6	34.29	45	1120	8	4	150	1.80	2250	4.80
Burrito Supreme, Steak, 8.75 Oz	1 Burrito	248	420	21	48	16	6	34.29	35	1140	8	4	150	2.70	2250	3.60
Chalupa Supreme, Beef, 5.5 Oz	1 Chalupa	156	380	14	29	23	8	54.62	40	580	3	3	150	1.80	300	4.80
Chalupa Supreme, Chicken, 5.5 Oz	1 Chalupa	156	360	17	28	20	7	50	45	490	2	3	100	1.80	200	4.80
Chalupa Supreme, Steak, 5.5 Oz	1 Chalupa	156	360	17	27	20	7	50.56	35	500	2	3	150	2.70	100	3.60
Enchirito, Beef, 7.5 Oz	1 Enchirito	213	370	18	33	19	9	45.60	50	1300	9	2	300	1.80	5000	1.20
Enchirito, Chicken, 7.5 Oz	1 Enchirito	213	350	21	32	16	8	40.45	55	1210	7	2	250	1.80	5000	1.20
Enchirito, Steak, 7.5 Oz	1 Enchirito	213	350	22	31	16	8	40.45	45	1220	7	2	250	2.70	4500	0
Gordita Supreme, Beef, 5.5 Oz	1 Gordita	156	300	17	27	14	5	41.72	35	550	3	4	150	1.80	100	3.60
Gordita Supreme, Chicken, 5.5 Oz	1 Gordita	156	300	16	28	13	5	39.93	45	530	3	4	150	1.44	200	3.60
Gordita Supreme, Steak, 5.5 Oz	1 Gordita	156	300	17	27	14	5	41.72	35	550	3	4	150	1.80	100	3.60
Grilled Stuft Burrito, Beef, 10.3 Oz	1 Burrito	292	730	27	75	35	11	43.57	65	2090	11	4	350	5.40	1500	9
Grilled Stuft Burrito, Chicken, 1C.3 Oz	1 Burrito	292	690	33	73	29	8	38.10	70	1900	8	4	300	5.40	1250	9
Grilled Stuft Burrito, Steak, 10.4 Oz	1 Burrito	295	690	30	72	30	8	39.82	60	1970	8	4	300	6.30	1250	6
Mexican Pizza, 6.75 Oz	1 Pizza	191	390	18	28	25	8	55.01	45	930	8	2	250	2.70	1750	6
Mexican Rice, 4.75 Oz	1 Order	135	190	5	23	9	3.50	41.97	15	750	1	1	150	1.44	5000	1.20
Nachos, 3.5 Oz	1 Order	99	320	5	34	18	4	50.94	5	560	3	2	100	0.72	300	0
Nachos Bellgrande, 11 Oz	1 Order	312	760	20	83	39	11	46	35	1300	17	4	200	3.60	500	4.80
Nachos Mucho Grande, 18 Oz	1 Order	510	1320	31	116	82	25	55.66	75	2670	18	6	250	5.40	1000	12
Nachos Supreme, 7 Oz	1 Order	198	440	14	44	24	7	48.21	35	800	9	3	150	2.70	0	3.60

Name	Serving Size	Gram weight	Calories	Protein (g)	Carb. (g)	Total Fat (g)	Sat Fat. (g)	% Calories from Fat	Chol. (mg)	Sodium (mg)	Fiber (g)	Sugar (g)	Calcium (mg)	Iron (mg)	Vit. A (IU)	Vit. C (mg)
Pintos 'n Cheese, 4.5 Oz	1 Order	128	180	9	18	8	4	40	15	640	10	1	150	1.80	2250	0
Quesadilla, Cheese, 4.25 Oz	1 Quesadilla	170	350	16	31	18	9	46.29	50	860	3	2	350	0.72	400	0
Quesadilla, Chicken, 6 Oz	1 Quesadilla	170	400	25	33	19	9	42.43	75	1050	3	2	350	0.72	500	1.20
Seven-Layer Burrito, 10 Oz	1 Burrito	283	520	16	65	22	7	37.93	25	1270	13	4	200	3.60	1500	6
Soft Taco Supreme, Beef, 5 Oz	1 Taco	142	260	11	22	13	6	46.99	40	590	3	3	100	1.08	400	3.60
Soft Taco Supreme, Chicken, 4.75 Oz	1 Taco	135	240	14	21	11	5	41.42	45	490	2	3	100	0.72	300	3.60
Soft Taco Supreme, Steak, 4.75 Oz	1 Taco	135	240	15	20	11	5	41.42	35	510	2	2	100	1.08	200	3.60
Soft Taco, Beef, 3.5 Oz	1 Taco	99	210	11	20	10	4	42.06	30	570	3	1	80	1.08	400	0
Soft Taco, Chicken, 3.5 Oz	1 Taco	99	190	13	19	7	2.50	32.98	35	480	2	1	80	0.72	200	1.20
Soft Taco, Steak, 3.5 Oz	1 Taco	99	190	14	18	7	3	32.98	25	490	1	1	100	1.08	200	0
Double Decker Taco, 7 Oz	1 Taco	198	330	14	37	15	5	39.82	30	740	9	2	100	1.80	400	0
Double Decker Taco Supreme, 7 Oz	1 Taco	200	380	15	39	18	7	42.86	40	760	9	3	150	1.80	400	3.60
Taco Supreme, 4 Oz	1 Taco	113	210	9	14	14	6	57.80	40	350	3	2	100	1.08	400	3.60
Taco Salad w/Salsa, 19 Oz	1 Salad	539	850	30	69	52	14	54.17	70	2250	16	12	300	6.30	1450	30
Taco, 2.75 Oz	1 Taco	78	170	9	12	10	4	51.72	30	330	3	1	80	0.72	400	0
Tostada, 6.25 Oz	1 Tostada	177	250	10	27	12	4.50	42.19	15	640	11	2	150	1.80	2500	1.20

Taco Bell – Dessert and Snacks

Name	Serving Size	Gram weight	Calories	Protein (g)	Carb. (g)	Total Fat (g)	Sat Fat. (g)	% Calories from Fat	Chol. (mg)	Sodium (mg)	Fiber (g)	Sugar (g)	Calcium (mg)	Iron (mg)	Vit. A (IU)	Vit. C (mg)
Cinnamon Twists, 1.25 Oz	1 Order	35	150	1	27	4.50	1	26.56	0	190	1	13	0	0.36	0	0

Source: CyberSoft, Inc. *The NutriBase Nutrition Facts Desk Reference.* 2nd ed. Avery, a member of Penguin Putnam, Inc. © 2001 by CyberSoft

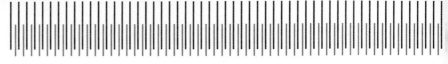

acclimatize Refers to the physiological adaptations that occur to assist the body in adjusting to environmental extremes. Exercise in a hot or even moderately hot environment will cause the body to adapt to these conditions.

acute muscle soreness This condition may develop during or immediately following an exercise bout that has been too long or too intense. Acute muscle soreness is likely caused by alterations in the chemical balance within muscle, increased fluid accumulation in muscle, or injury to muscle tissue.

adenosine triphosphate (ATP) A high-energy compound that is synthesized and stored in small quantities in muscle and other cells. The breakdown of ATP results in a release of energy that can be used to fuel muscular contraction. ATP is the only compound in the body that can provide this immediate source of energy.

aerobic Means "with oxygen"; as pertains to energy-producing biochemical pathways in cells that use oxygen to produce energy.

aerobics A common term to describe all forms of low-intensity exercise designed to improve cardiorespiratory fitness (e.g., jogging, walking, cycling, and swimming). Because aerobic exercise has proved effective in promoting weight loss and reducing the risk of cardiovascular disease, many exercise scientists consider cardiorespiratory fitness to be one of the most important components of health-related physical fitness.

AIDS A fatal disease that develops from infection by the human immunodeficiency virus, or HIV.

amino acids The basic structural unit of proteins. Twenty different amino acids exist and can be linked end to end in various combinations to create different proteins with unique functions.

anabolic steroids Hormones produced by the body which enhance muscle growth. Usually refers to the synthetic form of the hormone testosterone.

anaerobic threshold The work intensity during graded, incremental exercise at which there is a rapid accumulation of blood lactic acid. This usually occurs at 50% to 60% of $\dot{V}O_2$ and contributes to muscle fatigue.

anaerobic Means "without oxygen"; as pertains to energy producing biochemical pathways in cells that do not require oxygen to produce energy.

anorexia nervosa A common eating disorder that is unrelated to any specific physical disease. The end result of extreme anorexia nervosa is a state of starvation in which the individual becomes emaciated due to a refusal to eat.

antagonist The muscle on the opposite side of the joint.

antioxidants Substances that remove free radicals (also called oxygen radicals) from cells and thus prevent DNA damage. Although free radicals are constantly produced by the body, excess production of these compounds has been implicated in cancer, lung disease, heart disease, and even the aging process.

arteries The blood vessels that transport blood away from the heart.

arteriosclerosis A group of diseases characterized by a narrowing or "hardening" of the arteries. The end result of any form of arteriosclerosis is that blood flow to vital organs may be impaired due to a progressive blockage of the artery.

arthroscopic surgery A common type of surgery that can repair joint injuries without causing undue trauma to the joint.

asthma A disease that reduces the size of airways leading to the lungs and can result in a sudden difficulty in breathing. It is promoted by a number of factors, such as air pollution, pollen, and exercise.

atherosclerosis A special type of arteriosclerosis that results in arterial blockage due to collection of a fatty deposit (called *atherosclerotic plaque*) inside the blood vessel.

behavior modification A technique used in psychological therapy to promote desirable changes in behavior.

body composition The relative amounts of fat and lean body tissue (muscle, organs, bone) found in the body.

body mass index (BMI) A useful technique for categorizing people with respect to their degree of body fat. The body mass index is simply the ratio of the body weight (kilograms; kg) divided by the height squared (meters^2).

breathing exercises A simple means of achieving relaxation.

bulimia An eating disorder that involves overeating (called *binge eating*) followed by vomiting (called *purging*).

calorie The unit of measure used to quantify food energy or the energy expended by the body. Technically, a calorie is the amount of energy necessary to raise the temperature of 1 gram of water 1°C.

cancer A class of over 100 different diseases that can influence almost every body tissue. Cancer is caused by the uncontrolled growth and spread of abnormal cells.

capillaries Thin-walled vessels that permit the exchange of gases (oxygen and carbon dioxide) and nutrients to occur between the blood and tissues.

carbohydrates One of the macronutrients that is especially important during many types of physical activity because they are a key energy source for muscular contraction. Dietary sources of carbohydrates are breads, cereals, fruits, and vegetables.

carbon monoxide A gas produced during the burning of fossil fuels such as gasoline and coal; also contained in cigarette smoke. This pollutant binds to hemoglobin in the blood and reduces the blood's oxygen carrying capacity.

carcinogens Cancer-causing agents which include radiation, chemicals, drugs, and other toxic substances.

cardiac output The amount of blood the heart pumps per minute.

cardiovascular disease Any disease that affects the heart or blood vessels.

cartilage A tough, connective tissue that forms a pad on the end of bones in certain joints, such as the elbow, knee, and ankle. Cartilage act as a shock absorber to cushion the weight of one bone on another and to provide protection from the friction due to joint movement.

cellulite The "lumpy" hard fat that often gives skin a dimpled look. Cellulite is just plain fat and not a special category of fat.

chemical dependency A term for drug addiction.

chlamydia The most common sexually transmitted disease among heterosexuals in the United States. The disease is caused by a bacterial infection within the reproductive organs and is spread through vaginal, anal, and oral sex.

cholesterol A type of derived fat in the body which is necessary for cell and hormone synthesis. Can be acquired through the diet or can be made by the body.

chondromalacia Sometimes called "runner's knee"; it is a common exercise-induced injury which is manifest as pain behind the knee cap. In sports injury clinic, chondromalacia may account for almost 10% of all visits, or 20% to 40% of all knee problems.

cocaine Cocaine is a powerful stimulant derived from the leaves of the South American coca shrub, which grows primarily in the Andes mountains. Cocaine is extracted from the coca leaves using a multistep process to produce a white powder.

complete proteins Contain all the essential amino acids and are found only in foods of animal origin (meats and dairy products).

complex carbohydrates A term that refers to carbohydrates that provide both micronutrients and the glucose necessary for producing energy. They are contained in starches and fiber.

concentric contractions Isotonic muscle contractions that result in muscle shortening.

contributory risk factors; also called secondary risk factors Factors that increase the risk of CHD, but their direct contribution to the disease process has not been precisely determined.

convection Heat loss by the movement of air (or water) around the body.

cool-down The cool-down (sometimes called a *warm-down*) is a 5- to 15-min period of low-intensity exercise that immediately follows the primary conditioning period.

coronary artery disease See *coronary heart disease.*

coronary heart disease (CHD); also called *coronary artery disease* CHD is the result of atherosclerotic plaque forming a blockage of one or more coronary arteries (the blood vessels supplying the heart).

creeping obesity A slow increase in body fat collected over a period of several years.

cross training The use of a variety of activity modes for training the cardiorespiratory system.

cryokinetics A relatively new rehabilitation technique which is implemented after the acute injury and healing period have been completed. It incorporates varying periods of treatment using ice, rest, and exercise.

cycle ergometer fitness test A submaximal exercise test designed to evaluate cardiorespiratory fitness.

delayed-onset muscle soreness (DOMS) This condition develops within 24 to 48 hours after a bout of exercise that is excessive in duration or intensity. It is common following new or unique physical activities that use muscle groups unaccustomed to exercise.

derived fats A class of fats which does not contain fatty acids but are classified as fat because they are not soluble in water.

diabetes A metabolic disorder characterized by high blood glucose levels. Chronic elevation of blood glucose is associated with increased incidence of heart disease, kidney disease, nerve dysfunction, and eye damage.

diastolic blood pressure The pressure of the blood in the arteries at the level of the heart during the resting phase of the heart (diastole).

duration of exercise The amount of time invested in performing the primary workout.

dynamic Means "movement"; in reference to muscle contractions, dynamic is synonymous with isotonic contraction.

eccentric contractions Isotonic contractions in which the muscle exerts force while the muscle lengthens (also called *negative contractions*).

ergogenic aid A drug or nutritional product that improves physical fitness and exercise performance.

essential amino acids Amino acids which cannot be manufactured by the body and, therefore, must be consumed in the diet.

eustress A stress level that results in improved performance.

evaporation The conversion of water (or sweat) to a gas (water vapor). The most important means of removing heat from the body during exercise.

exercise metabolic rate (EMR) The energy expenditure during any form of exercise.

exercise prescription The correct dosage of exercise to effectively promote physical fitness. Exercise prescriptions should be tailored to meet the needs of the individual and include fitness goals, mode of exercise, a warm-up, a primary conditioning period, and a cool-down.

exercise stress test A diagnostic test designed to determine if the patient's cardiovascular system has a normal response to exercise. The test is generally performed on a treadmill while a physician monitors heart rate, blood pressure, and EKG.

fartlek training *Fartlek* is a Swedish word meaning "speed play," and it refers to a popular form of training for long-distance runners. It is much like interval training, but it is not as rigid in its work-to-rest interval ratios. It consists of "free-form" running done out on trails, roads, golf courses, and so on.

fast-twitch fibers Muscle fibers that contract rapidly but fatigue quickly. These fibers are white and have a low aerobic capacity, but they are well equipped to produce ATP anaerobically.

fat An efficient storage form for energy, because each gram of fat holds over twice the energy content of either carbohydrate or protein. Excess fat in the diet is stored in fat cells (called *adipose tissue*) located under the skin and around internal organs.

fatty acids The basic structural unit of triglycerides that are important nutritionally, not only because of their energy content, but also because they play a role in cardiovascular disease.

fiber A stringy, nondigestible carbohydrate found in whole grains, vegetables, and fruits in its primary form, cellulose.

flexibility The ability to move joints freely through their full range of motion.

frequency of exercise The number of times per week that one intends to exercise.

fructose Also called *fruit sugar;* a naturally occurring sugar found in fruits and in honey.

galactose A simple sugar found in the breast milk of humans and other mammals.

glucose The most noteworthy of the simple sugars because it is the only sugar molecule that can be used by the body in its natural form. All other carbohydrates must first be converted to glucose to be used for fuel.

glycogen The storage form of glucose in the liver and skeletal muscles.

gonorrhea A common sexually transmitted disease. The infection can be transmitted through vaginal, anal, and oral sex. Gonorrhea is caused by a bacterial infection and is curable by antibiotics.

heart attack; also called *myocardial infarction* Stoppage of blood flow to the heart, resulting in the death of heart cells.

heart rate Number of heart beats per minute.

heat injuries; also called *heat illness* Bodily injury that can occur when the exercise heat load exceeds the body's ability to regulate body temperature. They are serious and can result in damage to the nervous system and, in extreme cases, death.

herpes A general term for a family of diseases that are also caused by viral infections. Herpes is highly contagious and can be transmitted through any form of sexual contact (e.g., hand-to-genital contact, oral sex, or intercourse).

high-density lipoproteins (HDL) A combination of protein, triglycerides, and cholesterol in the blood, composed of relatively large amounts of protein. Protects against fatty plaque accumulation in the coronary arteries of the heart that leads to heart disease. Research has shown individuals with high blood HDL-cholesterol levels have less risk of CHD. Often called "good cholesterol."

homeotherms Animals that regulate their body temperature around a constant level; that is, body temperature is regulated around a set point. Humans regulate their body temperature around the set point of 98.6°F or 37°C.

humidity The amount of water vapor in the air. If the relative humidity is high, meaning the air is relatively saturated with water, and the air temperature is high, evaporation is retarded and body heat loss is drastically decreased.

hydrostatic weighing A method of determining body composition that involves weighing the individual both on land and in a tank of water.

hyperplasia An increase in the number of muscle fibers.

hypertension (high blood pressure) Usually considered to be a blood pressure of greater than 140 for systolic or 100 for diastolic.

hypertrophy An increase in muscle fiber size.

incomplete proteins Proteins that are missing one or more of the essential amino acids; can be found in numerous vegetable sources.

intensity of exercise The amount of physiological stress or overload placed on the body during exercise.

intermediate fibers Muscle fibers that possess a combination of the characteristics of fast- and slow-twitch fibers. They contract rapidly and are fatigue resistant due to a well-developed aerobic capacity.

interval training Repeated bouts or intervals of relatively intense exercise. The duration of the intervals can be varied, but a 1- to 5-minute duration is common. Each interval is followed by a rest period, which should be equal to or slightly greater than the interval duration.

isocaloric balance Food energy intake that equals energy expenditure.

isokinetic contractions A muscle contraction that is a subtype of isotonic contraction; isokinetic contractions are concentric or eccentric isotonic contractions performed at a constant speed.

isometric Refers to muscle contractions in which muscular tension is developed but no movement of body parts takes place.

isotonic Refers to muscle contractions in which there is movement of a body part. Most exercise or sports skills use isotonic contractions.

lactic acid A by-product of glucose metabolism. Produced primarily during intense exercise (i.e., greater than 50%–60% of maximal aerobic capacity.). Results in inhibition of muscle contraction and, therefore, fatigue.

lactose A simple sugar found in milk products; it is composed of galactose and glucose.

ligaments Connective tissue within the joint capsule which holds bones together.

lipoproteins Combinations of protein, triglycerides, and cholesterol in the blood that are important because of their role in promoting heart disease.

long, slow distance training The term utilized to indicate continuous exercise which requires a steady, submaximal exercise intensity (i.e., the intensity is generally around 70% HRmax).

low-density lipoproteins (LDL) A combination of protein, triglycerides, and cholesterol in the blood, composed of relatively large amounts of cholesterol. Promotes the fatty plaque accumulation in the coronary arteries of the heart that leads to heart disease. The association between elevated total blood cholesterol and the increased risk of CHD is due primarily to LDL cholesterol. Research has shown that individuals with high blood LDL cholesterol levels have an increased risk of CHD. Because of this relationship, LDL cholesterol has been labeled "bad cholesterol."

macronutrients Carbohydrates, fats, and proteins, which are necessary for building and maintaining body tissues and providing energy for daily activities.

major risk factors; also called *primary risk factors* Factors considered to be directly related to the development of CHD and stroke.

maltose A simple sugar found in grain products; it is composed of two glucose molecules linked together.

marijuana A plant mixture (stems, leaves, or seeds) from either the *Cannabis sativa* or *Cannabis indica* (hemp) plants. The active chemical in marijuana that produces physical effects is tetrahydrocannabinol (THC); the higher the THC concentration in marijuana, the greater the effect.

meditation A method of relaxation that has been practiced for ages in an effort to produce relaxation and achieve inner peace. There are many types of meditation, and there is no scientific evidence that one form is superior to another.

micronutrients Nutrients in food, such as vitamins and minerals, that regulate the functions of the cells.

minerals Chemical elements (e.g., sodium and calcium) that are required by the body for normal functioning.

mode of exercise The specific type of exercise to be performed. For example, to improve cardiorespiratory fitness, one could select from a wide variety of exercise modes, including running, swimming, or cycling.

motor unit A motor nerve and each of the muscle fibers that it innervates.

muscular endurance The ability of a muscle to generate force over and over again.

muscular strength The maximal ability of a muscle to generate force.

myocardial infarction (MI) Damage to the heart due to a reduction in blood flow, resulting in the death of heart muscle cells.

negative caloric balance Expending more calories than are consumed.

nonessential amino acids Eleven amino acids that the body can make and are therefore not necessary in the diet.

nutrients Substances contained in food which are necessary for good health.

obesity A term applied to individuals with a high percentage of body fat, generally over 25% for men and over 30% for women.

omega-3 fatty acid A type of unsaturated fatty acid that lowers both blood cholesterol and triglycerides and is found primarily in fresh or frozen mackerel, herring, tuna, and salmon.

1-mile walk test A fitness test designed to evaluate cardiorespiratory fitness. The objective of the test is to complete a 1 walking mile distance (preferably on a track) in the shortest possible time.

1.5-mile run test A fitness test designed to evaluate cardiorespiratory fitness. The objective of the test is to complete a 1.5-mile distance (preferably on a track) in the shortest possible time.

one-repetition maximum (1 RM) test Measurement of the maximum amount of weight that can be lifted one time.

organic Refers to foods that are grown without pesticides.

osteoporosis The loss of bone mass and strength, which increases the risk of bone fractures.

overload principle A basic principle of physical conditioning. The overload principle states that in order to improve physical fitness, the body or specific muscles must be stressed. For example, for a skeletal muscle to increase in strength, the muscle must work against a heavier load than normal.

overtraining Failure to get enough rest between exercise training sessions. Overtraining may lead to chronic fatigue and/or injuries.

overtraining syndrome A phenomenon resulting from improper training techniques which results in exercise-related injuries. Overtraining results from too much exercise and not enough recovery time between workouts. The symptoms may include increased resting heart rate, reduced appetite, weight loss, irritability, disturbed sleep, elevated blood pressure, frequent injuries, increased incidence of infectious, and chronic fatigue.

ozone A gas produced by a chemical reaction between sunlight and the hydrocarbons emitted from car exhausts. This form of pollution is extremely irritating to the lung and airways. It causes tightness in the chest, coughing, headaches, nausea, throat and eye irritation, and, worst of all, bronchoconstriction.

palpation Touching the skin in order to feel the pulse.

passive exercise Movement performed on a motor-driven device designed to move or vibrate the body without any muscular activity. Passive exercise devices come in many forms, including rolling machines, vibrating belts, pillows, and passive motion tables. Passive exercise devices do not improve physical fitness or promote weight loss.

patella-femoral pain syndrome (PFPS) A common exercise-induced injury that is manifest as pain behind the knee cap (patella).

pelvic inflammatory disease An inflammatory infection of the lining of the abdominal and pelvic cavities. Common symptoms of pelvic inflammatory disease include pain in the lower abdominal cavity, fever, and menstrual irregularities.

positive caloric balance Consuming more calories than are expended.

principle of progression A principle of training which dictates that overload should be increased gradually during the course of a physical fitness program.

principle of recuperation The principle of recuperation states that the body requires recovery periods between exercise training sessions in order to adapt to the exercise stress. Therefore, a period of rest is essential to achieve maximal benefit from exercise.

principle of reversibility The loss of fitness due to inactivity.

principle of specificity The principle that the exercise training effect is specific to those muscles involved in the activity.

progressive resistance exercise (PRE) The application of the overload principle applied to strength and endurance exercise programs. Even though the overload principle and PRE can be used interchangeably, PRE is preferred when discussing weight training.

proprioceptive neuromuscular facilitation (PNF) Combines stretching with alternating contracting and relaxing of muscles to improve flexibility. There are two common types of PNF stretching. One is called contract-relax (CR) stretching, while the second is called contract-relax/antagonist contract (CRAC) stretching.

pulmonary circuit The blood vascular system which circulates blood from the right side of the heart, through the lungs, and back to the left side of the heart.

push-up test A fitness test designed to evaluate muscular endurance of shoulder and arm muscles.

R.I.C.E. An acronym representing a treatment protocol for exercise-related injuries. It stands for a combination of rest-*R*, ice-*I*, compression-*C*, and elevation-*E*.

recovery index Measurement of heart rate during three 30-second recovery periods following a submaximal step test.

recruitment The process of involving more muscle fibers to produce increased muscular force.

repetition maximum (RM) The measure of the intensity of exercise in both isotonic and isokinetic weight training programs. The RM is the maximal load that a muscle group can lift a specified number of times before tiring. For example, 6 RM is the maximal load that can be lifted six times.

resting metabolic rate (RMR) The amount of energy expended during all sedentary activities.

saturated fatty acid A type of fatty acid that comes primarily from animal sources (meat and dairy products) and is solid at room temperature.

set The number of repetitions performed consecutively without resting.

set point theory A theory of weight regulation that centers around the concept that body weight is controlled at a set point by a weight-regulating control center within the brain.

sexually transmitted diseases (STDs) A group of more than 20 diseases that are generally spread through sexual contact.

sit and reach test A fitness test that measures the ability to flex the trunk (i.e., stretching the lower back muscles and the muscles in the back of the thigh).

sit-up test A field test to evaluate abdominal muscles endurance.

skinfold test A field test to estimate body composition. The test works on the principle that over 50% of the body fat lies just beneath the skin. Therefore, measurement of representative samples of subcutaneous fat provides a means of estimating overall body fatness.

slow-twitch fibers Muscle fibers that contract slowly and are highly resistant to fatigue. Red in appearance, they have the capacity to produce large quantities of ATP aerobically, making them ideally suited for low-intensity, prolonged exercise like walking or slow jogging.

specificity of training That development of muscular strength and endurance, as well as cardiorespiratory endurance, is specific to the muscle group that is exercised and the training intensity.

SPF Abbreviation for "sun protection factor." A sunscreen with an SPF of 15 provides you with 15 times more protection than unprotected skin.

spot reduction The false notion that exercise applied to a specific region of the body will result in fat loss in that region.

sprain Damage to a ligament that occurs if excessive force is applied to a joint.

starches Long chains of sugars commonly found in foods such as corn, grains, potatoes, peas, and beans. Starch is stored in the body as glycogen and is used for that sudden burst of energy often needed during physical activity.

static Stationary; in reference to muscle contractions, static is synonymous with isometric contraction.

static stretching Stretching that slowly lengthens a muscle to a point where further movement is limited.

step test A submaximal exercise test designed to evaluate cardiorespiratory fitness. The step test works on the principle that individuals with a high level of cardiorespiratory fitness will have a lower heart rate during recovery from 3 minutes of standardized exercise (bench stepping) than less-conditioned individuals.

strain Damage to a muscle that can range from a minor separation of fibers to a complete tearing of fibers.

stress A physiological and mental response to something in the environment that causes people to become uncomfortable.

stress fractures Tiny cracks or breaks in bone. Although stress fractures can occur in any leg bone, the long bones of the foot extending from the ankle to the toes are especially susceptible.

stressor A factor that produces stress.

stretch reflex Involuntary contraction of muscle that occurs due to rapid stretching of a muscle.

stroke Brain damage that occurs when the blood supply to the brain is reduced for a prolonged period of time.

stroke volume The amount of blood pumped per heart beat (generally expressed in milliliters).

sucrose; also called *table sugar* A molecule composed of glucose and fructose.

syphilis A sexually transmitted disease that can be transmitted through direct sexual contact. Syphilis is caused by a bacterial infection and can be cured by antibiotics.

systemic circuit The blood vascular system which circulates blood from the left side of the heart, throughout the body, and back to the right side of the heart.

systolic blood pressure The pressure of the blood in the arteries at the level of the heart during the contractile phase of the heart (systole).

target heart rate (THR) The range of heart rates that corresponds to an exercise intensity of approximately 50%–85% $\dot{V}O_{2max}$. This is the range of training heart rates that results in improvements in aerobic capacity.

tendonitis Inflammation or swelling of a tendon. One of the most common exercise-related injuries.

tendons Connective tissue that connects muscles to bones.

ten percent rule A rule of training that states that the training intensity or duration of exercise should not be increased more than 10% per week.

threshold for health benefits The minimum level of physical activity required to achieve some of the health benefits of exercise.

training threshold The training intensity above which there is an improvement in cardiorespiratory fitness. This intensity is approximately 50% of $\dot{V}O_{2max}$.

triglycerides The form of fat that is broken down and used to produce energy to power muscle contractions during exercise. Triglycerides constitute approximately 95% of the fats in the diet and are the storage form of body fat.

tumor A group of cancer cells.

unsaturated fatty acid A type of fatty acid that comes primarily from plant sources and is liquid at room temperature.

valsalva maneuver Breath holding during an intense muscle contraction that can reduce blood flow to the brain and cause dizziness and fainting.

veins Blood vessels that transport blood toward the heart.

venereal warts; also known as *genital warts* Warts caused by a small group of viruses called *human papilloma viruses*. Infection generally occurs through sexual contact with an infected individual; after exposure, the virus penetrates the skin or mucous membranes of the genitals or anus, and warts appear within 6 to 8 weeks.

visualization; also called *imagery* A relaxation technique that uses mental pictures to reduce stress. The idea is to create appealing mental images that promote relaxation and reduce stress.

vitamins Small molecules that play a key role in many body functions, including the regulation of growth and metabolism. They are classified according to whether they are soluble in water or fat.

$\dot{V}O_{2max}$ The highest oxygen consumption achievable during exercise. Practically speaking, $\dot{V}O_{2max}$ is a laboratory measure of the endurance capacity of both the cardiorespiratory system and exercising skeletal muscles.

waist-to-hip circumference ratio An index for determining the risk of disease associated with high body fat. The rationale for this technique is that a high percentage of fat in the abdominal region is associated with an increased risk of disease (e.g., heart disease or hypertension). Therefore, an individual with a large fat deposit in the abdominal region would have a high waist-to-hip ratio and would have a higher risk of disease than someone with a lower waist-to-hip ratio.

warm-up A brief (5 to 15 minute) period of exercise that precedes the workout. The purpose of a warm-up is to elevate muscle temperature and increase blood flow to those muscles that will be engaged in the workout.

wellness A state of healthy living. This state is achieved by the practice of a healthy lifestyle, which includes regular physical activity, proper nutrition, eliminating unhealthy behaviors, and maintaining good emotional and spiritual health.

INDEX

Page references followed by *fig* indicate a figure; by *t* a table; by *ph* a photograph.

abdominal curl, 118
accident prevention, 251–252*t*
aerobic ATP production, 77, 78*fig*
aerobic exercise
  body adaptation to, 91–94
  burning fat and, 204
  described, 76–77
  frequently asked questions about, 92
Aerobics (Cooper), 76
age/aging
  CHD risk and, 229
  exercise, physical working capacity and,
    3–4*fig*
  guidelines for evaluating health status
    and, 18
  norms for push-up tests, 32*t*
ages/aging, THR (target heart rate) and,
    86*fig*
AI (adequate intake), 166
alarm stage, 242–243
American Heart Association, 226, 228
amino acids, 154–155
anabolic steroids, 109
anaerobic ATP production, 77, 78*fig*
anaerobic exercise, 76
anaerobic threshold, 83
anorexia nervosa, 208–209*ph*
antagonist muscle contraction, 134
antioxidants, 166, 174
antioxidant vitamins, 231
appetite
  coffee and reduced, 210
  exercise and, 205
  leptin and, 197
arm circles (palms down), 141
arm circles (palms up), 141
arteries, 79
arteriosclerosis, 222, 223*fig*
Assessment of Your Risk of Heart Disease,
    237–238
ATP (adenosine triphosphate), 76, 77, 78*fig*

back/hip isotonic exercises, 121
basketball, 69*ph*
behavior modification
  accident prevention and, 251–252*t*
  for changing unhealthy behavior,
    249–250
  general steps in, 249*t*
  smoking and, 250
  specific goals of
    smoking cessation, 250–251
    weight loss/control, 205–206, 251
Behavior Modification Contract
  illustration of, 257
  illustration for smoking cessation, 258
bench press, 119
BIA (bioelectric impedance analysis), 197
biceps curl, 118
binge eating, 109
blood cholesterol, 154, 168*t*, 227–228*fig*
blood pressure, 80, 81*fig*
BMI (body mass index), 40, 41*t*, 61,
    215–216

body composition
  aerobic exercise and adaptation of, 94
  assessment of
    BMI (body mass index), 40, 41*t*, 61
    field techniques for, 37
    hydrostatic weighing, 36
    Metropolitan Life Insurance Company
      height/weight tables, 40
    skinfold test, 36–37*fig*, 61, 197
    waist-to-hip circumference ratio,
      37–39, 40*fig*, 41*t*, 61
  commercial devices for measuring, 197
  described, 7
  fitness categories for men/women, 40*t*
  rating your, 40–41
  See also human body
body fat
  aerobic exercise and burning, 204
  area of body affected by reduced, 200*fig*
  body mass index (BMI), 40, 41*t*, 61
  cellulite, 207–208
  determining ideal weight using BMI and,
    215–216
  estimates for men, 39*t*
  estimates for women, 38*t*
  estimating caloric expenditure required to
    lose 1 lb. of, 217
  exercise to gain, 210
  myth of spot reduction of, 207
  optimal weight based on percent of,
    195*fig*
  regulating stores of, 197*fig*
  waist-to-hip circumference ratio and,
    37–39, 40*fig*, 41*fig*, 61
  See also obesity
body weight
  daily caloric expenditure based on exercise
    and, 199
  determining ideal, 215–216
  optimal, 194
  optimal weight based on percent fat,
    195*fig*
  See also weight control
bone mass, 3
botulism, 179
Bouchard, Claude, 196
breathing exercises, 245–246
bulimia, 209
B vitamins, 166

calcium, 166, 172
caloric expenditure estimation, 199*t*
calories, 151, 163
capillaries, 79
carbohydrates, 150–153, 152*t*, 172–173
cardiac output, 80
cardiorespiratory fitness
  benefits of, 76
  described, 5–6
  exercise prescription for
    popular activities used in, 84*t*
    steps in, 91–92
  exercise program
    body adaptation to aerobic, 91–94

    starting and maintaining, 87–88
    training techniques for, 88–91*t*
  link between dehydration and, 25
  measuring
    classification for 1-mile walk test, 20*t*
    cycle ergometer fitness test, 20–22,
      21*t*, 23*t*, 51
    maximum oxygen uptake (VO2), 23,
      24*t*, 81, 82*fig*
    1.5-mile run test, 19–20, 47
    process of, 18–19
    the step test, 22*fig*, 24, 25*t*, 53
  motivation to maintain, 94–95
  physiological basis for developing, 76–77
  rating your, 24–25
cardiorespiratory fitness program
  exercise prescription
    developing individualized, 87–88
    motivation to maintain, 94–95
    for people with average/good fitness,
      90
    for people with excellent fitness, 91
    for people with poor fitness, 89*t*
    sample of, 88
  training techniques
    how body adapts to aerobic, 91–94
    listed, 88–91
cardiorespiratory system
  exercise and
    blood pressure, 80
    circulatory system, 78–80
    maximal cardiorespiratory function
      (VO2max), 81, 82*fig*
    respiratory system, 81
  physiological responses to exercise
    circulatory responses, 81–82
    respiratory responses, 82
    responses of energy-producing
      systems, 82
Cardiorespiratory Training Log, 101–102
cardiovascular diseases
  arteriosclerosis, 222, 223*fig*
  heart attack (myocardial infarction), 223,
    224*fig*, 225
  hypertension, 80, 225–226*fig*, 230
  stroke, 223, 224*fig*, 225
  in the United States, 222*fig*
  who is at risk for, 223
  See also CHD (coronary heart disease)
cardiovascular system
  aerobic exercise and adaptation of, 92–93
  responses to exercise by, 81–82
cartilage, movement and, 132
cellulite, 207–208
CHD (coronary heart disease)
  assessing your risk (RISKO score) of,
    237–239
  body composition and, 7
  described, 2, 223
  frequently asked questions about diet,
    exercise and, 233
  heredity/gender/increasing age, 229
  reducing risk of
    final word on, 233

306

PHOTO CREDITS

All photos by Anthony Neste except the following:

p. 1: Myrleen Ferguson Cate /PhotoEdit; p. 8; p. 17: Stone/Getty Images; p. 63; p. 69, left; p. 103: Alan Jacubek/CORBIS; p. 112: Courtesy of William J. Kraemer, Ph.D.; p. 113: Courtesy of Biodex; p. 131: Frank Siteman/Stock Boston; p. 149: Foodpix; p. 152: Mark Tomalty/Masterfile; p. 167: Michael Newman/PhotoEdit; p. 176: Courtesy Janice L. Thompson, Ph.D.; p. 177: Doug Martin/Photo Researchers, Inc.; p. 191; p. 192: Bob Daemmrich/Tony Stone; p. 195: Jeff Greenberg/PhotoEdit; p. 196: Courtesy of Claude Bouchard, M.D.; p. 206: Peter Johnson/CORBIS; p. 208: Janet Durran/Black Star ; p. 209: Nina Berman/Sipa Press; p. 224, 9.3a, b; p. 231: Bob Daemmrich/Stock Boston; p. 225: Matthew McVay/Stock Boston; p. 241: Jeff Greenberg/Visuals Unlimited; p. 243: Jeff Greenberg/Visuals Unlimited; p. 251: P. H. Dickenson/Sipa Press; p. 259: Bonnie Kamin/Photo Edit; p. 262: Courtesy Rod Dishman, Ph.D.; p. 263: A.Ramey/ Woodfin Camp & Associates; p. 266: Jeffrey Aaronson/Network Aspen